NUTRITION AND DIET RESEARCH PROGRESS

# GRAPE POMACE IN HEALTH AND DISEASE PREVENTION

# NUTRITION AND DIET RESEARCH PROGRESS

Additional books and e-books in this series can be found on Nova's website under the Series tab.

NUTRITION AND DIET RESEARCH PROGRESS

# GRAPE POMACE IN HEALTH AND DISEASE PREVENTION

VERONICA SANDA CHEDEA
EDITOR

nova
Medicine & Health
New York

DOI: https://doi.org/10.52305/HINI5835



## NOTICE TO THE READER



**Library of Congress Cataloging-in-Publication Data**

ISBN: 978-1-68507-409-8

*Published by Nova Science Publishers, Inc. † New York*

# Contents

# PREFACE

*Vitis vinifera L.* (common grapevine) cultivars are the most widely planted around the world and have a high commercial value for fresh table grapes, dried fruit, and wine. In the winemaking process, besides the free-run and pressed juice obtained from the berries, an important quantity of a byproduct -grape pomace (GP)- is generated. The GP represents on average 20% from the total mass of grapes taken for winemaking and typically consists of skins, stalks, and seeds. The valorization of grape pomace is based on the concept that this matrix has good nutritional and medicinal properties for human health and disease prevention. In this framework, the book aims to provide up to date information on grape pomace (GP) and its valorization through medicinal applications.

From the point of view of GP generation the stages of grapes ' crushing and pressing are the most important ones. Pressing in winemaking is the process of juice extraction from the grapes with the aid of a wine press, by hand, or even by the weight of the grape berries and clusters. There is a difference between white vinification and red vinification, resulting in fresh GP or fermented GP respectively. In order to extend the shelf life of GP for off-season use of its bioactive compounds (in medicine, cosmetics and food applications) the dehydration, as opposed to fermentation (ensiling), is by far the most common method used. From the chemical point of view GP contains organic acids and polyphenols, residual sugars, pectins, cellulose and some quantities of alcohol (ethanol) in case of red GP. Chapter 1 of the book aims to review some aspects of GP generation by winemaking, the processes of pressing and drying, as well as its biochemical composition.

In the last few years, the non-conventional technology known as "green technology", Pulsed Electric Field (PEF), has been developed, in order to reuse agricultural residues and this technique has been currently proposed for extracting the bioactive compound. The mechanism and optimal parameters of this technology are described in the first part of the chapter two. In addition, an innovative PEF device developed to promote the extraction of phenols and pigments from red grapes is presented. Most often, this technology has been used in the wine industry in order to obtain a product (usually, wine) with a pronounced color intensity and a high content of phenols and anthocyanin pigments. In recent years, the literature has shown that the PEF technique is effective in extracting phenolic compounds from various raw materials, especially from grape pomace.

The nutraceutical role of grape pomace's polyphenols is conditioned by the absorption and bioavailability of these compounds. In order to study these processes chapter three presents research results in rats, pigs and humans related to GP. The studies show that during the last few years, an increasing interest has been paid to the metabolism and microbial biotransformation of dietary polyphenols and bioactivity of their metabolites vs. parent compounds because these metabolites elicit significant intrinsic bioactivities that could explain the effects observed for the parent compounds The actual research has also emphasised the need for a new generation of intervention studies designed to show the variation at individual level in response to the consumption of the plant food bioactive compounds, regarding their bioavailability and bioefficacy. Furthermore the nutraceuticals impact the composition of the intestinal microbiota and its relationship to various pharmacological effects. Many studies have examined the effect of GP and its active compounds on the intestinal microbiota and found that they can modulate the intestinal microbiota and thus prevent or treat various diseases and this is presented in chapter four. However, further studies are needed to better understand the complex relationship between GP, its pharmacological effects and the microbiota.

There is a wide variety of diseases that are characterized by oxidative stress and inflammation like diabetes, hypertension and cardiovascular diseases, alcoholic liver disease, chronic kidney disease, neurodegenerative diseases, cancer, and aging. The classical treatment used for these diseases, besides their therapeutic effects comes along with numerous side effects. Many studies show the benefic effects of bioactive molecules in counteracting these side effects and therefore a lot of focus is directed toward identifying alternative sources of these compounds. In this context, chapter 5 aims to present the most recent studies that show the antioxidant and anti-inflammatory effects GP evidenced so far by the *in vitro* and *in vivo* studies. According to the most recent *in vitro* and *in vivo* animal studies, GP showed to have promising results on inflammation and oxidative stress associated with various chronic diseases. Few studies existing *in vivo* on humans show that more research is needed to demonstrate its potential in chronic conditions prevention and/or treatment in humans.

Current studies show that nutrition can be considered a two-way road towards reducing or increasing the risk factors for several chronic conditions such as metabolic diseases, cardiovascular disease (CVD) and certain types of cancer. Worldwide, at the forefront, CVD remains the leading cause of mortality, with 26% out of total deaths. It was already demonstrated that diets low in saturated fat, salt, and cholesterol, with high intakes of fruit, vegetables and fish are protective factors against CVD. Grapes are a rich source of bioactive phenolic compounds and some of them have been associated with a reduction in CVD risk. Therefore, the aim of the chapter six is to review grape pomace effects on cardiovascular risk factors in both *in vivo* and *in vitro* studies. The effects will be discussed starting from the molecular mechanisms of action of the main polyphenols found in the composition, focusing on the cellular effects that could influence the CVD risk factors: lipid profile, anti-atherosclerotic effect, antioxidant status, effects on blood pressure. The second part of the chapter six discusses epidemiological and interventional studies in humans, comparing the results obtained on resveratrol, the most studied component, and different grape products, to highlight the idea that the observed beneficial effects are not due to a single component, but that it is an accumulation of effects of the grape as a whole.

Grape pomace has demonstrated its beneficial effects for the prevention and progress of Non-Alcoholic Steato Hepatitis (NASH), from simple steatosis to steatohepatitis and even severe cirrhosis and its complications, as well as prevention in people with or without metabolic syndrome or associated disorders. Fatty liver disease encompasses a wide spectrum of pathologies mainly characterized by fatty infiltration of liver cells in the absence of excessive alcohol intake or in the presence of moderate alcohol consumption. This spectrum includes simple fatty liver, fatty infiltration with elevated transaminase levels, fibrosis and cirrhosis of the liver. It is assumed that most cases of liver cirrhosis of unknown origin are the direct consequence of NAFLD (Non-Alcoholic Fatty Liver Disease). There is a wide variety of drugs and supplements used in this condition. Among them, GP has occupied a unique place due to its beneficial effects on oxidative stress and lipid metabolic balance. The chapter seven reviews the main challenges in order to obtain clinical and biochemical effects in NASH using GP products and presents the most recent advances regarding the effects of these kinds of products in hepatic steatosis. We also discuss potential toxicity and drug interactions, considering that NASH is often associated with other medical and metabolic disorders that require treatment with certain drugs.

Finally in chapter 8 the existing knowledge on the anticancer activity of grape pomace is summarised. The possible use of grape pomace as chemoprevention and chemotherapeutic agent has considerable potential, and could be of great interest in the cancer research field.

# ACKNOWLEDGMENTS

The book *Grape Pomace in Health and Disease Prevention* is published in the year 2022 in which the Research Station for Viticulture and Enology (Stațiunea de Cercetare Dezvoltare pentru Viticultură și Vinificație Blaj-SCDVV Blaj) celebrates 75 years since being established in 1946. This period represents three-quarters of a century conducting sound and interdisciplinary scientific research to examine viticulture and winemaking in Târnave vineyards, Transylvania, România. I would like to sincerely congratulate all SCDVV Blaj employees on their outstanding work accomplished so far from the time of its establishment.

## Strugurele

Am ținut în palma mea un ciorchine de strugure
Ca pe un copilaș,
Ca pe un început și ca pe un sfârșit
Gălbui și dulce
Asteptând să fie zdrobit
De teascurile dure
Ale lumii în care
Strugurii se zdrobesc pentru vin
Iar oamenii sunt apăsați de suspin.

## The Grapes

I held a bunch of grapes in my palm
Like I held a little child,
As a beginning and as an end
Yellow and sweet,
Waiting to be crushed
By the hard presses
Of the world, in which
The grapes are crushed for wine
And people are tormented by dreams and wishes.

In: Grape Pomace in Health … ISBN: 978-1-68507-409-8
Editor: Veronica Sanda Chedea 

*Chapter 1*

# Grape Pomace Generation, Conditioning, and Biochemical Composition-General Aspects

***Crinuta Maria Vosloban and Veronica Sanda Chedea****

Research Station for Viticulture and Enology Blaj, (SCDVV Blaj), Romania

## Abstract

*Vitis vinifera L.* (common grapevine) cultivars are the most widely planted worldwide and have a high commercial value as fresh table grapes, dried fruit, and wine. During the winemaking process, in addition to the free-run and pressed juice obtained from the berries, a significant quantity of residue -grape pomace (GP)- is generated. The GP represents on average 20% of the total mass of grapes taken for winemaking and typically consists of skins, stalks, and seeds. The stages in which the grapes are crushed and pressed are the most crucial concerning GP generation. In winemaking, pressing is the process of juice extraction from the grapes using a wine press, by hand, or the

* Corresponding Author's E-mail: chedeaveronica@yahoo.com.

weight of the grape berries and clusters. Differences exist between white vinification and red vinification, resulting in fresh GP or fermented GP being produced, respectively. To extend the shelf life of GP for the off-seasonal use of its bioactive compounds (in medicine, cosmetics, and food applications), they are more often dehydrated than fermented (ensiling). From a chemical perspective, GP contains organic acids and polyphenols, residual sugars, pectins, cellulose, and some quantities of alcohol (ethanol) in red GP. This chapter reviews different aspects of GP generation by winemaking, pressing, drying, and biochemical composition.

**Keywords:** grape pomace, white vinification, red vinification, drying methods, bioactive compounds

## INTRODUCTION

"The cultural landscape of viticulture is the scenery of civilization". Its impression extends beyond vine rows and terraces to the homes and buildings of the winegrowers, the artifacts of industry, even the lifestyles of those who create the wines. Entire regions are dominated, saturated by the imagery of the vine and its cultural history. "Wherever in the world, one enters a winegrowing region, the atmosphere is unmistakably unique, a combination of serenity and civility" (De Blij 1983; Tiefenbacher 2019).

More than 100 species of grapevines belonging to the *Vitis L.* genus ("The Plant List" 2013) are currently recognized. Globally, grapevines have been cultivated for over 7.000 years (Mullins, Bouquet and Williams 1992; Gramaje, Urbez-Torres and Sosnowski 2017), and the changing landscape of grapevine cultivation considers the changing location and distribution of the practices of viticulture (growing of wine grapes) and viniculture or oenology (wine production) over these millennia (Tiefenbacher 2019). Because of their high commercial value as fresh fruits, dried grapes, and wine, the cultivars of common grapevine (*Vitis vinifera L.*) are planted worldwide (Gramaje, Urbez-Torres and Sosnowski 2018). Important for juice, fresh table grapes, wine production, and especially for rootstock development, are the other *Vitis* species and their interspecific hybrids (Gramaje, Urbez-Torres and Sosnowski 2018). Today, commercial viticulture occurs within the Tropics at higher elevations in places such as Hawaii, Mexico, and Boli. All wine-grape varieties require periods of cooler temperatures and high daily temperature fluctuations to mature and ripen to produce sufficient concentrations of sugars that yield alcohol. Society's demands relating to wine consumption determine the permanent innovation and changes in the wine industry, specifically in relation to the implementation of technology and the development of new grape varieties. Thus, the boundaries of wine production have the potential to be advanced beyond what is currently known (Tiefenbacher 2019).

*V. vinifera* and *Vitis spp.* are cultivated on approximately 7.16 million ha cultivated which produced 79.1 million tons of fruit harvested in 2018 (Gramaje, Urbez-Torres, and Sosnowski 2018). These figures demonstrate that grapevines are among the most often grown perennial fruit crops globally and have established their economic importance (Gramaje, Urbez-Torres, and Sosnowski 2018). The European continent, with 3.63 million ha and 29.84 million t, has the most significant grape production worldwide, followed by Asia (2.03 million ha and 27.37 million t), South America (0.55 million ha and 7.48 million t), North America (0.39 million ha and 7.01 million t), Africa (0.35 million ha and 4.85 million t), and Oceania (0.17 million ha and 2.09 million t) FAOSTAT 2020 ("http://Www.Fao.Org/Faostat/En/#data/QC" 2020). Table 1 presents the first 20 countries in the world in terms of vineyards area, grapes, and wine production ("http://Www.Fao.Org/Faostat/En/#data/QC" 2020) and ("http://Www.Fao.Org/Faostat/En/#data/QD" 2020). About 80% of the annual production is used in the winemaking process (Fontana, Antoniolli, and Bottini 2013; Frum et al. 2018).

The European *V. vinifera*, also recognized as the bunch grape, is characterized by its broad morphological and physiological variability and attractive high-quality fruits (Alleweldt and Possingham 1988; Negrul 1938). Separated existing cultivars into three broad groups (Alleweldt and Possingham 1988). First, the orientalis group that produce large berries and bunches (clusters) but require high temperatures to be made into table grapes (Alleweldt and Possingham 1988). Secondly, the occidentalis group which possess small berries but many per shoot which are winter hardy and well-adapted to mild summers (Alleweldt and Possingham 1988). The fruit of the occidentalis group is used to produce the most famous wines (Alleweldt and Possingham 1988). The third group, pontica, is intermediate between groups 1 and 2, used both as table grapes or wine grapes (Alleweldt and Possingham 1988).

**Table 1. First 20 countries in the world in terms of vineyards area, grapes and wine production ('http://Www.Fao.Org/Faostat/En/#data/QC" 2020) and ('http://Www.Fao.Org/Faostat/En/#data/QD" 2020)**

| Place in the world | Area harvested in 2018 (ha) | Country | Grape Production in 2018 (t) | Country | Wine Production in 2014 (t) | Country |
|---|---|---|---|---|---|---|
| 1. | 1123644 | Spain | 13397012 | China, mainland | 4796600 | Italy |
| 2. | 795150 | China, mainland | 8513643 | Italy | 4607850 | Spain |
| 3. | 752837 | France | 6890970 | United States of America | 4293466 | France |
| 4. | 675818 | Italy | 6673481 | Spain | 3300000 | United States of America |
| 5. | 417041 | Turkey | 6198323 | France | 1700000 | China, mainland |
| 6. | 379190 | United States of America | 3933000 | Turkey | 1498380 | Argentina |
| 7. | 218233 | Argentina | 2920000 | India | 1214000 | Chile |
| 8. | 212000 | Chile | 2573311 | Argentina | 1186343 | Australia |
| 9. | 174976 | Portugal | 2500000 | Chile | 1146006 | South Africa |
| 10. | 173685 | Romania | 2032031 | Iran (Islamic Republic of) | 920200 | Germany |
| 11. | 165097 | Iran (Islamic Republic of) | 1901736 | South Africa | 603327 | Portugal |

| Place in the world | Area harvested in 2018 (ha) | Country | Grape Production in 2018 (t) | Country | Wine Production in 2014 (t) | Country |
|---|---|---|---|---|---|---|
| 12. | 139000 | India | 1759472 | Egypt | 378283 | Romania |
| 13. | 135533 | Australia | 1663557 | Australia | 334300 | Greece |
| 14. | 126873 | Republic of Moldova | 1591986 | Brazil | 327400 | Russian Federation |
| 15. | 111310 | South Africa | 1589784 | Uzbekistan | 320400 | New Zealand |
| 16. | 100915 | Uzbekistan | 1403597 | Germany | 273100 | Brazil |
| 17. | 100340 | Greece | 1144305 | Romania | 258520 | Hungary |
| 18. | 100182 | Germany | 984081 | Afghanistan | 199869 | Austria |
| 19. | 87517 | Afghanistan | 933150 | Greece | 198183 | Serbia |
| 20. | 78853 | Egypt | 13397012 | Portugal | 149850 | Republic of Moldova |

The chemical composition of grapes has excellent significance in producing high-quality wine during the winemaking process (Gallander 1974). Not only do chemical components within the raw product contribute directly to the sensory properties of the wine, but many are also required during the fermentation process (Gallander 1974). Within this context, concerning the weight of the grape, the berries represent 90-98%, of which 8-20% is skins, 75-85% kernel or pulp, and 2-5% seeds. For varieties used in the production of wine, a kilogram of grapes contains between 450 and 1,000 berries. Compared to the table varieties, the seeds and skin of grape varieties used in wine production possess a greater mass (Ţârdea, Sârbu and Ţârdea 2010; Pop and Pop 2015). The greater mass of seed and skins in grape varieties used in wine production is important to the winemaking process, as besides the free-run and pressed juice obtained from the berries, a substantial quantity of residue - grape pomace (GP)- is generated.

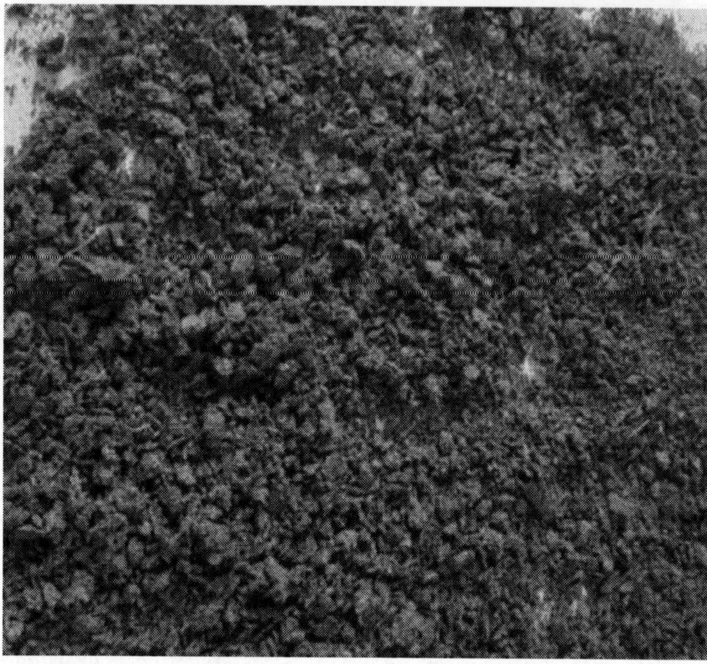

Figure 1. Dried grape pomace (from white grapes Neuburger cultivar).

## WINEMAKING PROCESS

When we discuss wine we are discussing civilization as the history of winemaking parallels that of civilization. The history of winemaking goes back to the year 6000 BC when wine is believed to have been produced in the Caucasus and Mesopotamia (Robinson 1994; Pretoria's 2000). One thousand years later, in 5000 BC, references to wine have been discovered in Egypt and Phoenicia and, by the year 2000 BC, wine was being produced in Greece and Crete (Pretorius 2000). The Roman Empire, with its colonization process, popularized winemaking throughout the Mediterranean countries and by 500 BC, wine was being produced in Sicily, Italy, France, Spain, Portugal, and northern Africa (Pretorius 2000). As the Empire advanced from the Balkan States in the south to Germany and Britain in the north, the cultivation of grapevine followed (Robinson 1994; Pretorius 2000).

From the old continent of Europe, the grapevine was introduced into the New World during the sixteenth century by European explorers. Thus, in Mexico and other South American countries such as Argentina, Peru, and Chile, the Spanish conquistadors planted *Vitis vinifera* in 1530, in South Africa, the Dutch settlers in 1655 planted French vine cuttings on the lower slopes of the Cape of Good Hope's majestic Table Mountain, in California the grapevine cultivation followed soon thereafter, and more than a century later, in 1813in Australia and New Zealand (Robinson 1994; Pretorius 2000). A turning point in grapevine history in the 1870s when the disaster struck the world of wine. Then, the root-eating insect Phylloxera vastatrix (*Dactylasphaera vitifoliae*) threatened almost all vine in Europe and the New World (Pretorius 2000). Salvation was achieved by grafting known grapevine varieties onto phylloxera-resistant rootstocks from the native American vine. All vineyards within the threatened zone removed the vulnerable vines before replacing them with the new grafted *V. vinifera* vines (Pretorius 2000).

Throughout the centuries of winemaking history, the basic principles have changed very little despite different techniques being used to produce various styles of wine (Pretorius 2000). However, during the previous170 years, winemaking has become a science and many practices and oenological processes once thought impossible have become routine (Pretorius 2000). Thus, now we speak about a wine industry that has been revolutionised through fundamental innovations in winemaking yet continues to be challenged by the tension between tradition and innovation as a process where the forces of market-pull and technology-push try to be balanced (Pretorius 1999; Pretorius 2000). This constitutes the premise for further improvements in winemaking through the refinement of viticultural and oenological practices with the aim of overall quality improvement and availability of endless varieties of wine (Pretorius 2000).

Winemaking processes differ depending on the variety of wine that is being produced. Firstly, there is an essential difference between making white or red wine: "white vinification" and "red vinification" respectively, fermented GP and sweet GP (Figure 2). Thus, the white vinification's stages includes destemming and crushing the grapes, maceration, pressing, fermentation, malolactic fermentation (if desired), clarification, maturation, fining/stabilization, filtration, and bottling. The stages of the red vinification includes destemming and crushing the grapes, fermentation, and maceration, pressing (early for rose wines and late for the red wines), malolactic fermentation (if desired), clarification, maturation, fining/stabilization, filtration, and bottling.

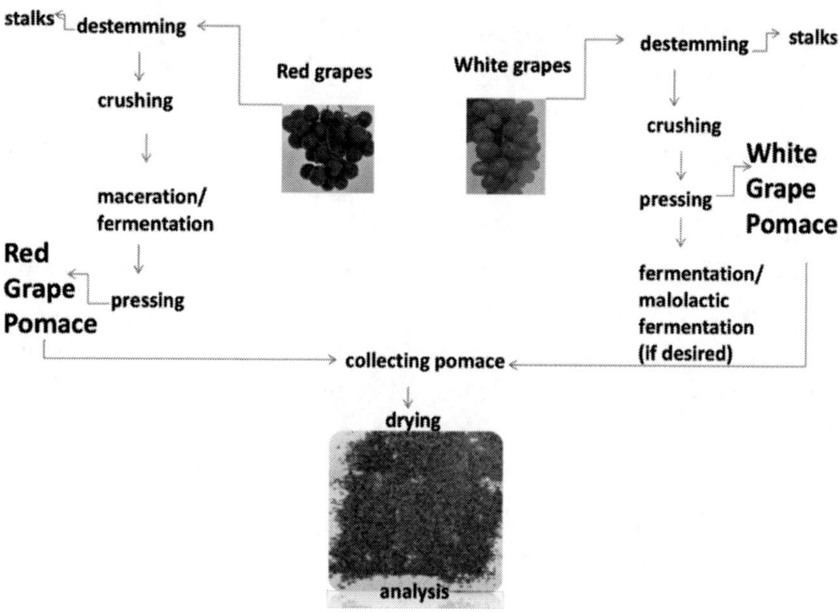


Figure 2. Technology for obtaining fermented grape pomace and sweet grape pomace, respectively.

Relating to GP generation, the crushing and pressing stages are the most significant. Pressing in winemaking is the process of extracting the juice from grapes with the aid of a wine presser, by hand, or even by the weight of the grape berries and clusters (Cox 1999). Historically, entire grape clusters were trodden on by feet but in most modern wineries the grapes are passed through a crusher/destemmer that removes individual grape berries from the stems and breaks the skins to release some juice before pressing ("https://Www.Wikiwand.Com/En/Pressing_(Wine)" 2020). Exceptions exist, such as sparkling wine production in regions such as Champagne, where grapes are traditionally whole-cluster pressed with their stems attached and this produces a lighter must that is low in phenolics (Robinson 2006).

Approximately 60-70% of the available juice within a grape berry recognized as the free-run juice and can be extracted during the crushing process without requiring the use of a presser (Robinson 2006). The remaining 30-40% that is extracted is done so using a presser and can have higher pH levels, lower titratable acidity, potentially higher volatile acidity, and higher phenolics compared to the free-run juice depending on the amount of pressure and skin tearing, producing more astringent and bitter wine (Boulton, Singleton, Bisson 1996).

The pressing of white grapes during white vinification is often performed immediately after harvest and crushing and before primary fermentation (Figure 1). After crushing the grapes, the free-run juice is obtained. The resulting matrix is then pressed with the most significant decision being how much pressure is applied and how much pressed juice and free-run juice the winemakers require. Certain grape varieties such as *Sémillon* (France and Australia), *Aurore* (USA and Canada), and *Fetească Regală* (Romania) have very "liquidy" pulps, requiring the application of very little pressure to avoid tearing the skins that release the juice. Other varieties such as *Catawba* (USA) and *Muscat Ottonel* (France, Romania), have significantly tougher pulps that must be pressed harder (Wagner 1996).

In red wine production, after crushing the grapes, the resulting mixture is allowed to ferment and it is and during this time that the contact between the skin and juice produces the color, tannins, and other phenolics that are to be extracted from the skin. Pressing usually occurs near the end or after fermentation with the must (Cox 1999). The maceration and phenolic extraction cease with pressing, and that's why in red wine production, the timing of when to press is one of the most critical decisions in the vinification. Generally, batch pressers are considered gentler, minimizing the movement and tearing of the grape skins. The more grape skins are torn or scoured, the more tannins and phenolic compounds are extracted, increasing the harshness of the wine ("https://Www.Wikiwand.Com/En/Pressing_(Wine)" 2020).

## GRAPE POMACE (GP) OBTAINING

Both red and white winemaking processes generate substantial quantities of solid organic waste named grape pomace (GP), and it is estimated that 1 kg of GP is generated for every 6 L of wine (Mendes et al. 2014). GP can be classified in different ways. Depending on the process and technology used during the vinification process (it is all referred to as wine grapes), the classifications that exist are:

- virgin, sweet or fresh GP: does not undergo fermentation and it has a relatively high sugar concentration (ex. GP coming from white vinification);
- fermented GP: has undergone a period of fermentation and therefore possesses variable alcoholic concentration (a main by-product of the red vinification) (Muhlack, Potumarthi and Jeffery 2018).

GP typically consists of skins, stalks, seeds, and moisture in addition to other components: among primary constituents such as organic acids and polyphenols, unfermented white GP contains residual sugars, whereas red GP has both residual sugars and some quantities of alcohol (ethanol) (Devesa-Rey et al. 2011; Hixson, Wilkes and Smith 2014; Muhlack, Potumarthi and Jeffery 2018). The concentration of residual sugars and alcohol in GP differs greatly according to the grapes 'source in addition to the processes, practices, and logistics involved when crushing the grapes and producing the wine (Zheng et al. 2012; Hixson, Wilkes and Smith 2014; Muhlack, Potumarthi and Jeffery 2018).

In the red vinification process, the stalks are generally removed from crushed grapes before the fermentation process and the grapes 'skins, and seeds are fermented using the must for several days to increase the phenolic content of the produced wine. The grape residues in the form of pomace still contain higher levels of polyphenols, especially within the skin matrix (Pinelo, Arenas and Meyer 2006; Nayak et al. 2018). As approximately 20% of the weight of processed grapes remain as GPs, the wine industry produces millions of tons of unused material that provide an ecological and economic waste management issue (Fontana, Antoniolli and Bottini 2013; Antoniolli et al. 2015).

During the winemaking process, after alcoholic fermentation, approximately 25% of the processed grape weight remains as organic solid waste, although this percentage varies (Balea et al. 2018). The mass of GP accounts for between 11% and 22% of the grapes crushed for red wine production and 12–25% for white wine production (Bacic 2003). For some grapes, the proportion of stalks is as high as 11% (Bacic 2003). The specific composition of GP's solid parts is dependent on the type of wine produced (Zhang et al. 2017). Pop and Pop (2015) reports that the solid parts of GP consist of 63% skins, 33% seeds, and 4% stalks (Pop and Pop 2015; Duba 2015) on a dry basis it is indicated a content of 51% skin, 47% seeds and 2% stalks (Duba 2015). The major by-product of the wine industry, GP equates to 250 g/kg of the pressed grapes and on a dry matter (DM) basis contains stalks (~20 g/kg), seeds (~470 g/kg), skin, and pulp (~510 g/kg) (Zhang et al. 2017; Beres et al. 2017; Chikwanha et al. 2018). Grape skins represent, on average, 82% of the wet weight of white GP (Deng, Penner and Zhao 2011; Jiang, Simonsen and Zhao 2011). These disparities can be linked to differences in the wine production process as well as to the grape varieties processed.

## GP CONDITIONING

Fresh GP has a high moisture content (~600 g/kg) and if unpreserved within a week after pressing, it spoils and results in the presence of pungent odors that attract flies and pests capable of transmitting pathogenic organisms (Zhang et al. 2017; Chikwanha et al. 2018). Generally, the high moisture content in feeds and foods is associated with elevated water reactions that accelerate microbial spoilage and deteriorative biochemical activity such as the oxidation of lipids and degradation of phenolic compounds (Choe and Oh 2013; Chikwanha et al. 2018).

Depending on the amount of GP processed and the required storage length, there can be different storage and preservation methods exist that allow for further analyses and applications. For small quantities, the storage for further experimental activity was performed at 4°C to prevent the enzymatic degradation of polyphenols in red GP with a moisture content of 76% (Nayak et al. 2018). This GP, *V.vinifera* L. cv. *Cabernet* was collected after the red vinification from the Experimental winery Mas Friars, the center linked to the Faculty of Oenology of Universitat Rovira I Virgilli at Tarragona, Spain (Nayak et al. 2018). In Romania, GP samples of the *Fetească neagră* grapes were stored at −22°C in vacuum bags before analysis (Balea et al. 2018). The grapes were harvested manually at full maturity level during the 2015 vintage (Balea et al. 2018). The GP samples were collected at two winemaking stages: one was supplied immediately after pressing the grapes to produce the fresh and unfermented GP, and the other was supplied after 20 days of fermentation at 20°C and following separation, the fermentation of GP (Balea et al. 2018). At -20°C, GP samples from *Cabernet Sauvignon* pomace from grapes collected from Carmen Vineyard, Region Metropolitana, Chile, were frozen until extraction (Vergara-Salinas et al. 2013). Before freezing after collection, GP was dried at ambient temperature for 2 days to reach equilibrium humidity (10% w/w) in a drying cabinet with forced ventilation and reduced to a particle size lower than 1 mm diameter (Vergara-Salinas et al. 2013). Two samples of the same pomace were taken at different stages of the winemaking process (Vergara-Salinas et al. 2013). At the beginning of the winemaking process just after the must was introduced into the fermentation tank, the first sample was taken (unfermented pomace) (Vergara-Salinas et al.

2013). The second sample was collected after the fermentation process had completed and produced fermented pomace (Vergara-Salinas et al. 2013). The pre-fermentation process was performed at 18°C for 10 days, and the must was loaded into a 10 $m^3$ fermentation tank (Vergara-Salinas et al. 2013). Fermentation was conducted between 25°C and 30°C for 21 days without pectolytic enzymes (Vergara-Salinas et al. 2013).

## DRYING

The most common method used to extend the shelf life of GP to make its bioactive compounds available for off-season is dehydration. This is used as an alternative to fermentation (ensiling) and decreases the amount of water available for deteriorative biochemical reactions and microbes (Gan et al. 2017; Chikwanha et al. 2018). Dehydration of wet pomace provides an initial step before developing further applications (Tseng and Zhao 2012). Reducing the bulkiness of GP through drying reduces the costs associated with its packaging, storage, and transportation (Gan et al. 2017; Chikwanha et al. 2018). However, dehydration also provides adverse effects on GP's quality, including the degradation of valuable nutrients (Tseng and Zhao 2012; Chikwanha et al. 2018) and loss of bioactive compounds due to their susceptibility to heat and oxygen. Consequentially, the importance of lowering the antioxidant and antimicrobial activities by drying should not be ignored (Tseng and Zhao 2012; Antoniolli et al. 2015; Gan et al. 2017; Chikwanha et al. 2018). These losses differ depending on the dehydration process (Çoklar and Akbulut 2017; Tseng and Zhao 2012; Chikwanha et al. 2018). Varietal differences among GP are also responsible for the varying content and composition of bioactive compounds (This, Lacombe and Thomas 2006) and subsequently the resultant biological properties (Chikwanha et al. 2018).

Due to the importance of this process, numerous studies evaluating different drying methods and biochemical changes caused to the agroindustrial residues have been performed (Shalini 2010; Jangam, Law and Mujumdar 2010; Khanal, Howard and Prior 2010; Vashisth, Singh and Pegg 2011; Tseng and Zhao 2012; Antoniolli et al. 2015; Martynenko and Kudra 2016; Taşeri et al. 2018). To fully benefit from GP, it is critical to develop drying conditions maximize the retention of bioactive properties while remaining economically feasible (Tseng and Zhao 2012).

Studies have been carried out on GP drying with different drying methods: electrohydrodynamic drying (Martynenko and Kudra 2016), infrared, convective and combined drying (Sui et al. 2014), hot air and sun drying (Maskan, Kaya and Maskan 2002), air-circulating oven (Larrauri, Rupérez and Saura-Calixto 1997), open sun and solar drying (Taşeri et al., 2016) and tray dryer (Goula, Thymiatis and Kaderides 2016; Taşeri et al. 2018).

A common and inexpensive method of drying the wine GP is by sun-drying; however, not only does GP become polluted and deteriorate, but sun drying is a lengthy process (Sui et al. 2014; Taşeri et al. 2018). Moreover, sun drying is heavily dependent on favorable weather conditions and the required product quality can never be guaranteed (Maskan, Kaya and Maskan 2002; Sui et al. 2014; Taşeri et al. 2018).

To study the polyphenolic content of *Fetească neagră* and *Italian Riesling* GPs, the pomaces were collected and transported in freezers before being stored for a short time until drying. Drying was performed at room temperature (20-22°C) and 40% humidity on polyethylene foils for 1 week (Muncaciu et al. 2017). To prevent the microbiological alterations, the material was turned manually several times a day (Muncaciu et al. 2017). GPs were later manually separated before being sampled in plastic bags under vacuum and stored at -18°C (Muncaciu et al. 2017).

*Quebranta* red GP and *Torontel* white GP were obtained from the Cite Agroindustrial Wine cellar (Guadalupe, ICA, PERÚ) and after pressing of fermentation must the peels and seeds were collected (Solari-Godiño, Lindo-Rojas, and Pandia-Estrada 2017). Two different drying methods were used for these GPs: (1) cool air-drying at 18°C for 24 h and (2) second is the freeze-drying for 28 h at a collector temperature of

−84°C in a vacuum at 0.021 mbar with 4 drying ramps (including freezing) (Solari-Godiño, Lindo-Rojas and Pandia-Estrada 2017). After drying, both GP varieties were milled at a particle size of 0.25 mm (Solari-Godiño, Lindo-Rojas and Pandia-Estrada 2017). The vacuum-packaged GP powders of *Quebranta* and *Torontel* varieties were then stored at −18°C, for the further extraction and analysis of polyphenols contents and antioxidant capacity (Solari-Godiño, Lindo-Rojas and Pandia-Estrada 2017).

High value-added natural products are preserved in the best conditions when the freeze-drying method is used but because this is too expensive, it is preferential to use other methods. Cool air drying is an example of a novel preservation method that provides a low-cost alternative to freeze-drying whilst sharing the same benefits (Ratti 2001; Solari-Godiño, Lindo-Rojas, and Pandia-Estrada 2017; Taşeri et al. 2018). To better preserve the polyphenolic fraction, freeze-drying is the ideal pre-treatment, although for the real industrial exploitation of GP, this is practically and economically not feasible (Antoniolli et al. 2015). In this case, an immediate extraction of the fresh GP or a drying pre-treatment may be performed, although it may be different for the later extraction yields (Antoniolli et al. 2015). Convective drying in hot air is a commonly used industrial method of drying fruit pomaces because it is less expensive compared to other dehydration methods such as freeze- or vacuum-drying (Teles et al. 2018), despite heat decreasing product quality (Che Ma 'et al. 1997; Chen and Martynenko 2013; Taşeri et al. 2018) and its energy consumption is large (Gabel et al. 2006; Sui et al. 2014).

The thermophysical properties of GP are dependent on the water content (Azzouz et al. 2016; Taşeri et al. 2018). During convective drying, the air is one of the most important variables (Teles et al. 2018). This can be responsible for the preservation or degradation of the thermo-sensitive compounds because it is directly related to mass and heat transfer in these molecules. (Teles et al. 2018).

Drying GP at high temperatures may cause significant reductions in the amount of extractable polyphenols available and consequently, the antioxidant and free radical scavenging activities are also affected (Larrauri, Rupérez, and Saura-Calixto 1997; Taşeri et al. 2018). Kataria (2007) suggested a maximum permissible drying temperature for GP of 65°C, but Goula, Thymiatis, and Kaderides (2016) stated that the air temperature of 60-85°C caused the loss of phenolic material by 87.0-95.4% (Kataria 2007; Goula, Thymiatis, and Kaderides 2016; Taşeri et al. 2018). A system for convective drying is described by Teles et al. 2018. This is composed of a dryer having input and output air flow moved by the rotation of an internal blower and with heated air by incandescent lamps (Teles et al. 2018). The dryer was a convective tray with perpendicular airflow having an air velocity of 0.42 m/s (Teles et al. 2018). GP was arranged in a layer with approximately 0.015 m in height, in one tray (0.50 × 0.75 m) (Teles et al. 2018). To model the experimental data, the sample behavior was considered as a semi-infinite plate because the sample thickness was considerably smaller than the tray dimensions (thickness: diameter ratio <0.1) (Azuara-Nieto, Gutierrez-Lopez and Beristain-Guevara 2003; Teles et al. 2018). Drying was carried out at the following temperatures: 40°C, 50°C, and 60°C (Teles et al. 2018). A heat-pump dryer can lower drying temperature; therefore, it is beneficial for quality products drying at a relatively lower cost (Guochen, Arason, and Árnason 2009; Aktaş et al. 2017; Taşeri et al. 2018). GP was placed in a tray inside an open-loop laboratory pilot heat pump (HP) dryer with a drying air temperature of 45°C and three air velocities (1.5, 2.0, and 2.5 m/s) (Taşeri et al. 2018). The drying system consisted of a compressor (frequency controlled), condenser, evaporator, expansion valve, frequency inverter (to adjust the drying air velocity), fans, drying chamber (manufactured for the drying of GP), mixing chamber, thermohygrometer, thermocouples, and the main control unit (Taşeri et al. 2018). The heat pump dryer (HPD) has an open cycle as follows: fresh air is actively circulated by a fan over the condenser acting as a heat source and sent to the drying chamber. According to thermodynamic calculations performed for R410A refrigerant, 25% of exhaust air high in moisture and temperature, and 75% of fresh air was mixed inside the mixing chamber to achieve the optimum evaporation temperature before being sent to the evaporator (Taşeri et al. 2018). The relative humidity and temperature measurements are performed using the thermo hygrometer placed in the fresh air inlet, condenser inlet, condenser outlet, and inside the mixing chamber. Changes in product weight was observed and recorded using a load cell mounted below the drying chamber (Taşeri et al. 2018). The total energy consumption of the drying system was measured during the experiments using an electrical meter (Taşeri et al. 2018).

In recent years, infrared drying has been applied to dehydrate materials such as onions, strawberries, apples, and almonds. This drying method has many advantages that include: rapid drying, high quality dried products, operational ease, and strong sterilizing ability (Shih et al. 2008; Yang et al. 2010; Zhu et al. 2010; Bingol et al. 2011). Infrared drying is fundamentally different from convective drying because infrared energy is absorbed directly by the product rather than requiring heat transfer from the air (Sui et al. 2014). Infrared energy is more energy-efficient than convective drying because heat is transferred directly from the heating element to the product surface without heating the surrounding air (Sui et al. 2014). As infrared provides a constant heat flux independent of the drying matrix's temperature, the product's temperature is not influenced by the temperature of the surrounding air, and will achieve a high temperature rapidly (Sui et al. 2014). Radiation impinges on the exposed material, penetrates it, and is converted to sensible heat; as a result, infrared drying can provide more uniform heating of the material and may reduce the moisture gradient during heating and drying (Sui et al. 2014).

The drying kinetics of GP and the drying characteristics, sterilizing efficacy, and effects on GP's polyphenols and pro-anthocyanidins content were assessed when the infrared drying or convective drying were applied (Sui et al. 2014). The highest drying rate was registered for infrared drying; the drying time is reduced by 47.3% (Sui et al. 2014). Therefore, infrared drying performs well in a product's drying treatment. It has been found that infrared drying was a better drying method for preserving phenolic compounds than hot air drying (Raksakantong et al.

2011), and recent studies also show that combining infrared and convective drying performs well, resulting in a higher drying rate and better sterilization efficacy (Yang et al. 2010; Supmoon and Noomhorm 2013; Sui et al. 2014). It also can enhance the retention of active content in dried products like phenolic compounds (Puente-Díaz et al. 2013; Sui et al. 2014).

Convective drying was found to have a lower drying rate than sequential infrared and convective drying (Sui et al. 2014). Infrared and convective drying at 90°C had the best sterilizing efficacy and minimized the survival of undesired organisms such as yeasts, molds, and bacteria. Higher drying temperatures performed better when assessing pasteurization (Sui et al. 2014). Sterilizing efficacy has not been enhanced by prolonging the infrared drying (Sui et al. 2014). The highest content of polyphenols and pro-anthocyanidins was registered when GP was dried using infrared and it was discovered that decreasing the drying temperature reduced the damage inflicted on both classes of bioactive molecules (Sui et al. 2014).

## DRYING TEMPERATURE

The drying temperatures of GP, as it was shown above, varies from 18°C to 90°C. It was reported that a minimum loss of bioactive compounds from fruit residues, when dried by heat, is reached at temperatures up to 50°C (Raghavan and Orsat 2007; Antoniolli et al. 2015). Thus, the polyphenols content and antioxidant activity of red GP peels dried at temperatures of 60°C, 100°C, and 140°C were studied, and in this case, freeze-dried samples have been used as reference (Larrauri, Rupérez and Saura-Calixto 1997). Drying at 60°C did not significantly affect the sample characteristics evaluated (Larrauri, Rupérez and Saura-Calixto 1997). It has been proved that grape polyphenols decompose during the drying process as it is known that both magnitude and duration of heating has a strong influence on phenolic stability (Larrauri, Rupérez and Saura-Calixto 1997; Chikwanha et al. 2018); the content of polyphenols did not decrease seriously when the temperature was under 60°C but significantly reduced at 100°C (Sui et al. 2014). Tseng and Zhao (2012) dried the GP at a temperature of 85°C (Tseng and Zhao 2012).

Also, in another recent study, the thermal degradation of GP was assessed at 80°C, 100°C and 150°C (Sólyom et al. 2014). To avoid excessively high operating pressures (above 10 bar), the temperature range was restricted to between 80°C and 150°C, corresponding to the boiling range of 50% vol. mixtures of ethanol-water mixtures between 1 and 10 bar (Sólyom et al. 2014). To this end, heating was performed at 80°C, 100°C and 150°C for up to 4 hours to study kinetic degradation in terms of total phenolic and anthocyanin contents and also of antioxidant activity (Sólyom et al. 2014). Finally, it can be concluded the process intensification methods for antioxidant extraction from GP may preserve at least 90% of the active compounds up to 150°C if the processing time does not exceed 1 minute at this temperature (Sólyom et al. 2014).

## GP Yield

Yield is an indicator that presents the percentage ratio between the total grape mass taken for winemaking and the quantity of must obtained (Balteş 2016). It is evaluated according to the variety, the degree of grapes ripening, the phytosanitary state of the grapes, and the level of the technical endowment of the vinification units (Balteş 2016). The tendency is for the yield to be lower in favor of wine quality (Balteş 2016). The theoretical yields of must and grape pomace obtained by processing the grapes are calculated following the below protocol (Ţârdea, Sârbu and Ţârdea 2010). The sample of grapes for analysis must weigh precisely 1 kg, and 3 – 4 samples of each grape variety available for analysis. The analysis of these samples must be performed in parallel to establish the uvological units 'variation limits. To determine the weight of the berries and stalks, the berries are cut from the stalks, and each category is weighed. The berries are then crushed, and the must is separated by pressing with laboratory pressers. The resulting quantity of must is determined by weighing and volume in liter measurements. An identical process is used with GP, where tweezers are used to collect the seeds and skins are before being weighed separately. The pulp amount is calculated by subtracting both the combined weight of the seeds and the skins from the weight of the berries. Based on this analytical data, the values of the uvological units that characterize the composition of the grapes are established (Ţârdea, Sârbu and Ţârdea 2010). The yield in the must is between 50% for traditional winepresses and 90% for continuous pressers. Hydraulic vertical or mechanical, or pneumatic horizontal pressers can achieve 75%, or even 80% efficiency.

Furthermore, depending on the type of presser used, the yield of the GP can be calculated. Calculating the amount of yield is crucial due to the growing interest in the re-use of this wine-product. It can be deduced that the yield of GP is inversely proportional to that of the must, and the most significant values are achieved when using traditional winepresses and vertical hydraulic pressers with percentages between 35% and 40% (Balteş 2016). However, GP accounts for approximately 10–30% of the mass of grapes after crushing (Muhlack, Potumarthi and Jeffery 2018), and on average 20% of the quantity of harvested grapes (Laufenberg, Kunz and Nystroem 2003; Solari-Godiño, Lindo-Rojas and Pandia-Estrada 2017). The lowest GP yield values are observed in pressers with a continuous action of only 12% because most of the elements of GP produce sludge in the must. The quantity of sludge in the must indicates wine quality and provides a specific taste: astringent, herbal, or unpleasant. It is beneficial to reduce the quantity of sludge in the must; not exceeding percentage values between 3-4% is recommended to be collected in GP. The highest amount is in the case of continuous action pressers (33%), and the lowest for the traditional winepresses, the vertical hydraulic, and the horizontal membrane pressers (2%) (Balteş 2016).

# GP Chemical Composition

Fresh GP possesses a chemical composition that varies depending on factors such as environmental conditions, place of provenance, vine variety, harvesting period, and winemaking technique (Rockenbach et al. 2007; Rockenbach et al. 2008; Burin et al. 2010; Ahmadi and Siahsar 2011; Muhlack, Potumarthi, and Jeffery 2018). The main chemical compounds present in GP are water, cellulose, sugars, organic acids, nitrogenous substances, pectins, fatty acids, sterols, aldehydes, esters, ketones, polyphenolic substances, coloring and aromatic substances, mineral salts (Rockenbach et al. 2007; Rockenbach et al. 2008; Burin et al. 2010; Ahmadi and Siahsar 2011). Substances that have beneficial effects on human health are present in GP in significant quantities: fibers (17-21%), tannins (16-27%) and other polyphenolic compounds (2-6.5), lipids (7-12%), sugars (3%) and tartaric acid salts (Amico et al. 2004; Bettio 2008).

## Water

Water is present in large quantities in GP and any plant tissue as it is indispensable for physiological activity. (De Rosa and Castagner 1994; Bettio 2008). GP is highly perishable due to its high moisture content and water activity (Vashisth, Singh and Pegg 2011). GP generally contains moisture in the range of 60-65% (Duba 2015) but its percentage differs between the ripening stage and the harvesting time due to the conditions in which the plant is found. The amount of water in GP is a parameter of its moisture value as the quantity of the must is affected. As a result, in sweet GP, the moisture and sugar content are closely correlated: the higher the humidity, the higher the value of GP (Bettio 2008).

Glucose and fructose are **sugars** present in GP in equal concentrations despite yeasts present within the carbohydrate demolition preferentially attack glucose and converting it into ethyl alcohol with a theoretical yield of 60% (Bettio 2008; Pizzichini, Agnelli and Mucciolo

2015). Concerning residual sugars, one technical report revealed fresh white GP contained up to 38% (based on dry weight, DW) glucose and fructose (Hixson, Wilkes, Smith 2014; Muhlack, Potumarthi and Jeffery 2018). In contrast, the residual sugar content in red GP varied depending on wine type; sparkling red winemaking yielded marc with 18–30% whereas still red winemaking had as low as around 1% glucose and fructose on a DW basis (Hixson, Wilkes and Smith 2014; Muhlack, Potumarthi and Jeffery 2018). One difference between white and red wine production is that red wine GP typically has a higher alcohol content but lower sugar content (Zhang et al. 2017). In the case of the pomace of the grape variety *Airen*, which is widely grown to produce white wine throughout central Spain, the profile of neutral sugars revealed glucose as the principal sugar (61.9% of total neutral sugars) while other neutral sugars found in lower concentrations included arabinose (9.1% of total), xylose, galactose and mannose, which are present in similar proportions (7.5%, 7.1% and 6.7%, respectively) (Valiente et al. 1995).

## Acids

Comparing it with the must, GP has lower titratable acidity and higher pH value. The fixed acidity (1-2%) is due primarily to tartaric acid and to a lesser extent to malic, citric, and succinic acids, primarily in potassium, calcium and magnesium salts (De Rosa and Castagner 1994; Bettio 2008). The degree of acidity depends on grape variety, the seasonal conditions (with years containing higher amounts of rain corresponding to higher pH values), and the amount of must that remains embedded in GP (Bettio 2008). As the pH of the must ranges between 2.8 and 3.2, the fermented GP with the must will possess lower pH values than the fresh GP, reaching pH levels between 3.8 and 5,5 (Bettio 2008). At pH levels between 3.8 and 5.5, pectin methylesterase enzymes become increasingly active, hydrolyzing the pectins and releasing methyl alcohol (Odello, Giomo, Versini 1997; Bettio 2008). Lipoxygenase also become more active and assault the polyunsaturated fatty acids present within the grape peel, leading to the formation of francid aldehydes (Odello, Giomo, Versini 1997; Bettio 2008). Having GP with an optimal acidity value is useful in the selection of the alcoholic fermentation yeasts and for inhibiting the actions of undesired organisms, primarily Gram-negative bacteria (Bettio 2008). Furthermore, extended periods of silage introduce a loss in fixed acidity due to the bacteria partially destroying the tartaric acid among other organic acids such as malic acid. The destruction of these acids increases the overall volatile acidity (Bettio 2008). Recovery of tartaric acid from wine lees and GP is a well-established process (Amerine 1980; Nurgel 1998; Devesa-Rey et al. 2011) involving its extraction with the use of dilute hydrochloric acid or hot water (Nurgel 1998) followed by tartrate precipitation with calcium salts (Amerine 1980; Versari et al. 2001; Muhlack, Potumarthi and Jeffery 2018).

## Polyphenolic Compounds

Polyphenols are secondary metabolites ubiquitously distributed in all higher plants and are characterized by more than one phenol group per molecule. Grapes, GP, and wines from red varieties of *Vitis vinifera L.* provide essential sources of natural antioxidants because of their high concentration of different phenolic compounds (Balea et al. 2018). In grapes, polyphenols accumulate in stalks, skins, and seeds and are extracted before being passed to the must and wine through a technological process recognized as maceration-fermentation (Ţârdea, Sârbu and Ţârdea 2010). The seeds and skin provide the most significant quantities of grape polyphenols, and these are the primary compounds available for extraction in grape processing (Kammerer et al. 2004; Deng, Penner, and Zhao 2011; Balea et al. 2018). The total extractable phenolics in grapes are present in a maximum yield of approximately 10% in the pulp, 60–70% in the seeds, and 28–35% in the skin (Shi et al. 2003; Chedea et al. 2011; Ribeiro et al. 2015). Polyphenols present in grapes and wine are generally classified into two main groups: non-flavonoids (hydroxybenzoic and hydroxycinnamic acids and their derivatives, stilbenes, and phenolic alcohols) and flavonoids (anthocyanins, flavanols, flavonols, dihydroflavonols, and procyanidins) (Kammerer et al. 2004; Deng, Penner, and Zhao 2011; Fanzone et al. 2012; Xu et al. 2016; Balea et al. 2018). For example, grape skins contain multiple types of polyphenols, including 39 types of anthocyanins, hydroxycinnamic acids, catechins, and flavonols (Kammerer et al. 2004; Deng, Penner, and Zhao 2011).

The total grape content contains quantities of polyphenols that vary between 2.9 and 5.7 g/kg (Țârdea, Sârbu and Țârdea2010). Approximately 70% of the phenolic compounds have been reported to remain in the pomace (Balea et al. 2018). Notably, the content of polyphenolic material varies considerably according to grape type, variety, environmental factors, and winemaking techniques (Solari-Godiño, Lindo-Rojas and Pandia-Estrada 2017). It has been well documented that different cultivars, harvest time, location, and growth environment affect the total polyphenolic content (TPC) of wine grapes (Alonso et al. 2002; Lee, Johnson and Talcott 2005; Chedea et al. 2011; Deng, Penner and Zhao 2011; Tseng and Zhao 2012; Jara-Palacios et al. 2015; Gerardi et al. 2020). TPC is measured using the Folin–Ciocalteu assay alongside a UV-Vis spectrophotometer (Chedea and Pop 2019). Below we present several examples that are available within the literature of the TPC content that is available in GP samples that have originated from different countries.

Thimothe et al. (2007) reported that for all the varieties studied GP, despite the pomace representing a waste material produced during the wine fermentation process, contained comparable or slightly higher TPC than whole fruit extracts; total phenols in GP was between 41.1 and 61.8 g of gallic acid equivalents (GAE)/100 g of extract (Thimothe et al. 2007). The tested grapevine variants were *Vitis vinifera* grapes (*Pinot Noir* and *Cabernet Franc*) and *Vitis* interspecific hybrids (*Baco Noir* and *Noiret*, a wine variety selected for its deep color resulting from a cross between NY65.0467.08 and Steuben) (Thimothe et al. 2007). Tseng and Zhao (2012) found that TPC in red GP *Vitis vinifera* L. from the Oregon

State University Research Winery (Corvallis, OR, USA), Pinot Noir contained 67.74 mg GAE/g GP. Dried GP consisting of stems, skins, and seeds derived from red grapes varieties from Valea Calugărească (Romania) had a TPC of 5.8 mg GAE/100 g dry GP (Chedea et al. 2018). Red and white wine GP from the vinification of *Vitis vinífera L. cv. Tempranillo* and *Verdejo* (Burgos, Spain) were analyzed for the polyphenolic content, and the sum of total phenolic composition was found to be 2176 μg/g for red GP and of 781 μg/g for white GP (Gerardi et al. 2020).

In the polyphenolic classes that were previously mentioned, the anthocyanins are the primary coloring pigments found in red grapes possess antioxidant properties that enable the long-term storage of the grapes (De Rosa and Castagner 1994; Odello, Giomo and Versini 1997; Bettio 2008). Red-violet pigments also exist within GP, emerging during the alcoholic fermentation of the wine (Pizzichini, Agnelli and Mucciolo 2015) when 30-40% of the anthocyanins content within grapes have been extracted from the skins (Luque-Rodríguez, Luque de Castro and Pérez-Juan 2007; Polovka et al. 2010; Teixeira et al. 2014; Pereira et al. 2019). Flavonoids provide white grapes with their color (Bettio 2008).

The importance of winemaking in many countries has encouraged the widespread availability of large quantities of grape skins containing high amounts of anthocyanin pigments. These pigments have been marketed under several trade names, such as Enocyanin in the United States, Italy, Germany, and France (Francis 1992; Larrauri, Rupérez and Saura-Calixto 1997). The beneficial health effects of consuming polyphenols extracted from GP such as anthocyanins (Fitzpatrick, Hirschfield, and Coffey 1993; Larrauri, Rupérez and Saura-Calixto 1997), for example, their antioxidant activity (Kanner et al. 1994; Larrauri, Rupérez and Saura-Calixto 1997; Chedea et al. 2019), could be useful in developing novel products such as dietary supplements capable of promoting improved health.

Due to challenges associated with extraction during the winemaking process, pomace retains high levels of condensed tannins, mainly proanthocyanidins composed of procyanidin and prodelphinidin units linked together by a C4–C8 bond in grapes (Ping et al. 2011; Bunea

2016). The tannins present in seeds differ from those in the skin (Hosu et al. 2010; Hosu et al. 2011; Pop 2015). Whereas seed tannins are only procyanidins (Prieur et al. 1994; Czochanska, Foo, and Porter 1979), grape skins contain procyanidin and prodelphinidin units (Souquet et al. 1996; Sarni-Manchado, Cheynier, and Moutounet 1999). The variation in tannin content between varieties, irrespective of the drying method, could be due to the number of seeds per berry rather than tannin per seed (Chikwanha et al. 2018).

Because of its well-acclaimed beneficial biological activities, the stilbene derivative (with a C6–C2–C6 structure) resveratrol (3,5,4′-trihydroxy-stilbene) has become the subject of many studies with links to the pharmaceutical industries (Chedea et al. 2017). The beneficial biological activities reported were its preventive role in cardiovascular health and disease, described as a phenomenon commonly known as the "French Paradox". Renaud (1992) observed that despite French people having a high saturated fat intake in their diet, they presented a lower incidence (about 40%) of coronary heart diseases than the rest of Europe (Renaud 1992). This was attributed to an increased red wine intake by the French population (Renaud 1992). Romero-Pérez et al. (1996; 1999) demonstrated that the amount of RESV varies depending on the wine type: it can reach even more than 580 μg per 100 mL in red wines, whereas its content is much lower (~68 μg per 100 mL) in white wines. This difference can be explained by considering that the skin is removed earlier during wine production in white wine, reducing the amount of resveratrol extracted. Furthermore, red wine contains more trans-resveratrol than white wine. In contrast, the latter has a higher concentration of cis-resveratrol, which is exceptionally light-sensitive (Chedea et al. 2017).

Different plants produce resveratrol, and this is most likely due to its antifungal properties. The level of this compound and its derivatives in plants depends on various factors such as environmental conditions, abiotic (light, UV radiation), or biotic stress (fungal infection, mainly by *Plasmopara viticola* and *Botrytis cinerea*) (Nour, Trandafir and Muntean 2012; Chedea et al. 2017).

In grapevine, resveratrol is synthesized in the leaf epidermis and in the skin of grapes, especially of the red varieties, and mostly when it is infected with *Botrytis cinerea* (Creasy 1988; Chedea et al. 2017). The compound is one of the essential polyphenols found in grapes, which can be extracted from grapes, red wine, and from different vegetative parts of the grapevine. The amount of resveratrol in grapevine cultivars varies widely. As grape skin is a good source of resveratrol (Fremont 2000; Gezer 2011; Taşeri et al. 2018) and all GP samples contain high amounts of skin, in addition to seeds and stems (Ribeiro et al. 2015), this compound is found in pomace in essential concentrations.

Fresh grape skins contain between 50 to 100 micrograms of resveratrol/g (Casas, Faraldi 2008; Bettio 2008). In red GP, Gerardi et al. (2020) found 4.58 μg resveratrol/g GP, and in the white GP 1.21 μg resveratrol/g GP (Gerardi et al. 2020). From red grape cultivar *Nerello Mascalese* grape stems, resveratrol was obtained in amounts of more than 130 mg kg−1 of the dried stem (Spatafora and Tringali 2012) and also from grape seeds, stems, skin, and pomace of the *Palomino fino* grape variety (Casas et al. 2010). Another potential and widely available source of resveratrol derived from the grapevine is the grapevine cane which is usually burned because it is a by-product of vine pruning and summer trimming (Çetin et al. 2011; Angelov, Boyadzhiev and Georgieva 2016). The cultivar and period of pruning have an important influence on the trans-resveratrol content in grapevine stems (Aaviksaar et al. 2003; Angelov, Boyadzhiev and Georgieva 2016). Therefore, depending on the variety, the amount of resveratrol was between 1 to 4.7 mg g−1 of the stem in canes collected during the autumn period, which is higher than the spring or summer harvest. *Pinot Noir* grape canes contained 3.45 mg per g dw trans-resveratrol and shoots 15.90 mg per kg dry matter (DM) (Lachman et al. 2016).

## The Pectic Substances

The pectic substances present in the skin consist of long, linear chains of galacturonic acid, whose carboxyls are either free or esterified with methyl groups. The enzymatic action of pectin methylesterase of plant origin during the storage period, favored by the fermentation and distillation temperatures, may contribute to releasing a high fraction of methyl alcohol. The presence of methyl alcohol in GP is influenced by grape variety (forming faster in white grapes than in red grapes), winemaking method, and conditioning (silage versus drying). In terms of gross composition, the residual winemaking products, GP (skin and seeds), contained more lipid, soluble sugar, and phenolic compounds than skin samples, which had a greater concentration of ash and pectin (Tseng and Zhao 2012). In fresh grapes and GP, pectic substances are the main polymer-type constituent of the cell walls, ranging from 38 to 49 mol% and 37 to 54 mol% of cell wall polysaccharides, respectively (González-Centeno et al. 2010). Pectins with a low degree of methyl-esterification were the primary cell wall polymer type in GP (González-Centeno et al. 2010). In contrast, cellulose was the predominant cell wall polysaccharide in grape stems (Beres et al. 2017).

## Cellulose

After pectin, cellulose is the second type of cell wall polysaccharide in GP, within the limits of 27 to 37 mol% of cell wall polysaccharides (González-Centeno et al. 2010). Cellulose is a linear polymer consisting of D-glucose molecules linked by 1,4 glucoside bonds. It has an average molecular weight of 400,000, corresponding to about 2800 units of glucose per molecule. Cellulose fibers consist of parallel strips of the polysaccharide chain, joined by hydrogen bonds between adjacent hydroxyl groups. This type of structure gives cellulose fiber a high mechanical strength. Other features of this molecule are insolubility in water and poor thermal conductivity, enabling it to be an insulating material (Bettio 2008). Deng, Penner and Zhao (2011) reported that total dietary fiber (TDF) was the predominant component in the red GP but not in the white GP in which soluble sugar took the most significant proportion. The percentage of TDF (51.1–56.3% on the dry matter) in the red GP was similar to those (about 50–60% of TDF) reported by Bravo (1998) and Valiente et al. (1995) (Valiente et al. 1995; Bravo 1998; Deng, Penner and Zhao 2011).

## Aromatic Substances

In GP, aromatic substances originate from the grape, but most of them are developed during pomace fermentation (Gerogiannaki-Christopolou et al. 2004). The inner layers of the grape's berry skin are home to the varietal or primary aromas, odorant molecules such as linalool (responsible for *Muscat*'s aroma), nerol, citronellol, and geraniol, which are terpenoids but also other chemical groups such as higher alcohols, esters, aldehydes, ketones, acids and sulfur compounds (Bettio 2008; Gerogiannaki-Christopolou et al. 2004). Some of these compounds are volatile or highly volatile, while others exhibit lower volatility (Gerogiannaki-Christopolou et al. 2004). Not all vine varieties possess aromatic molecules, which allows the distinction between non-aromatic and aromatic varieties such as *Muscat*, *Sauvignon*, *Traminer*. The aroma profile is influenced by factors such as environment, soil, climate, grape variety, degree of grape ripeness, enological methods used for pomace production, and pomace fermentation conditions (Carnacini 1986; Gerogiannaki-Christopolou et al. 2004; Bettio 2008). These aroma compounds exist in a wide concentration range. Some of them are present at high concentrations (hundreds of mg/L) (Mullins, Bouquet and Williams 1992), but most of them are found at a very low concentration range, from traces to l0 mg/L (Gerogiannaki-Christopolou et al. 2004).

## ACKNOWLEDGMENTS

The authors wish to thank Hesham Ahmed Kisher, University of the West of England, Bristol for his assistance with the reviewing and editing of the English for this manuscript.

## REFERENCES

Aaviksaar Aavo, Haga Mati, Pusssa Tonu, Roasto Matti. & Tsoupras George. (2003). "Purification of Resveratrol from Vine Stems." In *Proceedings of the Estonian Academy of Sciences*, Virve Kurnitski Hillar Aben eds., *52* (4) 155–164. Tallinn.

Ahmadi Seyed Mohammad. & Siahsar Barat Ali. (2011). "Analogy of Physicochemical Attributes of Two Grape Seeds Cultivars," *Food Technology Ciencia e Investigation Agraria*, *38* (2), 291–301.

Aktaş, Mustafa, Ataollah Khanlari, Ali Amini. & Seyfi Şevik. (2017). "Performance Analysis of Heat Pump and Infrared–Heat Pump Drying of Grated Carrot Using Energy-Exergy Methodology." *Energy Conversion and Management*, *132*, 327–338. https://doi.org/10.1016/j.enconman.2016.11.027.

Alleweldt, G. & Possingham, J. V. (1988). "Progress in Grapevine Breeding." *Theor Appl Genet.*, *75*, 669-673 Springer.

Alonso, Ángeles M., Dominico A. Guillén, Carmelo G. Barroso, Belén Puertas. & Alberto García. (2002). "Determination of Antioxidant Activity of Wine Byproducts and Its Correlation with Polyphenolic Content." *Journal of Agricultural and Food Chemistry*, *50* (21), 5832–5836. https://doi.org/10.1021/jf025683b.

Amerine M. A. (1980). *The Technology of Wine Making. 4th Ed.* https://agris.fao.org/agris-search/search.do?recordID=US19810706324#.XusdKqrDzmI.mendeley.

Amico, V., Napoli, E. M., Renda, A., Ruberto, G., Spatafora, C. & Tringali, C. (2004). "Constituents of Grape Pomace from the Sicilian

Cultivar 'Nerello Mascalese.'" *Food Chemistry, 88* (4), 599–607. https://doi.org/10.1016/j.foodchem.2004.02.022.

Angelov, George, Lubomir Boyadzhiev. & Silviya Georgieva. (2016). "Useful Bioactive Substances from Wastes: Recovery of Trans-Resveratrol from Grapevine Stems." *The Open Chemical Engineering Journal, 10* (1), 4–9. https://doi.org/10.2174/1874123101610010004.

Antoniolli, Andrea, Ariel R. Fontana, Patricia Piccoli. & Rubén Bottini. (2015). "Characterization of Polyphenols and Evaluation of Antioxidant Capacity in Grape Pomace of the Cv. Malbec." *Food Chemistry, 178*, 172–78. https://doi.org/10.1016/j.foodchem.2015.01.082.

Azuara-Nieto, E., Gutiérrez-Lopéz G. F. & Beristain-Guevara, C. I. (2003). "Mass transfer description osmodehydration of apple slabs" In: *Transport Phenomena in Food Processing.* G. V. Welti-Chanes, J.; Vélez-Ruiz, J. F.; Barbosa-Cánovas, Eds., 95-108, CRC Press.

Azzouz, Soufien, Imen Hermassi, Mohsen Toujani. & Ali Belghith. (2016). "Effect of Drying Temperature on the Rheological Characteristics of Dried Seedless Grapes." *Food and Bioproducts Processing, 100*, 246–254, https://doi.org/10.1016/j.fbp.2016.07.002.

Bacic, T. (2003). *Recovery of valuable products from lees and integrated approach to minimise waste and add value to wine production.* Report no. UM, University of Melbourne, Melbourne, Australia.

Balea, Ştefania Silvia, Alina Elena Pârvu, Nastasia Pop, Fernando Zamora Marín. & Marcel Pârvu. (2018). "Polyphenolic Compounds, Antioxidant, and Cardioprotective Effects of Pomace Extracts from Fetească Neagră Cultivar." Ada Popolo. 2018: 11. *Oxidative Medicine and Cellular Longevity.* https://doi.org/10.1155/2018/8194721.

Balteş Mihaela Virginia. (2016). *Valorificarea subproduselor vinicole cu obţinere de produşi valoroşi pentru industrie şi alimentaţie.* PhD thesis 6-8. Sibiu: Universitatea "Lucian Blaga" Sibiu. http://doctorate.ulbsibiu.ro/wp-content/uploads/REZUMAT-Baltes.pdf.

[*Capitalization of wine by-products with obtaining valuable products for industry and food*]

Beres, Carolina, Gislaine N. S. Costa, Ignacio Cabezudo, Nina K. da Silva-James, Aline S.C. Teles, Ana P. G. Cruz, Caroline Mellinger-Silva, Renata V. Tonon, Lourdes M. C. Cabral. & Suely P. Freitas. (2017). "Towards Integral Utilization of Grape Pomace from Winemaking Process: A Review." *Waste Management*. Elsevier Ltd., *68*, 581-594 https://doi.org/10.1016/j.wasman.2017.07.017.

Bettio Giacomo. (2008). *Utilizzo di batteri lattici per la produzione di composti bioattivi a partire da scarti vegetali.* Tesi di laurea. 9-13 Universita'degli studi di Padova, Italia. http://tesi.cab.unipd.it/24236/1/bettio_giacomo_tesi.pdf. [*Use of lactic bacteria for the production of bioactive compounds from vegetable waste*.]

Bingol, Gokhan, Jihong Yang, Maria T. Brandl, Zhongli Pan, Hua Wang. & Tara H. McHugh. (2011). "Infrared Pasteurization of Raw Almonds." *Journal of Food Engineering, 104* (3), 387–393. https://doi.org/10.1016/j.jfoodeng.2010.12.034.

Blij, J. Harm De. (1983). *Wine: A Geographic Appreciation*. Rowman & Littlefield Pub Incorporated.

Boulton, R., Singleton, V., Bisson, L. & Kunkee, R. (1996). *Principles and Practices of Winemaking*. New York.

Bravo, L. & Saura Calixto, F. (1998). "Characterization of Dietary Fiber and the *in Vitro* Indigestible Fraction of Grape Pomace." *American Journal of Enology and Viticulture*, *49* (2), 135–141.

Bunea Andrea. (2016). "Procyanidins: Structure and Occurrence." In *Procyanidins Characterisation, Antioxidant Properties and Health Benefits*, Chedea Veronica Sanda, 2–7. New York: Nova Science Publishers.

Burin, Vívian Maria, Leila Denise Falcão, Luciano Valdemiro Gonzaga, Roseane Fett, Jean Pierre Rosier. & Marilde Terezinha Bordignon-Luiz. (2010). "Colour, Phenolic Content and Antioxidant Activity of Grape Juice Cor, Conteúdo Fenólico e Atividade Antioxidante de Sucos de Uva." *Food Science and Technology*, *30* (4), 1027-1032, https://doi.org/10.1590/S0101-20612010000400030.

Carnacini, A. & Pozzo, A. (1986). "About the Volatile Compounds of Musts and Wines in Relation to the Obtaining Technologies." *Vignevini*, *13*.

Casas Elvira, Faraldi Marianna. & Bildstein Marie. (2008). *Guida Ai Composti Bioattivi Nei Residui Di Lavorazione Dell'uva.* Bioactive-Net. [*Guide to Bioactive Compounds in Grape Processing Residues.*]

Casas, L., Mantell, C., Rodríguez, M., Martínez de la Ossa, E. J., Roldán, A., De Ory, I., Caro, I. & Blandino, A. (2010). "Extraction of Resveratrol from the Pomace of Palomino Fino Grapes by Supercritical Carbon Dioxide." *Journal of Food Engineering*, *96* (2), 304–308. https://doi.org/10.1016/j.jfoodeng.2009.08.002.

Çetin, Emine Sema, Duygu Altinöz, Ecehan Tarçan. & Nilgün Göktürk Baydar. (2011). "Chemical Composition of Grape Canes." *Industrial Crops and Products*, *34* (1), 994–998. https://doi.org/10.1016/j.indcrop.2011.03.004.

Che Man', Yaakob B, Irwandi Jaswir, Yusof Salmah, Jinap Selamat, Hiroshi Sugisawa, Universiti Pertanian Malaysia, Upm Serdang. & Selangor De Malaysia. (1997). "Effect of different dryers and drying chemical characteristics of durian leather conditions on acceptability and physico." *Journal of Food Processing and Preservation.*, *21* (5), 425-441. https://doi.org/10.1111/j.1745-4549.1997.tb00794.x.

Chedea, Veronica S., Camelia Echim, Cornelia Braicu, Mirjana Andjelkovic, Roland Verhe. & Carmen Socaciu. (2011). "Composition in Polyphenols and Stability of the Aqueous Grape Seed Extract from the Romanian Variety 'Merlot Recas.'" *Journal of Food Biochemistry.*, *35* (1), 92–108. https://doi.org/10.1111/j.1745-4514.2010.00368.x.

Chedea, Veronica Sanda, Laurentiu Mihai Palade, Daniela Eliza Marin, Rodica Stefania Pelmus, Mihaela Habeanu, Mircea Catalin Rotar, Mihail Alexandru Gras, Gina Cecilia Pistol. & Ionelia Taranu. (2018). "Intestinal Absorption and Antioxidant Activity of Grape Pomace Polyphenols." *Nutrients*, *10* (5), 588. https://doi.org/10.3390/nu10050588.

Chedea, Veronica Sanda, Laurentiu Mihai Palade, Rodica Stefania Pelmus, Catalin Dragomir. & Ionelia Taranu. (2019). "Red Grape Pomace Rich in Polyphenols Diet Increases the Antioxidant Status in Key Organs— Kidneys, Liver, and Spleen of Piglets." *Animals*, *9* (4), 149. https://doi.org/10.3390/ani9040149.

Chedea, Veronica Sanda. & Raluca Maria Pop. (2019). "Total Polyphenols Content and Antioxidant DPPH Assays on Biological Samples." In *Polyphenols in Plants*, 169–183. Elsevier. https://doi.org/10.1016/b978-0-12-813768-0.00011-6.

Chedea, Veronica Sanda, Simona Ioana Vicaş, Claudia Sticozzi, Federica Pessina, Maria Frosini, Emanuela Maioli. & Giuseppe Valacchi. (2017). "Resveratrol: From Diet to Topical Usage." *Food and Function. Royal Society of Chemistry.*, *8* (11), 3879-3892. https://doi.org/10.1039/c7fo01086a.

Chen, Yougui. & Alex Martynenko. (2013). "Computer Vision for Real-Time Measurements of Shrinkage and Color Changes in Blueberry Convective Drying." *Drying Technology*, *31* (10), 1114–1123. https://doi.org/10.1080/07373937.2013.775587.

Chikwanha, Obert C., Emiliano Raffrenato, Umezuruike L. Opara, Olaniyi A. Fawole, Mathabatha E. Setati, Voster Muchenje. & Cletos Mapiye. (2018). "Impact of Dehydration on Retention of Bioactive Profile and Biological Activities of Different Grape (*Vitis Vinifera* L.) Pomace Varieties." *Animal Feed Science and Technology*, *244*, 116-127, https://doi.org/10.1016/j.anifeedsci.2018.08.006.

Choe, Eunok. & Soojung Oh. (2013). "Effects of Water Activity on the Lipid Oxidation and Antioxidants of Dried Laver (Porphyra) during Storage in the Dark." *Journal of Food Science*, *78* (8), 1144-1151. https://doi.org/10.1111/1750-3841.12197.

Çoklar, H. & Akbulut, M. (2017). "Effect of Sun, Oven and Freeze-Drying on Anthocyanins, Phenolic Compounds and Antioxidant Activity of Black Grape (Ekşikara) (*Vitis Vinifera* L.)." *South African Journal of Enology & Viticulture*, *38* (2). https://doi.org/10.21548/38-2-2127.

Cox Jeff. (1999). *Cox From Vines to Wines: The Complete Guide to Growing Grapes and Making Your Own Wine*.

Creasy, L. L. & Coffee, M. (1988). "Phytoalexin Production Potential of Grape Berries." *Journal of the American Society for Horticultural Science*, *113* (2), 230–234.

Czochanska, Zofia, Lai Yeap Foo. & Lawrence J Porter. (1979). "Compositional changes in lower molecular weight flavans during grape maturation." *Phytochemistry*, *18* (11), 1819-1822 C Pergamon Press Ltd. Printed m England.

Deng, Qian, Michael H. Penner. & Yanyun Zhao. (2011). "Chemical Composition of Dietary Fiber and Polyphenols of Five Different Varieties of Wine Grape Pomace Skins." *Food Research International*, *44* (9), 2712–2720. https://doi.org/10.1016/ j.foodres. 2011.05.026.

De Rosa, Tullio. & Castagner, Roberto. (1994). *Tecnologia delle grappe e dei distillati d'uva*. Edagricole. [*Grappa and grape distillates technology*.]

Devesa-Rey, R., Vecino, X., Varela-Alende, J. L., Barral, M. T., Cruz, J. M. & Moldes, A. B. (2011). "Valorization of Winery Waste vs. the Costs of Not Recycling." *Waste Management*, *31* (11), 2327–2335. https://doi.org/10.1016/j.wasman.2011.06.001.

Duba, Kurabachew Simon. (2015). *Supercritical Technologies for the Valorization of Wine Industry By-Products*.

Fanzone, Martín, Fernando Zamora, Viviana Jofré, Mariela Assof, Carmen Gómez-Cordovés. & Álvaro Peña-Neira. (2012). "Phenolic Characterisation of Red Wines from Different Grape Varieties Cultivated in Mendoza Province (Argentina)." *Journal of the Science of Food and Agriculture*, *92* (3), 704–718. https://doi.org/10.1002/ jsfa.4638.

Fitzpatrick, David F., Steven L Hirschfield. & Ronald G Coffey. (1993), *Endothelium-Dependent Vasorelaxing Activity of Wine and Other Grape Products.*, *265* (2), 774-778, www.physiology.org/ journal/ajpheart.

Fontana, Ariel R., Andrea Antoniolli. & Rubén Bottini. (2013). "Grape Pomace as a Sustainable Source of Bioactive Compounds: Extraction, Characterization, and Biotechnological Applications of Phenolics." *Journal of Agricultural and Food Chemistry*, *61* (38), 8987–9003. https://doi.org/10.1021/jf402586f.

Francis F. J. (1992). "*A New Group of Food Colorants*", *3*, 27-30, https://doi.org/10.1016/0924-2244(92)90112-A.

Fremont, Lucie. (2000). "Minireview biological effects of resveratrol." *Life Sciences.*, *66* (8), 663-673.https://doi.org/10.1016/S0024-3205(99)00410-5.

Frum, Adina, Cecilia Georgescu, Felicia G. Gligor, Ecaterina Lengyel, Diana I. Stegarus, Carmen M. Dobrea. & Ovidiu Tita. (2018). "Identification and Quantification of Phenolic Compounds from Red Grape Pomace." *Scientific Study and Research: Chemistry and Chemical Engineering, Biotechnology, Food Industry.*, *19* (1), 045-052.

Gabel, Michael M., Zhongli Pan, K. S. P. Amaratunga, Linda J. Harris. & James F. Thompson. (2006). "Catalytic Infrared Dehydration of Onions." *Journal of Food Science*, *71* (9), 351-357. https://doi.org/10.1111/j.1750-3841.2006.00170.x.

Gallander, James F. (1974). "Chemistry of Grapes and Other Fruits as the Raw Materials Involved in Winemaking." *American Chemical Society*, *137*(2), 11–49. https://doi.org/10.1021/ba-1974-0137.ch002.

Gan, Haozhe, Erin Charters, Robert Driscoll. & George Srzednicki. (2017). "Effects of Drying and Blanching on the Retention of Bioactive Compounds in Ginger and Turmeric." *Horticulturae*, *3* (1). https://doi.org/10.3390/horticulturae3010013.

Gerardi, Gisela, Mónica Cavia-Saiz, M. Dolores Rivero-Pérez, María Luisa González-Sanjosé. & Pilar Muñiz. (2020). "The Dose-Response Effect on Polyphenol Bioavailability after Intake of White and Red Wine Pomace Products by Wistar Rats." *Food and Function*, *11* (2), 1661–1671. https://doi.org/10.1039/c9fo01743g.

Gerogiannaki-Christopolou, Maria, Kyriakidis Nikolaos V. & Panagiotis E. Athanasopoulos. (2004). "Effect of Grape Variety (*Vitis Vinifera*

L.) and Grape Pomace Fermentation Conditions on Some Volatile Compounds of the Produced Grape Pomace Distillate." *J. Int. Sci. Vigne Vin*, *38* (4), 225-230.

Gezer, Pertvin Gizem. (2011). *Modeling Drying Kinetics of Grape Seeds and Skins from Turkish Cultivars*. Master thesis.

González-Centeno, M. R., Rosselló, C., Simal, S., Garau, M. C., López, F. & Femenia, A. (2010). "Physico-Chemical Properties of Cell Wall Materials Obtained from Ten Grape Varieties and Their Byproducts: Grape Pomaces and Stems." *LWT - Food Science and Technology*, *43* (10), 1580–1586. https://doi.org/10.1016/j.lwt.2010.06.024.

Goula, Athanasia M., Konstantinos Thymiatis. & Kyriakos Kaderides. (2016). "Valorization of Grape Pomace: Drying Behavior and Ultrasound Extraction of Phenolics." *Food and Bioproducts Processing*, *100*, 132–144. https://doi.org/10.1016/J.FBP.2016.06.016.

Gramaje, David, Jose Ramon Urbez-Torres. & Mark R. Sosnowski. (2018). "Managing Grapevine Trunk Diseases with Respect to Etiology and Epidemiology: Current Strategies and Future Prospects." *Plant Disease*, *102* (1), 12–39. https://doi.org/10.1094/PDIS-04-17-0512-FE.

Guochen, Zhang, Sigurjón Arason. & Sveinn Víkingur Árnason. (2009). "Dehydration Property of Shrimp (*Pandalus Borealis*) Undergoing Heat-Pump Drying Process." *International Journal of Agricultural and Biological Engineering*, *2* (4), 92–97. https://doi.org/10.3965/j.issn.1934-6344.2009.04.092-097.

Hixson, J., Wilkes, E., Smith, P. & Forsyth, K. (2014). "Understanding the Composition of Grape Marc and Its Potential as a Livestock Feed Supplement." *The Australian Wine Research Institute Technical Review*, *213*, 11–15.

Hosu, Anamaria, Claudia Cimpoiu, Vasile Miclaus, Grigore Damian, Irina Tarsiche. & Nastasia Pop. (2010). "Influence of Intermittent Heating during Maceration on the Antioxidant Capacity of Some Grape Seeds and Skins." *Hort. Agrobot. Cluj*, *38* (1), 41–43. www.notulaebotanicae.ro.

Hosu, Anamaria D., Claudia Cimpoiu, Vasile Miclaus. & Lorentz Jantschi. (2011). "Antioxidant Content of Three Different Varieties of Wine Grapes." *Biotechnology and Biotechnological Equipment*, *25* (1), 2217–2221. https://doi.org/10.5504/bbeq.2011.0005.

http://Www.Fao.Org/Faostat/En/#data/QC. 2020. 2020.

http://Www.Fao.Org/Faostat/En/#data/QD. 2020. 2020.

https://Www.Wikiwand.Com/En/Pressing_(Wine). 2020. 2020.

Jangam, S. V., Law, C. L. & Mujumdar, A. S. (2010). *Drying of Foods, Vegetables and Fruits*. Published in Singapore.

Jara-Palacios, M. José, Dolores Hernanz, Tania Cifuentes-Gomez, M. Luisa Escudero-Gilete, Francisco J. Heredia. & Jeremy P. E. Spencer. (2015). "Assessment of White Grape Pomace from Winemaking as Source of Bioactive Compounds, and Its Antiproliferative Activity." *Food Chemistry*, *183*, 78–82. https://doi.org/10.1016/ j.foodchem.2015.03.022.

Jiang, Yan, John Simonsen. & Yanyun Zhao. (2011). "Compression-Molded Biocomposite Boards from Red and White Wine Grape Pomaces." *Journal of Applied Polymer Science*, *119* (5), 2834–46. https://doi.org/10.1002/app.32961.

Kammerer, Dietmar, Achim Claus, Reinhold Carle. & Andreas Schieber. (2004). "Polyphenol Screening of Pomace from Red and White Grape Varieties (*Vitis Vinifera* L.) by HPLC-DAD-MS/MS." *Journal of Agricultural and Food Chemistry*, *52* (14), 4360–4367. https://doi.org/10.1021/jf049613b.

Kanner, Joseph, Edwin Frankel, J., Rina Granit, Bruce German. & John E Kinsellatss. (1994). "Natural Antioxidants in Grapes and Wines." *Journal of Agricultural and Food Chemistry*, *42* (1), 64-69. https://doi.org/10.1021/jf00037a010.

Kataria, S. S. & Shaikh, F. I. (2007). "Design of Drying Chamber for Grape Drying and Drying Process." *Bav Food World*, *34*, 56–60.

Khanal, Ramesh C., Luke R. Howard. & Ronald L. Prior. (2010). "Effect of Heating on the Stability of Grape and Blueberry Pomace Procyanidins and Total Anthocyanins." *Food Research International*, *43* (5), 1464–1469. https://doi.org/10.1016/j.foodres.2010.04.018.

Lachman, J., Kotikova, Z., Hejtmankova, A., Pivec, V., Psenienaja, O., Sulc, M., Stoalkova, R. & Didina, M. (2016). "Resveratrol and Piceid Isomers Concentrations in Grapevine Shoots, Leaves, and Tendrils." *Horticultural Science*, *43* (1), 25–32. https://doi.org/10.17221/258/2014-HORTSCI.

Larrauri, José A., Pilar Rupérez. & Fulgencio Saura-Calixto. (1997). "Effect of Drying Temperature on the Stability of Polyphenols and Antioxidant Activity of Red Grape Pomace Peels." *Journal of Agricultural and Food Chemistry*, *45*(4), 1390-1393. https://doi.org/10.1021/jf960282f.

Laufenberg, Gunther, Benno Kunz. & Marianne Nystroem. (2003). "Transformation of Vegetable Waste into Value Added Products: (A) the Upgrading Concept; (B) Practical Implementations." *Bioresource Technology*, *87*(2), 167-198. https://doi.org/10.1016/S0960-8524(02)00167-0

Lee, Joon Hee, Jodie V. Johnson. & Stephen T. Talcott. (2005). "Identification of Ellagic Acid Conjugates and Other Polyphenolics in Muscadine Grapes by HPLC-ESI-MS." *Journal of Agricultural and Food Chemistry*, *53* (15), 6003–6010. https://doi.org/10.1021/jf050468r.

Luque-Rodríguez, J. M., M. D. Luque de Castro. & Pérez-Juan, P. (2007). "Dynamic Superheated Liquid Extraction of Anthocyanins and Other Phenolics from Red Grape Skins of Winemaking Residues." *Bioresource Technology*, *98* (14), 2705–2713. https://doi.org/10.1016/j.biortech.2006.09.019.

Martynenko, Alex. & Tadeusz Kudra. (2016). "Electrohydrodynamic (EHD) Drying of Grape Pomace." *Japan Journal of Food Engineering* 17 (4): 123–129. https://doi.org/10.11301/jsfe.17.123.

Maskan, Aysun, Sevim Kaya. & Medeni Maskan. (2002). "Hot Air and Sun Drying of Grape Leather (Pestil)." *Journal of Food Engineering*, *54*, (1), 81-88. https://doi.org/10.1016/S0260-8774(01)00188-1.

Mendes Andressa Cristina Gaione, Daynna Miranda Rettore, Alcinéia de Lemos Souza Ramos, Simone de Fátima Viana Da Cunhalv, Luis Carlos de Oliveira. & Eduardo Mendes Ramos. (2014). "Salames

Tipo Milano Elaborados Com Libras de Subprodutos Da Produção de Vinho Tinto Milano." [Type Salami Elaborated with Fibers of Red Wine Byproducts]. *Ciência Rural, Santa Maria*, *44* (7), 1291-1296. https://doi.org/10.1590/0103-8478cr2013Q389.

Muhlack, Richard A., Ravichandra Potumarthi. & David W. Jeffery. (2018). "Sustainable Wineries through Waste Valorisation: A Review of Grape Marc Utilisation for Value-Added Products." *Waste Management.*, *72*, 99-118. https://doi.org/10.1016/ j.wasman. 2017.11.011.

Mullins Michael G., Bouquet Alain. & Williams Larry E. (1992). *Biology of the Grapevine*. Cambridge University Press.

Muncaciu, Maria L., Fernando Zamora Marín, Nastasia Pop. & Anca C. Babeş. (2017). "Comparative Polyphenolic Content of Grape Pomace Flours from 'Fetească Neagră' and 'Italian Riesling' Cultivars." *Notulae Botanicae Horti Agrobotanici Cluj-Napoca*, *45* (2), 532-539. https://doi.org/10.15835/nbha45210872.

Nayak, A., Brij Bhushan, A. Rosales, L. Rodriguez Turienzo. & Cortina, J. L. (2018). "Valorisation Potential of Cabernet Grape Pomace for the Recovery of Polyphenols: Process Intensification, Optimisation and Study of Kinetics." *Food and Bioproducts Processing*, *109*, 74-85. https://doi.org/10.1016/j.fbp.2018.03.004.

Negrul, A. M. (1938). "Evolution of Cultivated Forms of Grapes.," *CR Acad. Sci. URSS*, *18*, 585-588.

Nour, Violeta, Ion Trandafir. & Camelia Muntean. (2012). "Ultraviolet Irradiation of Trans-Resveratrol and HPLC Determination of Trans-Resveratrol and Cis-Resveratrol in Romanian Red Wines." *Journal of Chromatographic Science*, *50* (10), 920–927. https://doi.org/ 10.1093/chromsci/bms091.

Nurgel, C. & Canbas, A. (1998). "Production of Tartaric Acid From Pomace of Some Anatolian Grape Cultivars." *Amerian Journal of Enology and Viticulture*, *49*(1), 95–99.

Odello Luigi, Giomo, A., Versini, G. & Zironi, R. (1997). *Grappa: Analisi Sensoriale & Tecnologia*. Centro studi e formazione

Assaggiatori. Brescia. http://hdl.handle.net/10449/20525. [*Grappa: Sensory Analysis & Technology*.]

Pereira, Débora Tamires Vitor, Adriana Gadioli Tarone, Cinthia Baú Betim Cazarin, Gerardo Fernández Barbero. & Julian Martínez. (2019). "Pressurized Liquid Extraction of Bioactive Compounds from Grape Marc." *Journal of Food Engineering*, *240*, 105–113. https://doi.org/10.1016/j.jfoodeng.2018.07.019.

Pinelo, Manuel, Anis Arnous. & Anne S. Meyer. (2006). "Upgrading of Grape Skins: Significance of Plant Cell-Wall Structural Components and Extraction Techniques for Phenol Release." *Trends in Food Science and Technology*., *88*, 274-289. https://doi.org/10.1016/j.tifs.2006.05.003.

Ping, Lan, Antonio Pizzi, Zhou Ding Guo. & Nicolas Brosse. (2011). "Condensed Tannins Extraction from Grape Pomace: Characterization and Utilization as Wood Adhesives for Wood Particleboard." *Industrial Crops and Products*, *34* (1), 907–914. https://doi.org/10.1016/j.indcrop.2011.02.009.

Pizzichini, M., Agnelli, A. & Mucciolo, C. (2015). *Valorizzazione Dei Composti Chimici Bio-Attivi Dalle Vinacce Con Tecnologie Di Membrana*. Industre Alimentari., 5-11. [*Enhancement of Bio-Active Chemical Compounds from Pomace with Membrane Technologies*.]

Polovka, Martin, Lenka Šťavíková, Barbora Hohnová, Pavel Karásek. & Michal Roth. (2010). "Offline Combination of Pressurized Fluid Extraction and Electron Paramagnetic Resonance Spectroscopy for Antioxidant Activity of Grape Skin Extracts Assessment." *Journal of Chromatography A*, *1217* (51), 7990–8000. https://doi.org/10.1016/j.chroma.2010.08.003.

Pop Tiberia and Pop Nastasia. (2015). *Valorificarea Produselor Secundare Viti-Vinicole*. *71*. Cluj-Napoca: Academic Press. [*Valorization of Vine-Wine By-Products*.]

Pretorius, Isak S. (1999). "Oenology: Engineering Designer Genes for Wine Yeasts." *Australian and New Zealand Wine Industry Journal*, *14*, 42-54.

Pretorius, Isak S. (2000). *Tailoring Wine Yeast for the New Millennium: Novel Approaches to the Ancient Art of Winemaking.* 16 (8): 675-729. https://doi.org/10.1002/1097-0061(20000615) 16:8%3C675::AID-YEA585%3E3.0.CO;2-B.

Prieur, Corinne, Jacques Rigaud, Veronique Cheynier. & Michel Moutounet. (1994). "Oligomeric and polymeric procyanidins from grape seeds." *Phytochemistry*, *36* (3), 781-784. https://doi.org/10.1016/s0031-9422(00)89817-9.

Puente-Díaz, Luis, Kong Ah-Hen, Antonio Vega-Gálvez, Roberto Lemus-Mondaca. & Karina Di Scala. (2013). "Combined Infrared-Convective Drying of Murta (Ugni Molinae Turcz) Berries: Kinetic Modeling and Quality Assessment." *Drying Technology*, *31* (3), 329–338. https://doi.org/10.1080/07373937.2012.736113.

Raksakantong, Pornpimol, Sirithon Siriamornpun, Jiranan Ratseewo. & Naret Meeso. (2011). "Optimized Drying of Kaprow Leaves for Industrial Production of Holy Basil Spice Powder." *Drying Technology*, *29* (8), 974–983. https://doi.org/10.1080/ 07373937.2011.558649.

Raghavan, G. S. V. & Orsat, V. (2007). "Recent Advances in Drying of Biomaterials for Superior Quality Bioproducts." *Journal of Chemical Engineering Asia-Pac. J. Chem. Eng*, *2*, 20–29. https://doi.org/10.1002/apj.051.

Ratti, C. (2001). "Hot Air and Freeze-Drying of High-Value Foods: A Review." *Journal of Food Engineering*, *49* (4), 311-319. www.elsevier.com/locate/jfoodeng.

Renaud, S. & De Lorgeril M. (1992). "Wine, Alcohol, Platelets, and the French Paradox for Coronary Heart Disease." *The lancet*, *339* (8808), 1523-1526. https://doi.org/10.1016/0140-6736(92)91277-F.

Ribeiro, L. F., Ribani, R. H., Francisco, T. M. G., Soares, A. A., Pontarolo, R. & Haminiuk, C. W. I. (2015). "Profile of Bioactive Compounds from Grape Pomace (*Vitis Vinifera* and *Vitis Labrusca*) by Spectrophotometric, Chromatographic and Spectral Analyses." *Journal of Chromatography B: Analytical Technologies in the*

*Biomedical and Life Sciences.*, *1007*, 72-80. https://doi.org/10.1016/j.jchromb.2015.11.005.

Robinson Jancis. (2006). *The Oxford Companion to Wine*. Third edition Oxford.

Robinson Jancis. (1994). *The Oxford Companion to Wine*. Edited by Jancis Robinson. First Publ. Oxford University Press.

Rockenbach, Ismael Ivan, Graciela Lessa da Silva, Eliseu Rodrigues, Luciano Valdemiro Gonzaga. & Roseane Fett. (2007). "Atividade Antioxidante de Extratos de Bagaço de Uva Das Variedades Regente e Pinot Noir (*Vitis Vinifera*)." ["Antioxidant Activity of Grape Bagasse Extracts from Regente and Pinot Noir Varieties (*Vitis Vinifera*)"]. *Revista do Instituto Adolfo Lutz.*, *66.* [*Adolfo Lutz Institute Magazine*]

Rockenbach, Ismael Ivan, Graciela Lessa Da Silva, Eliseu Rodrigues, Eugênia Marta Kuskoski. & Roseane Fett. (2008). "Influência Do Solvente No Conteúdo Total de Polifenóis, Antocianinas e Atividade Antioxidante de Extratos de Bagaço de Uva (*Vitis Vinifera*) Variedades Tannat e Ancelota." [Solvent Influence on Total Polyphenol Content, Anthocyanins, and Antioxidant Activity of Grape (*Vitis Vinifera*) Bagasse Extracts from Tannat and Ancelota-Different Varieties of Vitis Vinifera Varieties."] *Ciênc. Tecnol. Aliment.*, *28*, 238-244. http://dx.doi.org/10.1590/S0101-20612008000500036.

Romero-Pérez, Ana I., Maite Ibern-Gómez, Rosa M. Lamuela-Raventós. & Carmen De La Torre-Boronat, M. (1999). "Piceid, the Major Resveratrol Derivative in Grape Juices." *Journal of Agricultural and Food Chemistry*, *47* (4), 1533–1536. https://doi.org/10.1021/jf981024g.

Romero-Pérez, Ana I., Rosa M Lamuela-Raventós, Andrew L Waterhouse, & De La Torre-Boronat, M. C. (1996). "Levels of Cis- and Trans-Resveratrol and Their Glucosides in White and Rosé Vitis Vinifera Wines from Spain." *Journal of Agricultural and Food Chemistry.*, *44* (8), 2124-2128. https://doi.org/10.1021/jf9507654.

Sarni-Manchado, Pascale, Véronique Cheynier. & Michel Moutounet. (1999). "Interactions of Grape Seed Tannins with Salivary Proteins." *Journal of Agricultural and Food Chemistry*, *47* (1), 42–47. https://doi.org/10.1021/jf9805146.

Shalini, R. (2010). Apple Pomace Drying: Drying Characteristics of Apple Pomace. By-Products Utilization. Saarbrücken: LAP Lambert Academic Publishing.

Shi, John, Jianmel Yu, Joseph E Pohorly. & Yukio Kakuda. (2003). "Polyphenolics in Grape Seeds-Biochemistry and Functionality." *Journal of medicinal food.*, *6* (4), 291-299.https://doi.org/ 10.1089/109662003772519831.

Shih, C., Pan, Z., Mchugh, T., Wood, D. & Hirschberg, E. (2008). "Sequential infrared radiation and freeze-drying method for producing crispy strawberries." *Transactions of the ASABE*, *51* (1), 205–216.

Solari-Godiño, A., Lindo-Rojas, I. & Pandia-Estrada, S. (2017). "Determination of Phenolic Compounds and Evaluation of Antioxidant Capacity of Two Grapes Residues (*Vitis Vinifera*) of Varieties Dried: Quebranta (Red) and Torontel (White)." *Cogent Food & Agriculture.*, *3* (1), https://doi.org/10.1080/ 23311932. 2017.1361599.

Sólyom, Katalin, Ruth Solá, María José Cocero. & Rafael B. Mato. (2014). "Thermal Degradation of Grape Marc Polyphenols." *Food Chemistry*, *159*, 361–366. https://doi.org/10.1016/j.foodchem.2014. 03.021.

Souquet, Jean-Marc, Veronique Cheynier, Franck Brossaud. & Michel Moutounet. (1996). *Polymeric proanthocyanidins from grape skins. 43* (2), 509-512. https://doi.org/10.1016/0031-9422(96) 00301-9.

Spatafora, Carmela. & Corrado Tringali. (2012). "Valorization of Vegetable Waste: Identification of Bioactive Compounds and Their Chemo-Enzymatic Optimization." *The Open Agriculture Journal.*, *6*, 9-16.http://dx.doi.org/10.2174/1874331501206010009.

Sui, Yinqiang, Jihong Yang, Qiuhong Ye, Hua Li. & Hua Wang. (2014). "Infrared, Convective, and Sequential Infrared and Convective

Drying of Wine Grape Pomace." *Drying Technology.*, *32* (6), 686-694. https://doi.org/10.1080/07373937.2013.853670.

Supmoon, Nattriya. & Athapol Noomhorm. (2013). "Influence of Combined Hot Air Impingement and Infrared Drying on Drying Kinetics and Physical Properties of Potato Chips." *Drying Technology*, *31* (1), 24–31. https://doi.org/10.1080/07373937.2012.711792.

Țârdea Constantin., Sârbu Gheorghe. & Țârdea Angela. (2010). *Tratat de Vinificație*. A II-A. Iași: Ion Ionescu de la Brad. 40-104. [*Vinification Treaty.*]

Taşeri, Levent, Mustafa Aktaş, Seyfi Şevik, Mehmet Güçlü, Gamze Uysal Seçkin. & Burak Aktekeli. (2018). "Determination of Drying Kinetics and Quality Parameters of Grape Pomace Dried with a Heat Pump Dryer." *Food Chemistry*, *260*, 152–159. https://doi.org/10.1016/j.foodchem.2018.03.122.

Teixeira, Ana, Nieves Baenas, Raul Dominguez-Perles, Ana Barros, Eduardo Rosa, Diego A. Moreno. & Cristina Garcia-Viguera. (2014). "Natural Bioactive Compounds from Winery By-Products as Health Promoters: A Review." *International Journal of Molecular Sciences.*, *15* (9), 15638-15678. https://doi.org/10.3390/ijms150915638.

Teles, Aline Soares Cascaes, Davy William Hidalgo Chávez, Flávia Dos Santos Gomes, Lourdes Maria Corrêa Cabral. & Renata Valeriano Tonon. (2018). "Effect of Temperature on the Degradation of Bioactive Compounds of Pinot Noir Grape Pomace during Drying." *Brazilian Journal of Food Technology.*, *21* https://doi.org/10.1590/1981-6723.5917.

"The Plant List." 2013.

Thimothe, Joanne, Illeme A. Bonsi, Olga I. Padilla-Zakour. & Hyun Koo. (2007). "Chemical Characterization of Red Wine Grape (Vitis Vinifera and Vitis Interspecific Hybrids) and Pomace Phenolic Extracts and Their Biological Activity against Streptococcus Mutans." *Journal of Agricultural and Food Chemistry*, *55* (25), 10200–10207. https://doi.org/10.1021/jf0722405.

This, Patrice, Thierry Lacombe. & Mark R. Thomas. (2006). "Historical Origins and Genetic Diversity of Wine Grapes." *Trends in Genetics.*, *22* (9), 511-519 https://doi.org/10.1016/j.tig.2006.07.008.

Tiefenbacher John P. & Townsend Christi. (2019). "The Semiofoodscape of Wine: The Changing Global Landscape of Wine Culture and the Language of Making, Selling, and Drinking Wine." In *Handbook of the Changing World Language Map.* Springer, Cham, Stanley D Brunn and Roland Kehrein eds., 4103–4145. https://doi.org/10.1007/978-3-030-02438-3_213.

Tseng, Angela. & Yanyun Zhao. (2012). "Effect of Different Drying Methods and Storage Time on the Retention of Bioactive Compounds and Antibacterial Activity of Wine Grape Pomace (Pinot Noir and Merlot)." *Journal of Food Science.*, *77* (9), 192-201. https://doi.org/10.1111/j.1750-3841.2012.02840.x.

Valiente, C., Arrigoni, E., Esteban, R. M. & Ft Amado. (1995). "Grape Pomace as a Potential Food Fiber." *Journal of Food Science*, *60*, 812–820.

Vashisth, Tripti, Rakesh K. Singh. & Ronald B. Pegg. (2011). "Effects of Drying on the Phenolics Content and Antioxidant Activity of Muscadine Pomace." *LWT - Food Science and Technology*, *44* (7), 1649–1657. https://doi.org/10.1016/j.lwt.2011.02.011.

Vergara-Salinas, José R., Pedro Bulnes, María Carolina Zúñiga, Jara Pérez-Jiménez, Josep Lluís Torres, María Luisa Mateos-Martín, Eduardo Agosin. & José R. Pérez-Correa. (2013). "Effect of Pressurized Hot Water Extraction on Antioxidants from Grape Pomace before and after Enological Fermentation." *Journal of Agricultural and Food Chemistry.*, *61* (28), 6929-6936. https://doi.org/10.1021/jf4010143.

Versari, A., Paola Parpinello, G., Battista Tornielli, G., Ferrarini, R. & Giulivo, C. (2001). "Stilbene Compounds and Stilbene Synthase Expression during Ripening, Wilting, and UV Treatment in Grape Cv. Corvina." *Journal of Agricultural and Food Chemistry*, *49* (11), 5531–5536. https://doi.org/10.1021/jf010672o.

Wagner, P. (1996). "The Wine Appreciation Guild." In *A Wine Growers Guild*, third, 15. San Francisco.

Xu, Yixiang, Sheanell Burton, Chyer Kim. & Edward Sismour. (2016). "Phenolic Compounds, Antioxidant, and Antibacterial Properties of Pomace Extracts from Four Virginia-Grown Grape Varieties." *Food Science and Nutrition, 4* (1), 125–133. https://doi.org/10.1002/fsn3.264.

Yang, Jihong, Gokhan Bingol, Zhongli Pan, Maria T. Brandl, Tara H. McHugh. & Hua Wang. (2010). "Infrared Heating for Dry-Roasting and Pasteurization of Almonds." *Journal of Food Engineering, 101* (3), 273–280. https://doi.org/10.1016/j.jfoodeng.2010.07.007.

Zhang, Nansen, Andrew Hoadley, Jim Patel, Seng Lim. & Chao'en Li. (2017). "Sustainable Options for the Utilization of Solid Residues from Wine Production." *Waste Management., 60*, 173-183. https://doi.org/10.1016/j.wasman.2017.01.006.

Zheng, Yi, Christopher Lee, Chaowei Yu, Yu Shen Cheng, Christopher W. Simmons, Ruihong Zhang, Bryan M. Jenkins. & Jean S. Vandergheynst. (2012). "Ensilage and Bioconversion of Grape Pomace into Fuel Ethanol." *Journal of Agricultural and Food Chemistry, 60* (44), 11128–11134. https://doi.org/10.1021/jf303509v.

Zhu, Yi, Zhongli Pan, Tara H. McHugh. & Diane M. Barrett. (2010). "Processing and Quality Characteristics of Apple Slices Processed under Simultaneous Infrared Dry-Blanching and Dehydration with Intermittent Heating." *Journal of Food Engineering, 97* (1), 8–16. https://doi.org/10.1016/j.jfoodeng.2009.07.021.

In: Grape Pomace in Health …
Editor: Veronica Sanda Chedea
ISBN: 978-1-68507-409-8


*Chapter 2*

# Grape Pomace Generation Using Pulsed Electric Field Technology

***Livia Bandici[1], Alin Cristian Teusdea[2], Adrian Cristian Oradan[3], Gheorghe Emil Bandici[2], Andreea Margareta Vlad[4] and Simona Ioana Vicaş[2,*]***

[1]Faculty of Electrical Engineering and Information Technology,
University of Oradea, Oradea, Romania
[2]Faculty of Environmental Protection,
University of Oradea, Oradea, Romania
[3]Doctoral School of Biomedical Science,
University of Oradea, Oradea, Romania
[4]Faculty of Medicine and Pharmacy,
University of Oradea, Oradea, Romania

* Corresponding Author's E-mail: sim_vicas@yahoo.com.

## ABSTRACT

In the last few years, the non-conventional technology known as "green technology", Pulsed Electric Field (PEF), has been developed, to reuse agricultural residues. The applications of pulsed electrical technologies such as PEF have been currently proposed for promoting bioactive compound extraction. The valorization of grape pomace is very promising because these residues are rich in phenols with antioxidant activity. The mechanism and optimal parameters of this technology are described in the first part of this chapter. Besides, an innovative PEF device is presented, developed to promote the extraction of phenols and pigments from red grapes. Most often, this technology has been used in the wine industry to obtain a product (usually, wine) with pronounced color intensity and a high content of phenols and anthocyanin pigments. In recent years, the literature has shown that the PEF technique is effective in extracting phenolic compounds from various raw materials, especially from grape pomace.

## INTRODUCTION: PRINCIPLES AND MECHANISM OF PEF

Mechanical pressing is the most common way of separating liquids from porous materials, completely or partially saturated with liquid. The procedure is used in various industrial applications, including wine production. However, mechanical compression manages to partially destroy the cell membranes, with much of the liquid remaining inside the cells. An expensive solution is to greatly increase the compressive strength, thus increasing the number of pores in the cell membrane. Other solutions are provided by chemical, biological, and ultrasound processes, which can rupture the cell membrane without an increase in temperature (Knorr et al., 2001; Donsì et al., 2010; Marsellés-Fontanet et al., 2013).

Electromagnetic methods promise to be the most efficient processes for improving liquid-solid separation. The injection of a direct current has been studied in the literature (López et al., 2008a; López et al., 2009) leading to the conclusion of increased efficiency, due to the combination between the effect of pressure and electroosmosis. Unfortunately, direct current can produce unwanted effects that degrade the quality of the product. Applying an alternating voltage of different shapes (most often in pulses) removes this disadvantage and has the effect of breaking the cell, a phenomenon called electroplasmolysis.

PEF technology is an alternative to traditional processing, as this application can preserve the sensory and nutritional qualities of the food while generating a microbiologically safe product but also an improvement in the extraction efficiency of intracellular compounds (Mosqueda-Melgar et al., 2012; Delsart et al., 2013; Boussetta et al., 2012a; Bandici et al., 2015; Bandici et al., 2017; Vicas et al., 2017).

In the winemaking process, PEF treatment involves the application of high intensity (20-80 kV) electric field pulses over a very short period (microseconds) to a grape matrix, which is located in a treatment chamber between two electrodes that allows the passage of electron flux through the sample (Clodoveo et al., 2016). The application of grape pomace to such a treatment results in the temporary or permanent formation of pores in the cell membrane (a process known as electroporation) (Boussetta et al., 2015). The PEF treatment causes damage to cell membranes and the presence of these pores allows for certain bioactive compounds to pass from inside the cell to the outside, enhancing the extraction process. Boussetta et al., 2009 found that the maximum cell damage of grape skins after applying PEF was attained after 1 s of treatment.

An innovative PEF device for treating grape pomace to obtain a wine with superior qualities in terms of bioactive compounds was developed by the National Institute for Research and Development in Electrical Engineering ICPE-CA Bucharest in collaboration with the Politehnica University of Bucharest, in the Partnerships Program in priority areas - PN II, developed with the support of MEN - UEFISCDI, project no. 170/2014 "Electromagnetic methods to improve wine processes" is shown in Figure 1.

The high voltage and frequency source generate high voltage pulses with amplitude up to 25kV and a duration of 0.5 ms. The voltage is limited by the discharge that occurs in the device to a value of 6-8 kV. These pulses are generated with certain repeatability over time, repeatability that can be adjusted so that the electricity transferred to the grapes can be controlled. The voltage transformer allows increasing the voltages provided by the power supply up to the maximum value of 8 kV.

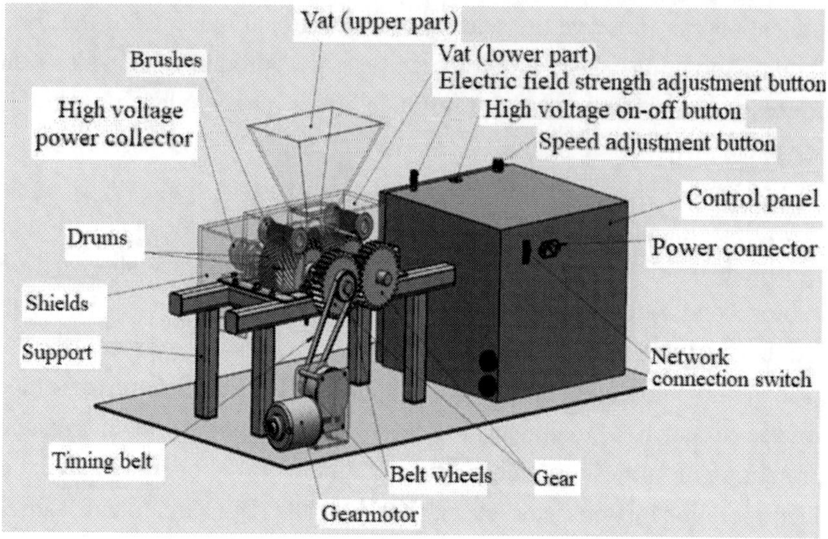


Figure 1. PEF device for the treatment of grape pomace.

The drive assembly of the drums with gears ensures the opposite rotation of the two pairs of drums (Figure 2). On the two shafts are mounted 4 drums with channels built according to a special geometry (30 channels at 12 degrees), so that the distance between the tips of the drums is kept constant at 5 mm during the rotational movement. The drums are supplied continuously (through aport brush-brush collector assembly) from the source of high voltage and variable frequency, the material (pomace) passing through the drums, the effect of electroplasmolysis by applying electrical impulses is obtained.

The rotational movement of the two axes on which the drums are mounted is performed using a gear with straight-toothed gears, with a distance between the axes of 80 mm and which ensures a distance between the tips of the drums of 5 mm, necessary to initiate and carry out the process of electroplasmolysis. The adjustment of the rotation speed of the drums utilizing the gear motor group ensures the normal development of the electroplasmolysis process through the corresponding amount of processed raw material (pomace).

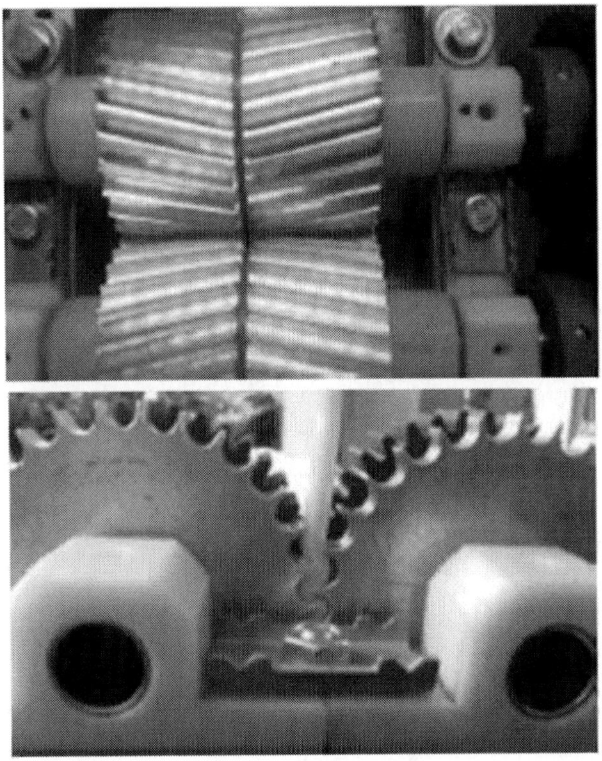

Figure 2. The shape of the drums used in the PEF treatment.

The experimental model is a new technology used to obtain quality wines. By using the experimental model a higher transfer of anthocyanins, volatile substances in a balanced register, an increase in the color intensity of the wine was obtained (Teusdea et al., 2017). The multivariate PCA analysis demonstrates that differences in the types of molecular matrices significantly influence the effect of electroporation by PEF treatments of musts (Vicas et al., 2017).

The package of programs designed to solve the problem of an electromagnetic field in the grape pomace coupled with the thermal diffusion problem provides a clear picture of how to use the equipment.

The influence of the pomace movement on the temperature is particularly important, the pomace mass is inhomogeneous and anisotropic from the point of view of the speed field. It results that a simplified but efficient calculation model can be chosen. The computing range is divided into subdomains separated by vertical lines joining two paired gears. After a period, the pomace in the subdomain on the left takes the place of the one in thc subdomain on the right. At each time step, the average temperature in the nodes inside each subdomain is determined and then transferred as the initial temperature to the adjacent subdomain on the right.

Electric field strength, temperature, treatment duration, and specific energy consumption are the main parameters that affect the degree of microbial inactivation (Corrales et. al. 2008). To ensure an efficient microbial inactivation, the electric field strength is recommended to be in the range of 20-50 kV/cm, the pulse duration between 1-10 μs, and the specific energy between 50-1000 kJ/kg (Boussetta et. al. 2012a). However, the multitude of variable parameters produced by the application of PEF, as well as the characteristics of food products require a systematic study of the individual influence of these parameters on the reactions that occur.

For the extraction of polyphenols, it is much more efficient to use two field levels, in the first phase 20 kV / cm, 0.37 J, exposure time 210 μS / cm, temperature obtained 13 °C, in the second phase 40 kV / cm, 5.2 J, exposure time 340 μS / cm, temperature obtained 25 °C (Delsart et. al., 2013).

## PEF Technology in Process of Making Red Wine

The conventional red winemaking systems include some stages (Figure 3). The most important and critical stage is maceration, a process of soaking crushed grapes (that include skins, seeds), and, sometimes, stems.

The maceration of the crushed grapes represents a critical point in obtaining a high-quality red wine. During maceration, the extraction of the compounds responsible for the color of the wine and tannin compounds takes place, but this step should not take too long because it can lead to a bitter and astringent taste in wine, that is not appreciated by consumers (Clodoveo et al., 2016). Research studies have demonstrated that the application of PEF treatment before the maceration stage to red grapes may help reduce the duration of maturation and may increase the content of bioactive compounds, such as phenols, in wine (Puértolas et al., 2010a; López- Puértolas et al., 2010b; López-Alfaro & Garde-Cerdán, 2015).

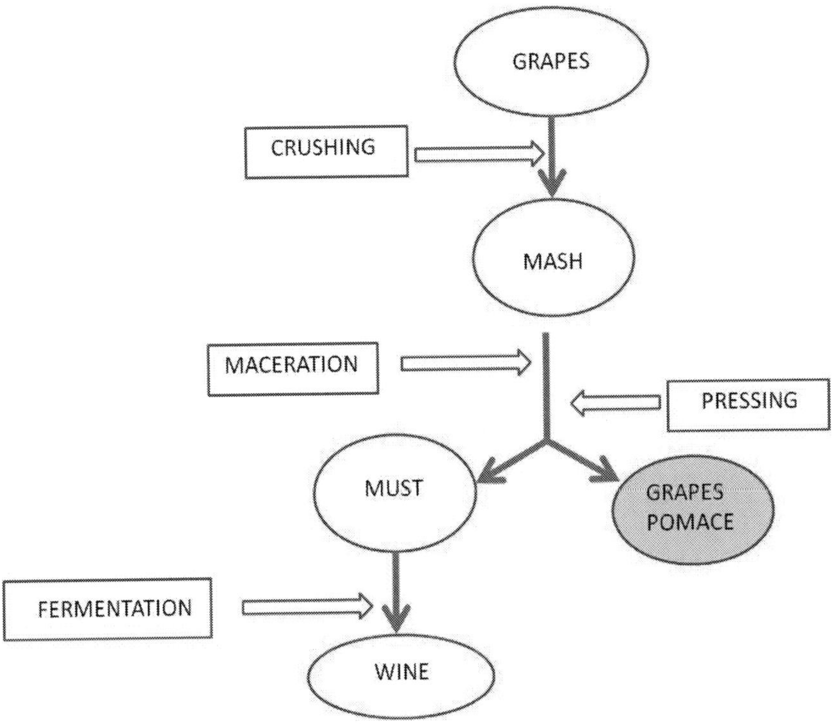


Figure 3. The general stages of red wine and grapes pomace production.

After maceration, the next stage is the pressing of grape mash, resulting in must and grape pomace. Finally, the alcoholic fermentation can be completed to obtain the red wine, or the wine by-products (grape pomace) can be valorized. Thereby, grape pomace is the solid residue remaining after the grapes have been pressed for winemaking.

The by-products of winemaking have attracted great attention as sources of bioactive compounds which are primarily phenolic compounds with various biological effects such as antioxidant, antitumor, antiaging, antimicrobial, and anti-inflammatory properties (Peixoto et al., 2018; Xia et al., 2010; Yu & Ahmedna, 2013). The phenolic compounds from grape pomace are used in the food industry as preservatives (antibacterial effects), antioxidants (by preventing lipid oxidation) (Yu & Ahmedna, 2013).

## THE EFFECT OF PEF ON WINE QUALITY

The quality of red wine depends on several factors including total phenol content, total antioxidant capacity, total monomeric anthocyanin content, color, aroma, and sensory perception.

Because most of the compounds responsible for wine quality (phenolic compounds, color precursors, tannins) are located in grape skin vacuoles, efficient extraction involves the use of vinification techniques that result in increased permeability of cytoplasmic membranes facilitating the release of bio-compounds.

In the case of PEF technology, intense electric pulses are applied to liquid or solid organic food matrices, resulting in the extraction of bioactive compounds, and this represents an innovative food processing system, especially in the oenological industry (Ricci et al., 2018).

PEF technology was recently introduced in the wine industry, as an alternative method to the maceration process, resulting in increased and accelerated extraction of bioactive compounds, without altering sensory properties, but improving the stability and color of wine (Morata et al., 2017).

One study (López et al., 2008b) investigated the effect of different PEF treatments on Tempranillo grape skin in terms of total phenol content, anthocyanins, and color parameters. For example, the maximum index of total phenols and anthocyanins was obtained after 50 hours of maceration in the case of samples treated with PEF compared to the untreated sample, where the same value of the index was reached after 96 hours. The color of the wine whose grapes were treated with PEF showed an intensity of color that increased with the increase of the electric energy irradiation (from 5 to 10 kV/cm).

PEF was used for increasing the extraction of anthocyanins and phenols during the maceration step of wine production (Puértolas et al., 2010c). The extraction of these compounds, at high levels, was achieved in half of the time compared to the control wine samples.

Vicas et al., 2017 investigated the effect of PEF treatment in the pre-maceration stage (pulses of 150μs, the electric field strength of 7 kV/cm, and a frequency of 178 Hz) on the content of total phenols, flavonoids, monomeric anthocyanin, antioxidant capacity, color intensity, and sensory quality of wines derived from three varieties of grapes (Muscat Ottonel, Pinot Noir, and Merlot). The high levels of total phenols and flavonoids were found in the wine obtained from PEF treated Pinot Noir grapes, followed by Merlot and Muscat Ottonel). The antioxidant capacity of wines depends both on the variety of grapes and the content of bioactive compounds. Also, in the PEF-treated red wines (Pinot Noir and Merlot), a high color intensity was recorded compared to the control wine samples.

Teusdea et al., (2017) used different PEF treatments in the pre-maceration stage of the mash of Pinot Noir and Merlot grapes, where the electrical and mechanical parameters were: the distance between the drums (Figure 2), different voltages (7-8 kV), and different frequencies (178-344 Hz). All PEF treatments resulted in an increase in bioactive compounds and color intensity of wines.

The five PEF treatments were tested and the best results were obtained when the distance between the drums of 2.5 mm, U = 8 kV, the frequency of 344 Hz, and the pulse durations of 300 s was applied to obtain quality red wines.

## THE EFFECT OF PEF ENERGY INPUT FOR THE VALORIZATION OF GRAPE POMACE

A wide variety of products can be obtained from grapes, such as grape juice, jams, raisins, and most often wine. During the winemaking process, a variety of phenolic compounds is extracted from grapes.

Grape pomace, as a residue of winemaking, is a good source of many bioactive compounds known for their cardioprotective, anticancer, anti-inflammatory, antioxidant, antiaging, and antimicrobial properties (Xia et al., 2010). The polyphenols from grape pomace can be used for different foods as colorants and antioxidants (Joana Gil-Chávez et al., 2013).

Finding alternatives for the extraction of bioactive compounds from grape pomace can increase the value of this by-product (Clodoveo et al., 2016; Kammerer et al., 2014). PEF treatment is an alternative way to improve phenol extraction from grape pomace.

A comparative study between enzyme (pectinase) and PEF treatments (5 kV, 1 μFarad, 20 Pulses) in term of extraction of phenols from three varieties of grapes (St. Croix, Frontenac, and St. Pepin) showed that PEF was more effective than pectinase treatment (Khalil, 2011).

In another study (Corrales et al., 2008), the efficiency of PEF treatment was demonstrated for the extraction of anthocyanins from grape by-products. Furthermore, the authors demonstrated a *selective extraction* of individual anthocyanins, where anthocyanin monoglucosides were more efficiently extracted by PEF.

PEF treatment does not modify the different groups of extracted polyphenols (Boussetta et al., 2015). Applying electric fields to grape pomace shows the presence of the main polyphenols in both treated and untreated samples (e.g., catechin, epicatechin, quercetin-3-O-glucoside, and kaempferol-3-O-glucoside) (Boussetta et al., 2012b).

The polyphenol composition of the PEF-treated grape skin extract was determined by HPLC, highlighting the presence of four major components, catechin, epicatechin, quercetin-3-O-glucoside, and kaempferol-3-O-glucoside (Boussetta et al., 2009).

In the case of vine-shoot, Rajha et al., 2014 found the same phenol composition in both PEF treatment and untreated samples (e.g., epicatechin, kaempferol, and resveratrol). In the PEF treated samples, the quantity of different phenol compounds is always higher than in the untreated ones. The effect of PEF treatment on *polyphenol functionality* has been studied by Boussetta et al., 2015).

The antioxidant capacity of PEF treated samples was evaluated. The antioxidant capacity of samples was higher than of the untreated samples, which proves that phenols remain active after the application of electric fields (Boussetta et al., 2015).

Barbara et al., 2015 used different alternative physical treatments, including PEF on fermented grape pomace to extract the bioactive compounds, such as polyphenols, especially, anthocyanins. For the PEF treatment, a custom-made pulsed high voltage power supply of 40 kV, 10 kA, and frequency of 0.5 Hz was used. From grape pomace total phenolic compounds, antioxidant capacity by DPPH method, and total and individual anthocyanins were evaluated in grape pomace samples. PEF treatment allowed the recovery of total phenolic compounds up to 47% compared to references extracted and antioxidant capacity increased with cell disintegration Index Z (an indicator of cell damages or treatment efficiency). From the point of view of anthocyanin extraction, yields were up to 5.3 times higher after PEF treatment compared to the reference extraction. Regarding the individual anthocyanins, malvidin-3-O-glucoside concentration was higher extracted than monoglucoside molecules peonidin, petunidin, and delphinidin, after applying electrical treatments.

The valorization of fermented grape pomace using PEF was investigated also by Brianceau et al., 2015. The effect of the apparent density of pre-compacted grape pomace on the efficiency of phenols extraction after PEF treatment is strongly correlated with the apparent density of grape pomace varying from 0.6 g·cm$^{-3}$ to 1.3 g·cm$^{-3}$. When the density of grape pomace was 1.0 g·cm$^{-3}$, the quantity of the extracted polyphenols was increased by 15%.

PEF treatment (E = 1.2 kV/cm−1; W=18 ± 2 kJ·kg−1) increased the extraction of total anthocyanin compounds and was depending on temperature. The temperature of 50 °C had a negative effect on the extraction of anthocyanins, probably because thesc compounds are not thermally stable at that temperature, and during a long duration of extraction (420 min), they are subjected to the polymerization process (Brianceau et al., 2015). The authors demonstrate the selective nature of PEF treatment in anthocyanin extraction.

The pulsed electrical technologies such as PEF and high voltage electrical discharges (HVED) have been proposed for bio-compounds extraction, both techniques are effective for the enhancement of polyphenol extraction from different raw materials as compared to untreated samples. Their principles of action are different. In the case of HVED, the tissue is fragmented, whereas the PEF treatment does not affect the tissue structure (Boussetta et al., 2015).

The effects of PEF treatments on grape skin structures and the organization of skin cell walls were investigated by Cholet et al., 2014. Two types of PEF treatment on Cabernet Sauvignon grapes were used. One of them used medium electric field strength (4 kV/cm); short duration (1 ms) and another applied low intensity (0.7 kV/cm), and longer duration (200 ms). The PEF treatments have significant consequences for the parietal structures of skin favoring phenols extraction.

In the last years, PEF was used in residues from the wine industry to improve extraction processes of compounds like phenols, including anthocyanins (Rocha et al., 2018). Boussetta et al., 2012c show that PEF treatment (8-20 kV/cm, 0-20 ms) used for extraction of phenols from grape seed increases the yield of phenol extraction. Additionally, a mixture of ethanol and water (50 g ethanol/100 g of the total amount of solvent) was more efficient during PEF extraction (7.2 ± 0.2 g GAE/100g Dow), at 50 °C compared to the solvent alone. These results can be explained by the fact that anthocyanins and proanthocyanins are more soluble in water, whereas others are more soluble in ethanol (catechin, epicatechin).

## CONCLUSION AND PERSPECTIVES

The pomace grape made of skin, seeds, and stems are an important source of bioactive compounds, especially in the phenol class, and can have applications in various industries (food, pharmaceutical, and cosmetics). The largest amount of phenolic compounds is found in grape seeds, and in grape skins, anthocyanin compounds are present in large quantities. There is a strong correlation between the presence of phenolic compounds and biological effects (antibacterial, antioxidant and cytotoxicity activity).

Recent studies in the literature have shown that PEF treatment applied to grape pomace is an effective method for extracting total phenols. Moreover, this treatment applied to grape pomace highlighted a selective extraction of total anthocyanins, thus offering possibilities to obtain different extracts with a specific phytochemical profile. This technology is an alternative process to conventional pre-treatments applied to raw materials with an impact on product quality.

Also, the effect of PEF treatment on polyphenol functionality has been studied, demonstrating that this type of treatment does not affect the biological activity of bioactive compounds.

Future studies should focus on the application of PEF technology on an industrial scale to capitalize on grape pomace, for example by recovering pigments (anthocyanins), thus laying the foundations for sustainable agriculture.

## REFERENCES

Bandici L., Leuca, T., Vicaş S, Bandici, Gh. E. "The influence of the high-frequency electromagnetic field on grape processing." *13th International Conference on Engineering of Modern Electric Systems* (EMES 2015): 1 – 4. 10.1109/EMES.2015.7158400.

Bandici L., Vicaş, S, Bandici, Gh. E., Teusdea, A. C., Popa, D. "The Effect of Pulsed Electric Field (PEF) Treatment on the Quality of Wine." *14th International Conference on Engineering of Modern Electric Systems* (EMES 2017): 17-22.

Barba, F. J., Brianceau, S., Turk M., Boussetta, N., Vorobiev, E. "Effect of Alternative Physical Treatments (Ultrasounds, Pulsed Electric Fields, and High-Voltage Electrical Discharges) on Selective Recovery of Bio-compounds from Fermented Grape Pomace." *Food Bioprocess Technol* (2015): 8:1139–1148. doi 10.1007/s11947-015-1482-3.

Boussetta, N., Lebovka, N., Vorobiev, E., Adenier H., Bedel-Cloutour C., Lanoisellé J. L. "Electrically Assisted Extraction of Soluble Matter from Chardonnay Grape Skins for Polyphenol Recovery." *J Agric Food Chem* (2009): 57 (4): 1491-1497.

Boussetta, N., Vorobiev E., Deloison V., Pochez F., Falcimaigne-Cordin A., Lanoisellé J. L. "Valorization of grape pomace by the extraction of phenolic antioxidants: application of high voltage electrical discharges." *Food Chem* (2012): 128 (2): 364-370.

Boussetta, N., Grimi N., Vorobiev, E." Pulsed Electrical Technologies Assisted Polyphenols Extraction from Agricultural Plants and Bioresources" A Review. *International Journal of Food Processing Technology* (2015): 2, 1-10.

Boussetta, N., Vorobiev, E., Reess, T., De Ferron, A., Pecastaing, L., Ruscassié, R., Lanoisellé J.-L. "Scale-up of high voltage electrical discharges for polyphenols extraction from grape pomace: Effect of the dynamic shock waves." *Innovative Food Science &Emerging Technologies,* (2012a):16, 129–136.

Boussetta, N., Vorobiev. E., Le, L. H., Cordin-Falcimaigne, A., Lanoiselle, J. L. "Application of electrical treatments in alcoholic solvent for polyphenols extraction from grape seeds". *LWT-Food Sci. Technol* (2012c): 46 (1), 127–134.

Brianceau, S., Turk M., Xavier Vitrac, X., Vorobiev, E. "Combined densification and pulsed electric field treatment for selective polyphenols recovery from fermented grape pomace." *Innovative Food Science and Emerging Technologies 29* (2015): 2–8.

Cholet, C., Delsart C., Petrel, M., Gontier, E., Grimi, N., L'Hyvernay, A., Ghidossi, R., Vorobiev, E., Mietton-Peuchot, M., Gény L. "Structural and Biochemical Changes Induced by Pulsed Electric Field Treatments on Cabernet Sauvignon Grape Berry Skins: Impact on Cell Wall Total Tannins and Polysaccharides." *J. Agric. Food Chem.* (2014): 62: 2925−2934. dx.doi.org/10.1021/jf404804d.

Clodoveo, M. L., Dipalmo, T., Rizzello, C. G., Corbo F., Crupi P. "Emerging technology to develop novel red winemaking practices: An overview." *Innovative Food Science and Emerging Technologies* (2016): 38, 41–56.

Corrales, M., ToepflS., Butz, P., Knorr, D., Tauscher, B. "Extraction of anthocyanins from grape by-products assisted by ultrasonics, high hydrostatic pressure or pulsed electric fields." *A comparison. Innovative Food Science and Emerging Technologies 9* (2008): pp. 85–91.

Delsart, C., Cholet, C., Ghidossi, R., Grimi, N., Gontier, E., Gény, L., et al., "Effects of pulsed electric fields on cabernet sauvignon grape berries and on the characteristics of wines." *Food and Bioprocess Technology* (2013): 1–13.

Donsì, F., Ferrari, G., & Pataro, G. "Applications of pulsed electric field treatments for the enhancement of mass transfer from vegetable tissue." *Food Engineering Reviews* (2010): 2, 109–130.

Joana Gil-Chávez, G., Villa, J. A., Fernando Ayala-Zavala, J., Basilio Heredia, J., Sepulveda, D., Yahia, E. M., & González-Aguilar, G. A. "Technologies for extraction and production of bioactive compounds to be used as nutraceuticals and food ingredients: an overview."

*Comprehensive Reviews in Food Science and Food Safety* (2013): 12 (1), 5–23.

Kammerer, D. R, Kammerer, J., Valet, R, Carle, R. "Recovery of polyphenols from the by-products of plant food processing and application as valuable food ingredients." *Food Research International 65 (A),* (2014): 2-12.

Khalil, (2011). *Pulsed Electric Field (P.E.F) and Pectinase for the Extraction of Polyphenols from Grape Pomace and Peel.* (https://www.researchgate.net/publication/267379360_Pulsed_electric_field_pef_and_pectinase_for_the_extraction_of_polyphenols_from_grape_pomace_and_peel).

Knorr, D., Angersbach, A., Eshtiaghi, M. N., Heinz, V., & Lee, D. U. "Processing concepts based on high intensity electric field pulses." *Trends in Food Science & Technology* (2001), 12, 129–135.

López, N., Puértolas, E., Condón, S., Álvarez, I., & Raso, J. "Application of pulsed electric fields for improving the maceration process during vinification of red wine: Influence of grape variety." *European Food Research and Technology,* (2008a):227, 1099–1107.

López, N., Puértolas, E., Condón, S., Álvarez, I., Raso, J. "Effects of pulsed electric fields on the extraction of phenolic compounds during the fermentation of must of Tempranillo grapes." *Innov. Food Sci. Emerg. Technol.* (2008b): 9, 477–482.

López, N., Puértolas, E., Hernández-Orte, P., Álvarez, I., & Raso, J. "Effect of a pulsed electric field treatment on the anthocyanins composition and other quality parameters of Cabernet Sauvignon freshly fermented model wines obtained after different maceration times." *LWT— Food Science and Technology*, (2008):42, 1225–1231.

López-Alfaro, I. & Garde-Cerdán, T. "Pulsed electric field treatment to improve the phenolic compound extraction from Graciano, Tempranillo and Grenache grape varieties during two vintages." *Innovative Food Science and Emerging Technologies* (2015): 28, 31–39.

Marsellés-Fontanet, A. R., Puig-Pujol, A., Olmos, P., Mínguez-Sanz, S., & Martín-Belloso, O. "A comparison of the effects of pulsed electric field and thermal treatments on grape juice." *Food and Bioprocess Technology* (2013): 6, 978–987.

Morata, A., Loira, I., Vejarano, R., González, C., Callejo, M. J., Suárez-Lepe, J. A. "Emerging preservation technologies in grapes for winemaking." *Trends Food Sci. Technol.* (2017): 67, 36–43.

Mosqueda-Melgar, J., Raybaudi-Massilia, R. M., & Martín-Belloso, O. "Microbiological shelf life and sensory evaluation of fruit juices treated by high-intensity pulsed electric fields and antimicrobials." *Food and Bioproducts Processing,* (2012): 90 (2), 205–214.

Peixoto, C. M., Maria, Inês Dias M. I., Alves M. J., Calhelha R. C., Lillian Barros L, Simão P. Pinho SP, Ferreira I ."Grape pomace as a source of phenolic compounds and diverse bioactive properties." *Food Chemistry 253* (2018) 132–138.

Puértolas E., Saldaña G., Condón S., Álvarez I. & Raso J. "Evolution of polyphenolic compounds in red wine from Cabernet Sauvignon grapes processed by pulsed electric fields during aging in bottle." *Food Chemistry* (2010b): 119, 1063- 1070.

Puértolas, E., López, N., Condón, S., Álvarez, I., & Raso, J. "Potential applications of pulsed electric fields on Cabernet Sauvignon grape berries and on the characteristics of wines." *Food and Bioprocess Technology* (2010a): 7, 426–436.

Puértolas, E., López, N., Saldaña, G., Álvarez, I., Raso, J. "Evaluation of phenolic extraction during fermentation of red grapes treated by a continuous pulsed electric fields process at pilot-plant scale." *J. Food Eng.* (2010c): 98 (1), 120–125.

Rajha, H. N., Boussetta, N, Louka N, Maroun RG, Vorobiev E. "A comparative study of physical pretreatments for the extraction of polyphenols and proteins from vine shoots." *Food Research International*, (2014): 65 (C), 462-468..

Ricci, A, Parpinello, G. P., Versari, A. "Recent Advances and Applications of Pulsed Electric Fields (PEF) to Improve Polyphenol

Extraction and Color Release during Red Winemaking." *Beverages* (2018): 4, 18; 1-12.

Rocha, C. M. R., Genisheva, Z, Ferreira-Santos, P., Rodrigues, R., Vicente, A. A., Teixeira, J. A., Pereira, R. N. "Electric field-based technologies for valorization of bioresources." *Bioresource Technology 254* (2018): 325–339.

Teusdea, A. C., Bandici, L., Kordiaka. R., Bandici, G. E., Vicas, S. I. "The Effect of Different Pulsed Electric Field Treatments on Producing High Quality Red Wines." *Not Bot Horti Agrobo* (2017): 45 (2):540-547..

Vicaş, S. I., Bandici, L., Teuşdea, A. C., Turcin, V., Popa, D., Bandici, Gh. E."The bioactive compounds, antioxidant capacity, and color intensity in must and wines derived from grapes processed by pulsed electric field." *CyTA - Journal of Food.* (2017): Volume 15, 553-562.

Xia, E., Deng, G., Guo, Y., & Li, H. "Biological activities of polyphenols from grapes." *International Journal of Molecular Sciences* (2010): 11, 622–646.

Yu, J., & Ahmedna, M. "Functional components of grape pomace: Their composition, biological properties, and potential applications." *International Journal of Food Science & Technology* (2013): 48, 221-237.

In: Grape Pomace in Health …
Editor: Veronica Sanda Chedea ISBN: 978-1-68507-409-8


*Chapter 3*

# ABSORPTION AND BIOAVAILABILITY OF GRAPE POMACE POLYPHENOLS

***Veronica Sanda Chedea[1,*]***
***and Raluca Maria Pop[2]***
[1]Research Station for Viticulture and Enology, Blaj, (SCDVV Blaj), Romania
[2]Department of Pharmacology, Toxicology and Clinical Pharmacology, "Iuliu Hatieganu" University of Medicine and Pharmacy, Cluj-Napoca, Romania

## ABSTRACT

The nutraceutical role of grape pomace (GP) polyphenols is conditioned by the absorption and bioavailability of these compounds. This review presents results from research in rats, pigs, and humans related to GP to study these processes. These studies highlight an increasing interest in the metabolism and microbial biotransformation of dietary polyphenols and their metabolites' bioactivity compared to their parent compounds. These metabolites elicit significant intrinsic bioactivities that could explain the effects observed for the parent compounds. This research has also emphasized a requirement for a new

[*] Corresponding Author's E-mail: chedeaveronica@yahoo.com.

generation of intervention studies designed to investigate the variation in bioavailability and bioefficacy within individuals in response to the consumption of bioactive compounds present in plant food material.

**Keywords**: grape pomace polyphenols, bioavailability, polyphenol metabolites

## Introduction

The primary byproduct of the wine and grape juice production, grape pomace (GP), can be classified as a nutraceutical due to containing high quantities of bioactive molecules, flavonoids (anthocyanins, flavan-3-ols, flavonols, and flavanones), non-flavonoids (phenolic acids and their derivatives, stilbenes, lignans) and dietary fibers (Castello et al. 2018; Martin-Carron et al. 1997; Guendez et al. 2005; Chedea et al. 2011; Chedea et al. 2018). In 1997, Martin-Carron et al. stated that despite the composition of GP being known, its physiological effects and bioavailability remained poorly understood (Martin-Carron et al. 1997). By the year 2020, *in vitro* (Chedea, Braicu, and Socaciu 2010; Chedea et al. 2014; Ignea et al. 2013; Chedea et al. 2011), *in vivo* (Chedea et al. 2017, 2018, 2019), and epidemiological studies had revealed that polyphenols, which are among the most important bioactive components in GP, are associated with multiple health benefits. These health benefits are attributed to their extensive range of physiological properties, e.g., antiallergenic, anti-inflammatory, antimicrobial, antioxidant, and cardioprotective effects (Haminiuk et al. 2012; Bordiga, Travaglia, and Locatelli 2019), the prevention of cerebrovascular, neurodegenerative, and intestinal diseases (Halake, Birajdar, and Lee 2016; Cueva et al. 2017; Nagar, Okun, and Shpigelman 2020) and anti-ageing and anti-diabetic properties (Xia et al. 2010; Torres et al. 2002; Alonso et al. 2002).

Therefore, promoting the increased inclusion of polyphenols within the human diet has been described as an essential objective for promoting improved public health (Eran Nagar, Okun, and Shpigelman 2020). In recent years, increased interest in the digestive fate of polyphenolic compounds has mounted due to developments in understanding the significant influence of digestive processes on the bioactive properties of food components within the body (Eran Nagar, Okun, and Shpigelman 2020; Chedea et al. 2018, 2019). However, the currently available data regarding the bioavailability of polyphenols is insufficient for an evidence-based discussion regarding their health-promoting properties (Eran Nagar, Okun, and Shpigelman 2020).

The bioavailability of a compound is influenced by its properties and the metabolic events that allow them to be made available for use in the body. Examples of these properties and events include solubility, digestion, absorption, tissue distribution and retention, and enzymatic transformation in addition to secretion and excretion mechanisms (Packer, Rimbach, and Virgili 1999; Chedea and Pop 2016). While various mechanisms related to the possible activation of cellular signaling pathways have been proposed for polyphenols, it's unclear if these pathways occur *in vivo*. Questions arise due to the reported (very) low bioavailability of the original compounds (Zhang and Tsao 2016), which are believed to be strongly influenced by the different chemical structures within various polyphenol groups (Santhakumar, Battino, and Alvarez-Suarez 2018; G. Williamson 2017; Bohn et al. 2015; Eran Nagar, Okun, and Shpigelman 2020). Low phenolic bioavailability is also dependent on the complex formation, which is influenced by their physicochemical stability and food interactions during gastrointestinal absorption in addition to hepatic and gut metabolism (Xiao 2018; Sies 2010; Luca et al. 2020). Data acquired from *in vitro* and *in vivo* experiments investigating the bioavailability of natural phenols has also provided evidence to suggest that stability issues arise in these molecules (Luca et al. 2020).

Furthermore, despite their poor oral bioavailability, polyphenols exert many biological effects, creating a low bioavailability and high bioactivity paradox (Luca et al. 2020). However, there is significant evidence to support the proposition that it is the relatively high polyphenol content that influences these biological effects, which include anti-oxidative effects and the modulation of gastrointestinal enzyme activity (Martinez-Gonzalez et al. 2017; Terra et al. 2017; Domínguez-Avila et al. 2017; Eran Nagar, Okun, and Shpigelman 2020). Phenolic compounds also contain antioxidants and possess anti-inflammatory properties, providing intestinal cells protection from oxidative and inflammatory injuries (Soobrattee et al. 2005; Oz, Chen, and de Villiers 2013; Mosele, Macià, and Motilva 2015; Rodríguez-Ramiro et al. 2013).

Alongside their bioavailability, the inter-individual variability that may exist in the production of phenolic metabolites has not yet been comprehensively researched (Castello et al. 2018). However, it is known that their intrinsic activity is dependent on the intestinal absorption and bioactive metabolites, and this differs from native polyphenols whose metabolites are instead produced via digestive and hepatic metabolic processes (Manach et al. 2004; Del Rio et al. 2013; Rodriguez-Mateos et al. 2014; Gerardi et al. 2020). Therefore, studying the chemical transformations that phenolic compounds undergo during their passage through the human body can help to establish a more accurate understanding of their biological effects (Selma, Espín, and Tomás-Barberán 2009; Manach et al. 2004; Castello et al. 2018).

Research groups have in the past used simulations of human digestion to study the chemical transformations that phenolic compounds undero (Gomes et al. 2019). Although it is challenging to mimic the natural physiological conditions using *in vitro* assays based on digestion models, they are a primary tool that is essential for studying food systems and behaviors due to their advantages which include their reliability, simplicity, and broad applicability (Lucas-González et al. 2018; Gomes et al. 2019). Simulated human digestion models have been used to assess changes in the macro-, microelements, and polyphenols found in the peel, pulp, and seeds of *Vitis labrusca L.* grapes (Gomes et al. 2019). It is well known that the composition and bioaccessibility of grape polyphenols and minerals are influenced by grape variety and matrix. The pulp and seeds were characterized by flavanols, while peels were found to be high in phenolic acids (Gomes et al. 2019). After the simulated human digestion, anthocyanins diglucosides became more bioaccessible during the gastric phase (153% and 113% for malvidin and cyanidin, respectively), while the greatest bioaccessibility was found for quercetin (85%) (Gomes et al. 2019). The simulated human digestion of grape peels has shown a higher bioaccessibility of most minerals, suggesting that the nutritional value of this matrix is most significant (Gomes et al. 2019). Although simulated human digestion models provide information relating to the metabolic transformation of polyphenols, studies using animal models and human clinical trials can provide more accurate data on polyphenol metabolization, absorption, and bioaccessibility.

## Grape Pomace Polyphenols Metabolites in Rats

When male Wistar rats were fed a standard diet supplemented with 10% GP for 8 weeks, it was discovered that 68% of soluble polyphenols were absorbed within the gastrointestinal tract, while 99% of insoluble polyphenols remained undegraded and were excreted in faeces, improving the high bulking capacity of dietary fiber (Martin-Carron et al. 1997). More recently, Del Pino-García et al. (2016) observed that high levels of phenolic acids in Wistar rats plasma are associated with the increased prevention of lipid peroxidation and a high nitric oxide bioavailability following the administration of red GP product in a single oral dose of 300 mg/kg BW (Del Pino-García et al. 2016). The red GP product was a seedless wine pomace used as raw material to produce a powdered seasoning (Del Pino-García et al. 2016). After administrating the oral dose, dihydroferulic acid followed by 4-hydroxyphenylacetic acid, homovallinic, protocatechuic, syringic, gentisic, caffeic, dihydro-3-coumaric, and ferulic acids were the phenolic acids that were present in rat plasma samples (Del Pino-García et al. 2016). Gerardi et al. (2020) also reported that hydroferulic, p-hydroxyphenylacetic, syringic, and vanillic acids were the most abundant phenolic acids in Winstar rats plasma samples after red GP intake, in addition to significant concentrations of m-hydroxyphenylacetic, protocatechuic, homovanillic, gentisic, and caffeic acids (Gerardi et al. 2020) (Table 1). Anthocyanins constitute a substantial group of flavonoids found in red GP (Gerardi et al. 2020; Chedea and Pop 2016) and are metabolized in the upper gastrointestinal tract. 4-Hydroxyhippuric and ferulic acids derivates are the primary metabolites of anthocyanin and reach their highest concentration in plasma following a 1-1.5-hour period after consumption (Gerardi et al. 2020). Following the administration of white GP, the same study found thc primary phenolic acids in the plasma to be m-hydroxyphenylacetic, p-hydroxyphenylacetic, protocatechuic, 4-O-methylgallic acids, ferulic, homovanillic, vanillic, homoprotocatechuic, syringic, and hydroferulic acids (Gerardi et al. 2020).

Catechin, epicatechin, and procyanidin B2 were predominant in white GP (García-Lomillo and González-SanJosé 2017; Gerardi et al. 2020; Cueva et al. 2017), and there were generated by their microbial catabolism hydrophenylvalerolactones and dihydroxyphenylpropionic acids, which by further metabolization produce m-hydroxyphenylacetic and protocatechuic acids. In rat urine samples, 4-hydroxyphenylacetic, dihydroferulic, dihydro-3-coumaric, vallinic, ferulic and syringic acids were found after the red GP seasoning product consumption (Del Pino-García et al. 2016). In terms of absorption rate, an increased presence of total phenolic acid metabolites in the plasma samples was observed at 2h (43% of the phenolic metabolites of red GP and 55% of the white GP), 4h (55% of the phenolic metabolites of red GP and 24% of white GP), and 6h (20% of white GP) after their consumption (Castello et al. 2018; Gerardi et al. 2020). A 2% increase in the amount of these metabolites was observed beyond 6h, and this provides an indication that their formation occurs via microbial metabolism in the large intestine (Del Rio et al. 2013; Gerardi et al. 2020). To acquire the results described in the previously paragraph, Gerardi et al. (2020) measured the concentration of phenolic acids using gas chromatography (GC) coupled with a triple quadrupole mass spectrometer (MS). The identification and quantification of stilbenes, flavanols, and flavonols were performed using high-performance liquid chromate-graphy-diode-array detection (HPLC-DAD) (Gerardi et al. 2020).

**Table 1. Grape pomace metabolites determined in rats and humans**

| Grape Pomace (GP) | GP polyphenolic component | Specie | Metabolite | Reference |
|---|---|---|---|---|
| Red GP | Anthocyanins | Wistar rats | 4-hydroxyhippuric and ferulic acids, hydroferulic and dihydroferulic acids | (Del Pino-García et al. 2016; Gerardi et al. 2020) |
| Red GP | malvidin and peonidin | Wistar rats | syringic and vanillic acids | (Del Pino-García et al. 2016; Gerardi et al. 2020) |
| Red GP | ferulic and other cinnamic acids | Wistar rats | hydroferulic, isoferulic, dihydroferulic acids, | (Del Pino-García et al. 2016; Gerardi et al. 2020) |
| Red GP | | Wistar rats | m-hydroxyphenylacetic, protocatechuic, homoprotocatechuic, homovanillic, gentisic, and caffeic acids | (Del Pino-García et al. 2016; Gerardi et al. 2020) |
| Red GP | | Wistar rats | Dihydro-3-coumaric acid | (Del Pino-García et al. 2016) |
| White GP, Red GP | | Wistar rats | m(3)-hydroxyphenylacetic, p-hydroxyphenylacetic, protocatechuic, homoprotocatechuic, 4-O-methylgallic acids | (Del Pino-García et al. 2016; Gerardi et al. 2020) |

## Table 1. (Continued)

| Grape Pomace (GP) | GP polyphenolic component | Specie | Metabolite | Reference |
|---|---|---|---|---|
| White GP | flavanols such as catechin, epicatechin, and procyanidin B2 | Wistar rats | m-hydroxyphenylacetic and protocatechuic acids, ferulic, homovanillic, vanillic, homoprotocatechuic, syringic, and hydroferulic acids | (Gerardi et al. 2020) |
| GP seed extract, GP skin extract | catechin and epicatechin; procyanidin dimers B1, B2, B3, and B4; Procyanidin Trimer C1, Procyanidin oligomers, Delphinidin-3-O-monoglucoside; Cyanidin-3-O-monoglucoside; Petunidin-3-O-monoglucoside; Peonidin-3-O- monoglucoside; Malvidin-3-O-monoglucoside; petunidin-3-O-acetylmonoglucoside, peonidin-3-O-acetylmonoglucoside, malvidin-3-O- acetylmonoglucoside; peonidin-3-(6-O-p-coumaroyl)monoglucoside malvidin-3-(6-O-p- coumaroyl)monoglucoside | Spontaneously hypertensive rats (SHR) | (Epi)catechin-O-glucuronide, O-methyl-(epi)catechin-O-glucuronide, 5-(Hydroxyphenyl)--valerolactone-O-glucuronide, 5-(Hydroxyphenyl)--valerolactone-O-sulphate, 5-(Hydroxyphenyl)--hydroxyvaleric acid-O-sulphate, 5-(Phenyl)--hydroxyvaleric acid-O-sulphate, Isoferulic acid-4-O-sulfate, 5-(Hydroxyphenyl)--valerolactone-O-glucuronide, (Epi)catechin-O-glucuronide, O-methyl-(epi)catechin-O-glucuronide, 5-(Hydroxyphenyl)--valerolactone-O-glucuronide, Methyl-(epi)catechin-O-glucuronide, Di-methyl-(epi)catechin-O-glucuronide, 1-5-(Hydroxyphenyl)-4-hydroxyvaleric acid-O-sulphate, 5-(Hydroxyphenyl)--valerolactone sulphate, 5-(Hydroxyphenyl)--valerolactone-O-glucuronide, | (Rasines-Perea et al. 2018; Ky et al. 2014) |

| Grape Pomace (GP) | GP polyphenolic component | Specie | Metabolite | Reference |
|---|---|---|---|---|
| Red GP aqueous extract | Gallic acid, Catechin, Epicatechin, Galloyl glucose, Quercetin rhamnoside, Quercetin-3-O-glucoside, Quercetin-3-O-glucuronide<br>Myricetin hexoside, Syringetin hexoside<br>Quercetin rutinoside, Procyanidin dimer B-type, Procyanidin dimer B-type, Procyanidin B2, Procyanidin dimer gallate B-type, Procyanidin trimer B-type, Procyanidin trimer B-type, Procyanidin trimer B-type, Cyanidin-3-O-glucoside, Delphinidin-3-O-glucoside, Petunidin-3-O-glucoside, Malvidin-3-O-glucoside, Malvidin-3-O-acetylglucoside, Petunidin-3-p-coumaroylglucoside, Malvidin-3-p-coumaroylglucoside, Malvidin-diglucoside | Humans | Gallic acid,<br>Vanillic acid-4-glucuronide,<br>Protocatechuic acid-3-glucuronide, Protocatechuic acid, 4-Hydroxyhippuric acid, Catechol-sulphate, Methylpyrogallol-sulphate, Methylcatechol-sulphate, Protocatechuic acid-3-sulphate,<br>Benzoic acid-4-sulphate, (Epi)catechin glucuronide-sulphate, Ferulic acid-4-glucuronide, Vanillic acid-4-sulphate Hydroxyphenylpropionic acid-sulphate (3′,5′-Dihydroxyphenyl)-γ-valerolactone, Hippuric acid, 5-(3′-Hydroxyphenyl)-γ-valerolactone-4′-glucuronide, 5-(phenyl)-γ-valerolactone-sulphate-glucuronide, 5-(4′-Hydroxyphenyl)-γ-valerolactone-3′-glucuronide, (Epi)catechin-glucuronide, 5-(3′,4′-Dihydroxyphenyl)-γ-valerolactone, 5-(5′-Hydroxyphenyl)-γ-valerolactone-3′-sulphate, Dihydrocaffeic acid-sulphate, Feruloylglycine, 5-Phenyl-γ-valerolactone-3′-glucuronide, Dihydroferulic acid-sulphate, (Epi)catechin-sulphate, isomer, Ferulic acid-4-sulphate, 5-(Hydroxyphenyl)-γ-valerolactone-sulphate isomers, 5-Phenyl-valeric acid-sulphate-glucuronide, Methyl(epi)catechin-sulphate, isomer, sinapic acid-sulphate, Methyl(epi)catechin-sulphate isomer, 5-Phenyl-γ-valerolactone-3′-sulphate, 5-(phenyl)-γ-valerolactone-sulphate-methoxy | (Castello et al. 2018) |

Using HPLC ESI-MSn analysis, Rasines-Perea et al. (2018) were able to identify 18 metabolites in urine, 11 in plasma, and 2 in the heart, liver, and kidneys tissues (Table 1) of spontaneously hypertensive rats that had been administered with different GP extracts using a gavage (a tube leading down the throat and into the stomach).

To evaluate the *in vivo* effect of GP and its potential impact on hypertension, spontaneously hypertensive rats were administrated with three GP extracts at a dose of 21 mg/kg/day, which is the equivalent to a daily dose of 0.5 L of wine consumed by a 70 kg human (Rasines-Perea et al. 2018). The extracts were produced in 70:30, Ethanol: Water, *v*/*v* solution acquired from Grenache seed pomace, Mourvèdre skin pomace, and Alicante skin pomace. The study was conducted over six weeks of treatments with the fourth week of treatment resumption (Rasines-Perea et al. 2018).

Urine samples that had been collected between 0–8 h and 8–24 h on days 1 and 7 after ingestion did not contain any of the flavan-3-ols and procyanidins found in the original GP extract but did contain glucuronides and methylglucuronides of (epi)catechin in addition to valerolactone and valeric acid phase II glucuronide and sulphate metabolites (Rasines-Perea et al. 2018). In urine samples, 18 metabolites were identified (Table 1) with the most important being: (epi)catechin-*O*-glucuronide, *O*-methyl-(epi)catechin-*O*-glucuronide, 5-(hydroxyphenyl)--valerolactone-*O*-glucuronide, 5-(hydroxyphenyl)--valerolactone-*O*-sulphate, 5hydroxy-phenyl-4-hydroxyvaleric acid-*O*-sulphate, 5-(phenyl)-4-hydroxyvaleric acid-*O*sulfate and isoferulic acid-4-*O*-sulphate (Rasines-Perea et al. 2018). More *O*-methyl-(epi)catechin-*O*-glucuronide relative to (epi)catechin-*O*-glucuronide and sulphate derivatives of 5-(hydroxyphenyl)--valerolactone relative to glucuronides were detected (Rasines-Perea et al. 2018).

Between 0-8 h and 8-24 h on day 1, a decrease in 5-(hydroxyphenyl)-4-hydroxyvaleric acid-*O*-sulfate was observed alongside an increase in 5-(phenyl)-4hydroxyvaleric acid-*O*-sulphate at 8–24 h when compared to 0–8 h in all rat urine samples on days 1 and 7 (Rasines-Perea et al. 2018).

On day 1 after the gavage, substantial 0–8 h urinary excretion of metabolites was observed after the administration of Grenache seed pomace and Mourvèdre skin pomace in hypertensive rats. This observation was different from the group administered with Alicante skin pomace, in which the highest excretion occurred in 8–24 h period (Rasines-Perea et al. 2018). On day 7, no significant difference was observed between the different experimental groups. The authors highlighted that this observation could reduce the inter-individual variability of absorption and excretion in the same group (Rasines-Perea et al. 2018). In the plasma of hypertensive rats, 11 metabolites were detected. No polyphenols present in GP were found in plasma samples collected 4 h after the rats had ingested the GP extract. Still, their metabolites were detected, and these mainly included glucuronides as opposed to sulphates (glucuronide, methyl-glucuronide and di-methylglucuronide of (epi)catechin and glucuronide, sulphate and mono-substituted valerolactone and valeric acid) (Rasines-Perea et al. 2018). The same metabolites were detected in urine except for di-methyl-(epi)catechin-*O*-glucuronide (Rasines-Perea et al. 2018). Tsang et al. (2005) also observed similar patterns, with sulphate metabolites being most dominant in the urine of Sprague – Dawley male rats after the ingestion of grape seed extracts, while the glucuronidated forms of (epi)catechins were dominant in plasma samples (Tsang et al. 2005). No (epi)catechin conjugates were present in hypertensive rat tissues such as the kidneys and liver, but instead was the detection of a 5-(hydroxyphenyl)--valerolactone-*O*-glucuronide (*m*/*z* 383/207, 163) and 5-(hydroxyphenyl)--valerolactone-*O*-sulphate (*m*/*z* 287/207, 163) with the glucuronide being most dominant (Rasines-Perea et al. 2018). The liver contained the highest level of metabolites with the kidneys containing more 5-(hydroxyphenyl)--valerolactone-*O*-sulphate compared to liver (Rasines-Perea et al. 2018).

## Studies of GP Metabolites in Pigs

Despite the majority of polyphenol absorption and bioavailability studies use rats as the *in vivo* experimental model, these models are less effective at modelling humans compared to other models. Pigs are the most suitable non-primate animal models for use in nutritional studies due to similarities with humans in terms of their anatomy, physiology, digestion and gastrointestinal tract when compared to humans (Davis, Illum, and Hinchcliffe 2001; Rauw et al. 2007). Other similarities between pigs and humans include the population of intestinal microbiota (Rzeppa et al. 2012), the development of features of the intestine during fetal and postnatal development, including the small intestines being relatively mature at birth in addition to fat digestion and absorption (Innis, 1993; Burke and Weiler, 2002; Guilloteau et al. 2010). Furthermore, the digestive processes of a newborn piglet and a human infant is highly similar in terms of enzyme activity and digestive capacity (Guilloteau et al. 2010). Studies conducted in the past have revealed that body composition, presented in percentages and on a fat-free basis, is highly similar between humans and pigs at three stages in life. The stages of life at which humans and pigs have been shown to have similar body compositions at birth, 3 months, and at the ages of 3 years in pigs and 33 years in humans (Guilloteau et al. 2010; Chedea et al. 2019). All the aforementioned similarities between pigs and humans allow the pig to be regarded as a brilliant experimental model for simulating human digestive processes in nutritional studies (Langerholc et al. 2011; Lunney 2007; Chedea et al. 2018). Therefore, the findings of dietary studies investigating the absorption and activity of polyphenols using pigs as the experimental model can be more reliability applied to humans when compared to studies using alternative models (Rzeppa et al. 2012).

Few nutritional studies have investigated the absorption and activities of polyphenol metabolites in pig models due to the high monetary and time requirements associated with feeding and maintaining them. In this context, Chedea et al. (2019) described the beneficial health effects of replacing 5% of the corn content with GP in the diet of piglets. The total polyphenols content in plasma of the piglets fed the GP diet for 36 days was higher than in the previous diet that did not include GP; a significant interaction between diet and time was also observed ($p < 0.026$) (Chedea et al. 2019). Similar effects were observed when measuring the total phenol content in the plasma of dairy cows that had been fed a 15% GP diet (Chedea et al. 2017). The 5% GP diet of piglets also resulted in a significantly higher quantity of polyphenols being stored in the kidney ($p = 0.019$) (Chedea et al. 2019). In another investigation, Serra et al. (2011) detected a high number of polyphenol metabolites in the kidneys of rats (Serra et al. 2011; Chedea et al. 2019). The most important and interesting effect of introducing an increased amount of GP into the diet of the model organisms was the significant increased levels of antioxidant activity in the liver, spleen, and kidneys, which are vital organs in animal physiology that facilitate the animals' good health after weaning (Chedea et al. 2019).

The composition of polyphenols present in the duodenum and colon has been analyzed using liquid chromatography-mass spectrometry (LC-MS) to investigate the fate of the dietary GP in weaned piglets in the intestines (Chedea et al. 2018). In their investigation, only the procyanidin trimer C2 appeared to have accumulated in slightly significant concentration within the duodenum (14.4%) of piglets after being fed this diet for 36 days. This accumulation included all classifications of polyphenols identified (procyanidin trimer possibly C2, procyanidin dimer, caffeoylquinic acids, ferulic acid, and the isoflavones: daidzin, 6"-*O*-malonyldaidzin, genistin and 6"-*O*-malonylgenistin,). This finding may be critical because polyphenol bioactivity is heavily influenced by metabolization, and therefore the conserved activity of the free procyanidin dimers and trimers *in vivo* might partly compensate for their low absorption (Appeldoorn et al. 2009). Procyanidin dimers and trimers were also detected in the rats' intestines (Serra et al. 2011). Besides the procyanidin trimer C2 identified in the duodenum, catechin and procyanidin trimer C1 were found in colon tissue samples recovered from the piglets. This result indicates variation in the absorption of different isomers in the duodenum and colon that is not concentration-dependent but is instead based on minor structural differences (procyanidin trimer C1 versus procyanidin trimer C2) (Chedea et al. 2018).

To explain the presence of trimers in the colon and duodenum samples, their UV-Vis spectra were evaluated (Chedea et al. 2018). Examination of the UV-Vis spectra provided evidence to suggest that polyphenols were primarily structurally modified by metabolization, and in this form, they were absorbed in the duodenum and colon at λmax between 274.9 nm and 298.0 nm (Chedea et al. 2018). The UV-Vis absorption maxima between 315 nm and 588 nm might be explained by extensive oxidation at the intermolecular and intramolecular level between polyphenols, proteins, or other antioxidants and molecules with the formation of o-quinones and dimers-possibly trimers, as indicated by other LC-MS results (Chedea, Braicu, and Socaciu 2010; Choueiri et al. 2012; Chedea et al. 2012). These findings suggest that synergy exists between low and high degrees of polymerization oligomers occurs. Therefore the bioavailability of procyanidins might be understated as it only includes the ingested parent molecules while excluding their metabolites. Therefore, polyphenol-rich foods may provide beneficial health effects due to containing high amounts of procyanidin trimers (Chedea et al. 2018).

## Studies of GP Metabolites in Humans

The most relevant investigations into polyphenols bioavailability involve human clinical trials. Usually, polyphenols are administrated orally in a drink (Borges et al. 2010; Castello et al. 2018). Later, the urine and plasma are analyzed for the presence of the polyphenols. Few studies have investigated the bioavailability of GP polyphenols (and their metabolites) following ingestions. The most recent and representative investigation was conducted by Castello et al. (2018), who administrated a drink produced from red GP to ten volunteers. The polyphenolic composition of the drink was analyzed using LC-MS, leading to the identification and quantification of 25 phenolic compounds that includedanthocyanins, flavan-3-ol monomers procyanidins, small amounts of flavonols, galloyl glucose, and gallic acid (Castello et al. 2018) (Table 1). In urine and plasma samples collected from the volunteers, the same analysis was used to identify and quantify 35 phenolic metabolites, many of which were present in both physiological liquids. Specifically, 35 phenolic metabolites were present in the urine samples, while the plasma contained 28 (Castello et al. 2018) (Table 1).

Immediately after ingestion (0-3h), no anthocyanins were found in urine. Still, insignificant traces of several anthocyanin derivatives were detected in samples recovered from a small number of volunteers (Castello et al. 2018). Borges et al. (2010) did not investigate the presence of anthocyanins in plasma or urine (Borges et al. 2010). Instead, they studied the bioavailability of various phenolic compounds, principally flavonoids, following their acute ingestion of 350mL of a low-calorie, polyphenol-rich juice drink by human participants (Borges et al. 2010). Generally, anthocyanins are poorly absorbed and difficult to detect in plasma samples except for pelargonidin- 3-O-glucoside (Crozier, Jaganath, and Clifford 2009; Borges et al. 2010). Like anthocyanins, no procyanidin dimers, trimers, or pentamers were detected in plasma or urine samples despite the drink containing high quantities of procyanidins (Borges et al. 2010). In urine samples, high concentrations of hippuric acid and 4′-hydroxyhippuric acid were detected due to both metabolizing the GP drink and other dietary, endogenous sources (Manach et al. 2004; Rechner et al. 2002; Castello et al. 2018). Plasma samples were also found to contain 4′-hydroxyhippuric acid (Castello et al. 2018).

Phenyl-γ-valerolactones were the most abundant class of phenolic metabolites in circulation containing phase II glucuronide- and sulphate-conjugated isomers of 5-(3′,4′-dihydroxyphenyl)-γ-valerolactone identified in both plasma and urine samples (Castello et al. 2018). The phenyl-γ-valerolactones were quantitatively the most abundant, followed by simple phenols, hydroxybenzoic acids, hydroxyphenylpropionic, hydroxycinnamic acids, and (epi)catechins (Castello et al. 2018). The 9 simple phenols and hydroxybenzoic acids have all been detected in urine samples (the main ones: methylpyrogallol-sulphate, benzoic acid-4-sulphate, and the glucuronide and sulphate forms of vanillic acid) (Castello et al. 2018). In contrast, 10 simple phenols and hydroxybenzoic acids were present in plasma (the most important being methylpyrogallol-sulphate and protocatechuic acid-3-sulphate) (Castello et al. 2018). Protocatechuic acid-3-glucuronide was present in plasma samples but absent in urine (Castello et al. 2018). Hydroxyphenylpropionic acids and hydroxycinnamic acids (ferulic acid-4-glucuronide and feruloylglycine are the examples detected in the highest concentrations) were identified in quantities of 7 in urine and 5 in the plasma because sinapic acid-sulphate and hydroxyphenylpropionic acid-sulphate were not included (Castello et al. 2018). Finally, a total of 6 phase II (epi)catechin metabolites were detected in urine samples and 5 in plasma, with the difference existing due to the absence of one of the two methyl(epi)catechin-sulphate isomers in the plasma samples (Castello et al. 2018). As a percentage of intake, the excretion of flavan-3-ol metabolites by humans is much higher than other flavonoids (Borges et al. 2010). In terms of their excretion rate, these compounds are eliminated quickest in the first 3 hours (Castello et al. 2018). Concerning phenyl-γ-valerolactones, the most rapid excretion of simple phenols and hydroxybenzoic acids was achieved after 6 h following the ingestion of red GP drink with an additional peak after 36 h (Castello et al. 2018). The urinary excretion of phenyl-γ-valerolactones, simple phenols and hydroxybenzoic acids was much higher than that of hydroxyphenylpropionic and hydroxycinnamic acids, which was almost constant throughout the 48 h period except for a minor peak between 3-6 h (Castello et al. 2018).

## Aspects of Polyphenols Metabolites Generation

Various phenolic compounds are absorbed and excreted at the same rate whether consumed in isolation or amongst a combination of other phenolic compounds, demonstrating that there is no significant competition when being transported across the gastrointestinal mucosa and into the circulatory system (Borges et al. 2010). Tsang et al. (2005) found that the levels of the metabolites in the bloodstream were much higher than in the gastrointestinal tract. Most of the phenolic compounds are scarcely or not absorbed within the small intestine, unlike other phenolic compounds that are readily absorbed (De Ferrars et al. 2014; Clifford et al. 2017; Borges et al. 2018). In one study, human participants with an ileostomy (an opening in the abdominal wall that brings the small intestine to the skin surface) were provided with green tea flavan-3-ol, and it was found that (epi)gallocatechins are poorly absorbed, whereas (epi)catechins can continue to be absorbed despite increases in dosage (Auger et al., 2008; Rasines-Perea et al. 2018). In rats fed with red and white GP, the total phenolic acid content in plasma samples varied significantly, indicating that an increased intake of red GP will not increase the amount of these compounds present. Instead, it was found that the number of metabolites significantly increased after the consumption of higher doses of white GP (Gerardi et al. 2020). These results indicate that the bioavailability of phenolic acids in plasma was dose-dependent when sourced from white GP. However, the bioavailability of red GP does not appear to be dose-dependent, and this suggests that a saturation mechanism might exist for red GP and not for white GP (Gerardi et al. 2020). Rodriguez-Mateos, et al. (2016) also reported a dose-dependent enhancement in endothelial function by cranberry phenolic metabolites following the consumption of cranberry juice (Rodriguez-Mateos et al. 2016). The apparent saturation mechanism was also reported regarding specific plasma (poly)phenols after wild blueberry consumption (Rodriguez-Mateos et al. 2016). Over time, spontaneously hypertensive rats may be able to ingest higher doses of polyphenols, especially those contained in Mourvèdre skin pomace extract, as opposed to the other varieties that have been tested (Rasines-Perea et al. 2018).

The absorption of flavan-3-ols and procyanidins initially occurs during their passage through walls of the small intestine (Rasines-Perea et al. 2018). In the duodenum, a procyanidin trimer (C2) was identified using LC-MS in control and experimental samples, with the highest quantities being found in samples derived from the piglets that were fed the 5% GP diet (16.00 mg catechin equivalents (CE)/100 g) when compared to the samples recovered from piglets receiving the control diet (13.69 mg CE/100 g) (Chedea et al. 2018). The detection of small quantities of phenolic metabolites (or failure to detect them entirely) within the gastrointestinal tract may be attributed to their low-level efflux back into the lumen of the intestine or due to enterohepatic recirculation via the bile (Tsang et al. 2005). The methylation and glucuronidation of flavan-3-ols and procyanidins occur on the luminal side of the endoplasmic reticulum of the small intestine during transportation into the bloodstream (Kuhnle et al. 2000; Donovan et al. 2001; Tsang et al. 2005). Phenolic acid content reached its maximum amount at 2h after intake, suggesting that the absorption of these simple molecules occurs principally in the first regions of the gastrointestinal tract that they pass through. Approximately 24 and 20% of the metabolites had the peak plasma at 4h and 6h following the consumption of white GP in rats (Gerardi et al. 2020).

The passage of digesta through the small intestine is estimated to require around 2–4 h, but the transit time increases considerably (as long as 24 h or more) in the large intestine (González-Barrio et al. 2010; Cummings et al., 1978; Mosele, Macià, and Motilva 2015). Therefore, most dietary phenolic compounds will reach the large intestine, further metabolized into various phenol derivatives by the local gut microbiota (Aura 2008; Rechner et al. 2002). This time is probably sufficient to accumulate substantial amounts of phenolic compounds and induce both metabolic and microbial changes in the gut lumen. The presence of luminal phenolic compounds could also impact the metabolic profile, enhancing or inhibiting the generation of fermentation products derived from endogenous and dietary compounds (Mosele, Macià, and Motilva 2015). In this respect, it is known that the half-life of phenolic metabolites depends on both their stabilization by conjugation with plasma proteins and their eventual elimination through the biliary or urinary pathways (Gerardi et al. 2020).

The main phenolic catabolites are formed by the cleavage of ester and glycoside bonds, ring-fission, and chemical modifications of their more complex parent compounds (Bresciani et al. 2017; Aura 2008; Rechner et al. 2002; Ludwig et al. 2015; Ottaviani et al. 2016). It has been reported that partial dihydroxylation reactions occur gradually as colonic metabolism progresses because dihydroxylated derivatives have been found 6–10 h after the phenolic intake. Furthermore, monohydroxylated forms at 6–24 h, and unhydroxylated derivatives at 10–24 h, indicating a change in the hydroxylation pattern of the phenyl ring from di- to mono- and unhydroxylated forms (Rasines-Perea et al. 2018; Llorach et al. 2010). Once absorbed at the colonic level, the newly formed metabolites may undergo phase I/II transformations exerted by both gut epithelial cells and hepatocytes, and some may even undergo an intense enterohepatic recirculation (Ludwig et al. 2015; Aura 2008; Bresciani et al. 2017; Ottaviani et al. 2016; Rechner et al. 2002). For instance, in the case of GP, no anthocyanins have been identified in urine and plasma samples collected from rats (Gerardi et al. 2020) or humans (Borges et al. 2010; Castello et al. 2018), but the high concentration of hydroferulic acid in plasma proceeds from the colonic metabolism of several phenolic compounds, principally anthocyanins, ferulic and other cinnamic acids (G. Williamson 2017; Gerardi et al. 2020; Mosele, Macià, and Motilva 2015). Also, the high concentration of syringic and vanillic acids in rats 'urine could be a consequence of the microbial metabolism, in the large intestine, of the high content of malvidin and peonidin present in the red GP (Forester and Waterhouse 2010; Mosele, Macià, and Motilva 2015; Gerardi et al. 2020). It has been estimated that, along with some unabsorbed monomers, 90–95% of ingested procyanidins enter the colon unaltered (Griffin et al. 2017). In the colon, procyanidins and their (epi)catechin monomeric units are catabolized by the microflora into low molecular weight phenolic acids, and the health potential of these metabolites should also be studied as the original procyanidins are only found in low quantities in the plasma (Appeldoorn et al. 2009;

Chedea et al. 2018). The differences in the qualitative and quantitative absorption of catechins in the duodenum and colon might also be attributed to the modulation of gut microbiota by these compounds (Chedea et al. 2018). Thus, it has been found that the gut microbiota metabolizes unabsorbed procyanidins into smaller phenolic compounds that are highly bioavailable (Griffin et al. 2017; Chedea et al. 2018). In animal models, grape bioactive compounds have been found to have the ability to increase the abundance of beneficial bacterial species such as *Bifidobacterium* and *Lactobacillus* spp. (Cardona et al. 2013; Griffin et al. 2017; Chedea et al. 2018). As these changes could alter the overall health status of the host, the impacts of various compound structures and doses within this context must be given careful consideration (Cardona et al. 2013; Griffin et al. 2017; Chedea et al. 2018).

The liver appears to be the most important organ involved in the metabolization of phenolics, as the situs of the phase II transformation, because a high level of metabolites has been identified in rats (Rasines-Perea et al. 2018) in addition to a significantly high antioxidant activity in piglets (Chedea et al. 2019). Some conjugated metabolites may also be transported to other organs via the bloodstream as shown through their presence in the heart of rats (Rasines-Perea et al. 2018) and the significant antioxidant activity in the spleen and kidneys of piglets (Chedea et al. 2019). Metabolites have also been detected in the kidneys of rats and piglets because of renal excretion (Rasines-Perea et al. 2018; Chedea et al. 2019).

It is worth emphasizing that the timing of tissue sampling may be of the utmost importance when attempting to detect and quantify the presence of metabolites due to the kinetics associated with their accumulation and elimination within the tissues (Rasines-Perea et al. 2018). The presence of metabolites was detected in rat tissue samples 1 h and 4 h after the ingestion of a grape seed extract and 4 h after the ingestion of GP extracts. No metabolites were detected in the same samples at 6, 12, and 24 h after intake (Tsang et al. 2005; Rasines-Perea et al. 2018).

In rats and humans, generally, lower amounts of metabolites were observed in plasma than in urine, revealing that flavan-3-ols are rapidly turned over the circulatory system, and rather than accumulating, are quickly excreted via the kidneys and being treated as xenobiotics by the body (Chedea and Pop 2016; Rasines-Perea et al. 2018; Brenes et al. 2016). Inversely, a possible cumulative effect was observed for some flavonoid metabolites that could be responsible for maintaining high phenolic acids concentrations in plasma (Gerardi et al. 2020). Higher concentrations of metabolites are identified in humans compared to rats because humans ingest higher amounts of flavan-3-ol monomers and polymers than rats (Rasines-Perea et al. 2018).

## Conclusion

Research investigating the presence of polyphenol metabolites in different sample types following GP ingestion presents differing results regarding identified metabolites. These differences are due to the absorption, excretion, and metabolic pathways of GP, in addition to differences that exist in matrix compositions and the effects that ingested polyphenols have when interacting with plasma proteins and other matrix components. Amplifying or decreasing polyphenols absorption through selecting effective GP can modulate the formed metabolites and their beneficial effects on health. Substantial quantities of polyphenols remain in GP after the winemaking process, and these are sufficient for achieving these effects (Rasines-Perea et al. 2018). During the last few years, an increasing interest has existed surrounding the metabolism and microbial biotransformation of dietary polyphenols and the bioactivity of their metabolites versus parent compounds due to these metabolites eliciting significant intrinsic bioactivities that could provide explanations for the effects observed in their parent compounds (Luca et al. 2020).

Studies also show that the absence of appropriate reference standards and sample processing before analysis (Day et al. 2003; Rasines-Perea et al. 2018) are factors hampering the adequate identification and quantification of phenolic metabolites in biological fluids (Brindani et al. 2017). In human plasma and urine, several classes of phenolic compounds were detected, including simple phenols (catechol derivatives), hydroxybenzoic acids, hydroxyphenylpropionic acids, hydroxycinnamic acids, phenyl-valeric acids, phenyl-γ-valerolactones, and (epi)catechin phase II conjugates (Castello et al. 2018). Generally, dietary polyphenols are poorly absorbed or are extensively metabolized within enterocytes and the liver by phase I and phase II enzymatic reactions. In addition, dietary phenols undergo intensive biotransformation facilitated by the gut microbiota to form a wide variety of new chemical structures that can pass easily into the systemic blood circulation (Stevens and Maier 2016; Ozdal et al. 2016; Williamson and Clifford 2017; Luca et al. 2020). It is considered that less than 5% of the total polyphenolic intake is absorbed into the plasma unaltered (Cao, Xie, and Chen 2015). In addition to microbial products, phase I and II metabolites are dominant within the plasma, especially when compared to their parent molecule, which is often undetectable even when using the most sensitive analytical techniques. Alternatively, these parent compounds may be present in a plasmatic level so low that they are considered incapable of achieving a sufficient overall efficacy (Chiou et al. 2014; Carbonell-Capella et al. 2014; Luca et al. 2020).

In humans, there is a high inter-individual variability of GP ingested polyphenols metabolization. Different circulating metabolites patterns were unraveled due to the vast variability in the production of colonic microbial metabolites and phase II conjugates. These findings are essential to further understand the potential health benefits of phenolic metabolites at the individual level (Castello et al. 2018) as a premise of the personalized nutrition concept (Morand et al. 2020). As food phytochemicals are continuously demonstrated to play a critical role in the cardiometabolic health effects of plant foods, the heterogeneity in responsiveness to their intake frequently observed in clinical trials can hinder the beneficial effects of these compounds in specific subpopulations (Morand et al. 2020). These interindividual variations can be due to a range of factors, including genetic background, gut microbiota, age, sex, and health status. In this context, the current knowledge is limited and fragmented, despite the increasing amount of research in the field. It has been stated that the human subjects ' intervention studies published so far are not adequate for investigating the relevant determinants of absorption/metabolism and biological responsiveness (Manach et al. 2017; Morand et al. 2020). The European network, European Cooperation in Science and Technology (COST)-POSITIVe, has systematically analyzed the existing knowledge to better understand the factors responsible for the interindividual variation in response to the consumption of the major families of plant food bioactive compounds, regarding their bioavailability and bioefficacy. In conclusion, the need for a new generation of intervention studies designed to capture this intermediate variation is emphasized (Morand et al. 2020).

## ACKNOWLEDGEMENTS

The authors wish to thank Hesham Ahmed Kisher, University of the West of England, Bristol for his assistance with the reviewing and editing of the English for this manuscript.

## REFERENCES

Alonso, Ángeles M., Dominico A. Guillén, Carmelo G. Barroso, Belén Puertas, and Alberto García. 2002. "Determination of Antioxidant Activity of Wine Byproducts and Its Correlation with Polyphenolic Content." *Journal of Agricultural and Food Chemistry* 50 (21): 5832–36. https://doi.org/10.1021/jf025683b.

Appeldoorn, Maaike M., Jean-Paul Vincken, Harry Gruppen, and Peter C. H. Hollman. 2009. "Procyanidin Dimers A1, A2, and B2 Are Absorbed without Conjugation or Methylation from the Small

Intestine of Rats." *The Journal of Nutrition* 139 (8): 1469–73. https://doi.org/10.3945/jn.109.106765.

Auger, Cyril, William Mullen, Yukihiko Hara, and Alan Crozier. n.d. *Bioavailability of Polyphenon E Flavan-3-Ols in Humans with an Ileostomy 1-4.* https://academic.oup.com/jn/article-abstract/138/8/1535S/4750813.

Aura, Anna Marja. 2008. "Microbial Metabolism of Dietary Phenolic Compounds in the Colon." In *Phytochemistry Reviews*, 7:407–29. https://doi.org/10.1007/s11101-008-9095-3.

Bohn, Torsten, Gordon J. Mcdougall, Amparo Alegría, Marie Alminger, Eva Arrigoni, Anna Marja Aura, Catarina Brito, et al. 2015. "Mind the Gap-Deficits in Our Knowledge of Aspects Impacting the Bioavailability of Phytochemicals and Their Metabolites-a Position Paper Focusing on Carotenoids and Polyphenols." *Molecular Nutrition and Food Research*. Wiley-VCH Verlag. https://doi.org/10.1002/mnfr.201400745.

Bordiga, Matteo, Fabiano Travaglia, and Monica Locatelli. 2019. "Valorisation of Grape Pomace: An Approach That Is Increasingly Reaching Its Maturity – a Review." *International Journal of Food Science and Technology*. https://doi.org/10.1111/ijfs.14118.

Borges, Gina, William Mullen, Adam Mullan, Michael E.J. Lean, Susan A. Roberts, and Alan Crozier. 2010. "Bioavailability of Multiple Components Following Acute Ingestion of a Polyphenol-Rich Juice Drink." *Molecular Nutrition and Food Research* 54 (SUPPL. 2). https://doi.org/10.1002/mnfr.200900611.

Borges, Gina, Javier I. Ottaviani, Justin J.J. van der Hooft, Hagen Schroeter, and Alan Crozier. 2018. "Absorption, Metabolism, Distribution and Excretion of (−)-Epicatechin: A Review of Recent Findings." *Molecular Aspects of Medicine*. https://doi.org/10.1016/j.mam.2017.11.002.

Brenes, Agustín, Agustín Viveros, Susana Chamorro, and Ignacio Arija. 2016. "Use of Polyphenol-Rich Grape by-Products in Monogastric Nutrition. A Review." *Animal Feed Science and Technology*. Elsevier. https://doi.org/10.1016/j.anifeedsci.2015.09.016.

Bresciani, Letizia, Daniela Martini, Pedro Mena, Michele Tassotti, Luca Calani, Giacomo Brigati, Furio Brighenti, et al. 2017. "Absorption Profile of (Poly)Phenolic Compounds after Consumption of Three Food Supplements Containing 36 Different Fruits, Vegetables, and Berries." *Nutrients* 9 (3). https://doi.org/10.3390/nu9030194.

Brindani, Nicoletta, Pedro Mena, Luca Calani, Iris Benzie, Siu Wai Choi, Furio Brighenti, Franca Zanardi, Claudio Curti, and Daniele Del Rio. 2017. "Synthetic and Analytical Strategies for the Quantification of Phenyl-γ-Valerolactone Conjugated Metabolites in Human Urine." *Molecular Nutrition and Food Research* 61 (9). https://doi.org/10.1002/mnfr.201700077.

Burke, A, and H Weiler. n.d. *"The Effect of Prostaglandin E 2 (PGE 2) and Long-Chain Polyunsaturated Fatty Acids (LC PUFA) on Bone Formation in Piglets: A Model for Bone Growth in Nutritional Investigation."* http://www.idealibrary.com.

Cao, Hui, Yixi Xie, and Xiaoqing Chen. 2015. "Type 2 Diabetes Diminishes the Benefits of Dietary Antioxidants: Evidence from the Different Free Radical Scavenging Potential." *Food Chemistry* 186 (November): 106–12. https://doi.org/10.1016/j.foodchem.2014.06.027.

Carbonell-Capella, Juana M., Magdalena Buniowska, Francisco J. Barba, María J. Esteve, and Ana Frígola. 2014. "Analytical Methods for Determining Bioavailability and Bioaccessibility of Bioactive Compounds from Fruits and Vegetables: A Review." *Comprehensive Reviews in Food Science and Food Safety* 13 (2): 155–71. https://doi.org/10.1111/1541-4337.12049.

Cardona, Fernando, Cristina Andrés-Lacueva, Sara Tulipani, Francisco J. Tinahones, and María Isabel Queipo-Ortuño. 2013. "Benefits of Polyphenols on Gut Microbiota and Implications in Human Health." *Journal of Nutritional Biochemistry*. https://doi.org/10.1016/j.jnutbio.2013.05.001.

Castello, Fabio, Giuseppina Costabile, Letizia Bresciani, Michele Tassotti, Daniele Naviglio, Delia Luongo, Paola Ciciola, et al. 2018. "Bioavailability and Pharmacokinetic Profile of Grape Pomace

Phenolic Compounds in Humans." *Archives of Biochemistry and Biophysics* 646 (May): 1–9. https://doi.org/10.1016/j.abb.2018.03.021.

Chedea, Veronica S., Camelia Echim, Cornelia Braicu, Mirjana Andjelkovic, Roland Verhe, and Carmen Socaciu. 2011. "Composition in Polyphenols and Stability of the Aqueous Grape Seed Extract from the Romanian Variety 'Merlot Recas.'" *Journal of Food Biochemistry* 35 (1): 92–108. https://doi.org/10.1111/j.1745-4514.2010.00368.x.

Chedea, Veronica Sanda, Cornelia Braicu, Flore Chirilă, Ciprian Ober, and Carmen Socaciu. 2011. "Antibacterial Action of an Aqueous Grape Seed Polyphenolic Extract." *African Journal of Biotechnology* 10 (33): 6276–80. http://www.academicjournals.org/AJB.

Chedea, Veronica Sanda, Cornelia Braicu, Flore Chirilə, Henry Joseph Oduor Ogola, Rodica Ştefania Pelmuş, Loredana Georgeta Cəlin, and Carmen Socaciu. 2014. "Antioxidant/Prooxidant and Antibacterial/Probacterial Effects of a Grape Seed Extract in Complex with Lipoxygenase." *BioMed Research International* 2014. https://doi.org/10.1155/2014/313684.

Chedea, Veronica Sanda, Cornelia Braicu, and Carmen Socaciu. 2010. "Antioxidant/Prooxidant Activity of a Polyphenolic Grape Seed Extract." *Food Chemistry* 121 (1): 132–39. https://doi.org/10.1016/j.foodchem.2009.12.020.

Chedea, Veronica Sanda, Lamis Choueiri, Mitsuo Jisaka, and Panagiotis Kefalas. 2012. "O-Quinone Involvement in the Prooxidant Tendency of a Mixture of Quercetin and Caffeic Acid." *Food Chemistry* 135 (3): 1999–2004. https://doi.org/10.1016/j.foodchem.2012.06.094.

Chedea, Veronica Sanda, Laurentiu Mihai Palade, Daniela Eliza Marin, Rodica Stefania Pelmus, Mihaela Habeanu, Mircea Catalin Rotar, Mihail Alexandru Gras, Gina Cecilia Pistol, and Ionelia Taranu. 2018. "Intestinal Absorption and Antioxidant Activity of Grape Pomace Polyphenols." *Nutrients* 10 (5). https://doi.org/10.3390/nu10050588.

Chedea, Veronica Sanda, Laurentiu Mihai Palade, Rodica Stefania Pelmus, Catalin Dragomir, and Ionelia Taranu. 2019. "Red Grape Pomace Rich in Polyphenols Diet Increases the Antioxidant Status in Key Organs— Kidneys, Liver, and Spleen of Piglets." *Animals* 9 (4). https://doi.org/10.3390/ani9040149.

Chedea, Veronica Sanda, Rodica Stefania Pelmus, Cristina Lazar, Gina Cecilia Pistol, Loredana Georgeta Calin, Smaranda Mariana Toma, Catalin Dragomir, and Ionelia Taranu. 2017. "Effects of a Diet Containing Dried Grape Pomace on Blood Metabolites and Milk Composition of Dairy Cows." *Journal of the Science of Food and Agriculture* 97 (8): 2516–23. https://doi.org/10.1002/jsfa.8068.

Chedea, Veronica Sanda, and Raluca Maria Pop. 2016. "Procyanidins-Bioavailability and Metabolization." In *Procyanidins: Characterisation, Antioxidant Properties and Health Benefits*, edited by Veronica Sanda Chedea, 91–128. New York: Nova Scienca Publishers.

Chiou, Yi Shiou, Jia Ching Wu, Qingrong Huang, Fereidoon Shahidi, Ying Jan Wang, Chi Tang Ho, and Min Hsiung Pan. 2014. "Metabolic and Colonic Microbiota Transformation May Enhance the Bioactivities of Dietary Polyphenols." *Journal of Functional Foods* 7 (1): 3–25. https://doi.org/10.1016/j.jff.2013.08.006.

Choueiri, Lamis, Veronica Sanda Chedea, Antony Calokerinos, and Panagiotis Kefalas. 2012. "Antioxidant/pro-Oxidant Properties of Model Phenolic Compounds. Part II: Studies on Mixtures of Polyphenols at Different Molar Ratios by Chemiluminescence and LC-MS." *Food Chemistry* 133 (3): 1039–44. https://doi.org/10.1016/j.foodchem.2012.01.057.

Clifford, Michael N., Indu B. Jaganath, Iziar A. Ludwig, and Alan Crozier. 2017. "Chlorogenic Acids and the Acyl-Quinic Acids: Discovery, Biosynthesis, Bioavailability and Bioactivity." *Natural Product Reports*. Royal Society of Chemistry. https://doi.org/10.1039/c7np00030h.

Crozier, Alan, Indu B. Jaganath, and Michael N. Clifford. 2009. "Dietary Phenolics: Chemistry, Bioavailability and Effects on Health."

*Natural Product Reports* 26 (8): 1001–43. https://doi.org/10.1039/b802662a.

Cueva, Carolina, Irene Gil-Sánchez, Begoña Ayuda-Durán, Susana González-Manzano, Ana María González-Paramás, Celestino Santos-Buelga, Begoña Bartolomé, and M. Victoria Moreno-Arribas. 2017. "An Integrated View of the Effects of Wine Polyphenols and Their Relevant Metabolites on Gut and Host Health." *Molecules*. MDPI AG. https://doi.org/10.3390/molecules22010099.

Cummings, J H, H S Wiggins, D J A Jenkins, Helen Houston, T Jivraj, B S Drasar, and M J Hill. n.d. *"Influence of Diets High and Low in Animal Fat on Bowel Habit, Gastrointestinal Transit Time, Fecal Microflora, Bile Acid, and Fat Excretion."*

Davis, S. S., L. Illum, and M. Hinchcliffe. 2001. "Gastrointestinal Transit of Dosage Forms in the Pig." *Journal of Pharmacy and Pharmacology* 53 (1): 33–39. https://doi.org/10.1211/0022357011775163.

Day, Andrea J., Jennifer M. Gee, M. Susan DuPont, Ian T. Johnson, and Gary Williamson. 2003. "Absorption of Quercetin-3-Glucoside and Quercetin-4′-Glucoside in the Rat Small Intestine: The Role of Lactase Phlorizin Hydrolase and the Sodium-Dependent Glucose Transporter." *Biochemical Pharmacology* 65 (7): 1199–1206. https://doi.org/10.1016/S0006-2952(03)00039-X.

Domínguez-Avila, J. Abraham, Abraham Wall-Medrano, Gustavo R. Velderrain-Rodríguez, C. Y.Oliver Chen, Norma Julieta Salazar-López, Maribel Robles-Sánchez, and Gustavo A. González-Aguilar. 2017. "Gastrointestinal Interactions, Absorption, Splanchnic Metabolism and Pharmacokinetics of Orally Ingested Phenolic Compounds." In *Food and Function*, 8:15–38. Royal Society of Chemistry. https://doi.org/10.1039/c6fo01475e.

Donovan, Jennifer L, Vanessa Crespy, Claudine Manach, Christine Morand, Catherine Besson, Augustin Scalbert, Christian Ré, and Mé Sy. 2001. "Nutrient Metabolism Catechin Is Metabolized by Both the Small Intestine and Liver of Rats." *J. Nutr.* Vol. 131. https://academic.oup.com/jn/article-abstract/131/6/1753/4686825.

Eran Nagar, Eden, Zoya Okun, and Avi Shpigelman. 2020. "Digestive Fate of Polyphenols: Updated View of the Influence of Chemical Structure and the Presence of Cell Wall Material." *Current Opinion in Food Science*. Elsevier Ltd. https://doi.org/10.1016/j.cofs.2019.10.009.

Ferrars, R. M. De, C. Czank, Q. Zhang, N. P. Botting, P. A. Kroon, A. Cassidy, and C. D. Kay. 2014. "The Pharmacokinetics of Anthocyanins and Their Metabolites in Humans." *British Journal of Pharmacology* 171 (13): 3268–82. https://doi.org/10.1111/bph.12676.

Forester, Sarah C., and Andrew L. Waterhouse. 2010. "Gut Metabolites of Anthocyanins, Gallic Acid, 3-O-Methylgallic Acid, and 2,4,6-Trihydroxybenzaldehyde, Inhibit Cell Proliferation of Caco-2 Cells." *Journal of Agricultural and Food Chemistry* 58 (9): 5320–27. https://doi.org/10.1021/jf9040172.

García-Lomillo, Javier, and María Luisa González-SanJosé. 2017. "Applications of Wine Pomace in the Food Industry: Approaches and Functions." *Comprehensive Reviews in Food Science and Food Safety* 16 (1): 3–22. https://doi.org/10.1111/1541-4337.12238.

Gerardi, Gisela, Mónica Cavia-Saiz, M. Dolores Rivero-Pérez, María Luisa González-Sanjosé, and Pilar Muñiz. 2020. "The Dose-Response Effect on Polyphenol Bioavailability after Intake of White and Red Wine Pomace Products by Wistar Rats." *Food and Function* 11 (2): 1661–71. https://doi.org/10.1039/c9fo01743g.

Gomes, Trilícia Margarida, Isabela Maia Toaldo, Isabel Cristina da Silva Haas, Vívian Maria Burin, Vinicius Caliari, Aderval S. Luna, Jefferson Santos de Gois, and Marilde T. Bordignon-Luiz. 2019. "Differential Contribution of Grape Peel, Pulp, and Seed to Bioaccessibility of Micronutrients and Major Polyphenolic Compounds of Red and White Grapes through Simulated Human Digestion." *Journal of Functional Foods* 52 (January): 699–708. https://doi.org/10.1016/j.jff.2018.11.051.

González-Barrio, Rocío, Gina Borges, William Mullen, and Alan Crozier. 2010. "Bioavailability of Anthocyanins and Ellagitannins

Following Consumption of Raspberries by Healthy Humans and Subjects with an Ileostomy." *Journal of Agricultural and Food Chemistry* 58 (7): 3933–39. https://doi.org/10.1021/jf100315d.

Griffin, Laura E., Katherine A. Witrick, Courtney Klotz, Melanie R. Dorenkott, Katheryn M. Goodrich, Gabrielle Fundaro, Ryan P. McMillan, Matthew W. Hulver, Monica A. Ponder, and Andrew P. Neilson. 2017. "Alterations to Metabolically Active Bacteria in the Mucosa of the Small Intestine Predict Anti-Obesity and Anti-Diabetic Activities of Grape Seed Extract in Mice." *Food and Function* 8 (10): 3510–22. https://doi.org/10.1039/c7fo01236e.

Guendez, Ramila, Stamatina Kallithraka, Dimitris P Makris, and Panagiotis Kefalas. 2005. "An Analytical Survey of the Polyphenols of Seeds of Varieties of Grape (Vitis Vinifera) Cultivated in Greece: Implications for Exploitation as a Source of Value-Added Phytochemicals." *Phytochem. Anal* 16: 17–23. https://doi.org/10.1002.pca.804.

Guilloteau, Paul, Romuald Zabielski, Harald M. Hammon, and Cornelia C. Metges. 2010. "Nutritional Programming of Gastrointestinal Tract Development. Is the Pig a Good Model for Man?" *Nutrition Research Reviews* 23 (1): 4–22. https://doi.org/10.1017/S0954422410000077.

Halake, Kantappa, Mallinath Birajdar, and Jonghwi Lee. 2016. "Structural Implications of Polyphenolic Antioxidants." *Journal of Industrial and Engineering Chemistry*. Korean Society of Industrial Engineering Chemistry. https://doi.org/10.1016/j.jiec.2016.01.003.

Haminiuk, Charles W.I., Giselle M. Maciel, Manuel S.V. Plata-Oviedo, and Rosane M. Peralta. 2012. "Phenolic Compounds in Fruits - an Overview." *International Journal of Food Science and Technology*. https://doi.org/10.1111/j.1365-2621.2012.03067.x.

Ignea, Codruta, Cristina Mihaela Dorobantu, Christopher Paul Mintoff, Norica Branza-Nichita, Michael R. Ladomery, Panagiotis Kefalas, and Veronica Sanda Chedea. 2013. "Modulation of the Antioxidant/pro-Oxidant Balance, Cytotoxicity and Antiviral Actions of Grape Seed Extracts." *Food Chemistry* 141 (4): 3967–76. https://doi.org/10.1016/j.foodchem.2013.06.094.

Inhis2, Sheila M. n.d. *The Colostrum-Deprived Piglet as a Model for Study of Infant Lipid Nutrition 1.* https://academic.oup.com/jn/article-abstract/123/suppl_2/386/4723796.

Kuhnle, Gunter, Jeremy P.E. Spencer, Hagen Schroeter, Baskar Shenoy, Edward S. Debnam, S. Kaila S. Srai, Catherine Rice-Evans, and Ulrich Hahn. 2000. "Epicatechin and Catechin Are O-Methylated and Glucuronidated in the Small Intestine." *Biochemical and Biophysical Research Communications* 277 (2): 507–12. https://doi.org/10.1006/bbrc.2000.3701.

Ky, Isabelle, Bénédicte Lorrain, Natallia Kolbas, Alan Crozier, and Pierre Louis Teissedre. 2014. "Wine By-Products: Phenolic Characterization and Antioxidant Activity Evaluation of Grapes and Grape Pomaces from Six Different French Grape Varieties." *Molecules* 19 (1): 482–506. https://doi.org/10.3390/molecules 19010482.

Langerholc, Tomaz, Petros A. Maragkoudakis, Jan Wollgast, Lidija Gradisnik, and Avrelija Cencic. 2011. "Novel and Established Intestinal Cell Line Models - An Indispensable Tool in Food Science and Nutrition." *Trends in Food Science and Technology*. https://doi.org/10.1016/j.tifs.2011.03.010.

Llorach, Rafael, Ignacio Garrido, María Monagas, Mireia Urpi-Sarda, Sara Tulipani, Begoña Bartolome, and Cristina Andres-Lacueva. 2010. "Metabolomics Study of Human Urinary Metabolome Modifications after Intake of Almond (Prunus Dulcis (Mill.) D.A. Webb) Skin Polyphenols." *Journal of Proteome Research* 9 (11): 5859–67. https://doi.org/10.1021/pr100639v.

Luca, Simon Vlad, Irina Macovei, Alexandra Bujor, Anca Miron, Krystyna Skalicka-Woźniak, Ana Clara Aprotosoaie, and Adriana Trifan. 2020. "Bioactivity of Dietary Polyphenols: The Role of Metabolites." *Critical Reviews in Food Science and Nutrition*. Taylor and Francis Inc. https://doi.org/10.1080/10408398.2018.1546669.

Lucas-González, Raquel, Manuel Viuda-Martos, José Angel Pérez-Alvarez, and Juana Fernández-López. 2018. "In Vitro Digestion Models Suitable for Foods: Opportunities for New Fields of Application and Challenges." *Food Research International*. Elsevier Ltd. https://doi.org/10.1016/j.foodres.2018.02.055.

Ludwig, Iziar A., Pedro Mena, Luca Calani, Gina Borges, Gema Pereira-Caro, Letizia Bresciani, Daniele Del Rio, Michael E.J. Lean, and Alan Crozier. 2015. "New Insights into the Bioavailability of Red Raspberry Anthocyanins and Ellagitannins." *Free Radical Biology and Medicine* 89 (December): 758–69. https://doi.org/10.1016/j.freeradbiomed.2015.10.400.

Lunney, Joan K. 2007. "Advances in Swine Biomedical Model Genomics." *Int. J. Biol. Sci* 3 (3): 179–84. www.biolsci.org.

Manach, Claudine, Dragan Milenkovic, Tom Van de Wiele, Ana Rodriguez-Mateos, Baukje de Roos, Maria Teresa Garcia-Conesa, Rikard Landberg, et al. 2017. "Addressing the Inter-Individual Variation in Response to Consumption of Plant Food Bioactives: Towards a Better Understanding of Their Role in Healthy Aging and Cardiometabolic Risk Reduction." *Molecular Nutrition and Food Research*. Wiley-VCH Verlag. https://doi.org/10.1002/mnfr.201600557.

Manach, Claudine, Augustin Scalbert, Christine Morand, Christian Rémésy, and Liliana Jiménez. 2004. "Polyphenols: Food Sources and Bioavailability 1,2." *Am J Clin Nutr*. Vol. 79. https://academic.oup.com/ajcn/article-abstract/79/5/727/4690182.

Martin-Carron, N., A. Garcia-Alonso, I. Goñi, and F. Saura-Calixto. 1997. "Nutritional and Physiological Properties of Grape Pomace as a Potential Food Ingredient." *American Journal of Enology and Viticulture* 48 (3): 328–32. https://www.ajevonline.org/content/48/3/328.

Martinez-Gonzalez, Alejandra I., Ángel G. Díaz-Sánchez, Laura A. De La Rosa, Claudia L. Vargas-Requena, Ismael Bustos-Jaimes, and Emilio Alvarez-Parrilla. 2017. "Polyphenolic Compounds and

Digestive Enzymes: In Vitro Non-Covalent Interactions." *Molecules*. MDPI AG. https://doi.org/10.3390/molecules22040669.

Morand, Christine, Baukje De Roos, Maria Teresa Garcia-Conesa, Eileen R. Gibney, Rikard Landberg, Claudine Manach, Dragan Milenkovic, Ana Rodriguez-Mateos, Tom Van de Wiele, and Francisco Tomas-Barberan. 2020. "Why Interindividual Variation in Response to Consumption of Plant Food Bioactives Matters for Future Personalised Nutrition." *Proceedings of the Nutrition Society* 79 (2): 225–35. https://doi.org/10.1017/S0029665120000014.

Mosele, Juana I., Alba Macià, and Maria José Motilva. 2015. "Metabolic and Microbial Modulation of the Large Intestine Ecosystem by Non-Absorbed Diet Phenolic Compounds: A Review." *Molecules*. MDPI AG. https://doi.org/10.3390/molecules200917429.

Ottaviani, Javier I., Gina Borges, Tony Y. Momma, Jeremy P.E. Spencer, Carl L. Keen, Alan Crozier, and Hagen Schroeter. 2016. "The Metabolome of [2-14C](-)-Epicatechin in Humans: Implications for the Assessment of Efficacy, Safety, and Mechanisms of Action of Polyphenolic Bioactives." *Scientific Reports* 6 (July). https://doi.org/10.1038/srep29034.

Oz, Helieh S., Theresa Chen, and Willem J.S. de Villiers. 2013. "Green Tea Polyphenols and Sulfasalazine Have Parallel Anti-Inflammatory Properties in Colitis Models." *Frontiers in Immunology* 4 (JUN). https://doi.org/10.3389/fimmu.2013.00132.

Ozdal, Tugba, David A. Sela, Jianbo Xiao, Dilek Boyacioglu, Fang Chen, and Esra Capanoglu. 2016. "The Reciprocal Interactions between Polyphenols and Gut Microbiota and Effects on Bioaccessibility." *Nutrients*. MDPI AG. https://doi.org/10.3390/nu8020078.

Packer, L, G Rimbach, and F Virgili. 1999. "Antioxidant activity and biologic properties of a procyanidin-rich extract from pine (Pinus maritima) bark, pycnogenol." *Free Radical Biology and Medicine* 27, (5-6): 704-724.

Pino-García, Raquel Del, María D. Rivero-Pérez, María L. González-SanJosé, Kevin D. Croft, and Pilar Muñiz. 2016. "Bioavailability of Phenolic Compounds and Antioxidant Effects of Wine Pomace

Seasoning after Oral Administration in Rats." *Journal of Functional Foods* 25 (August): 486–96. https://doi.org/10.1016/j.jff.2016.06.030.

Rasines-Perea, Zuriñe, Isabelle Ky, Gérard Cros, Alan Crozier, and Pierre-Louis Teissedre. 2018. "Grape Pomace: Antioxidant Activity, Potential Effect Against Hypertension and Metabolitcs Characterization after Intake." *Diseases* 6 (3): 60. https://doi.org/10.3390/diseases6030060.

Rauw, W. M., O. Portolés, D. Corella, J. Soler, J. Reixach, J. Tibau, J. M. Prat, I. Diaz, and L. Gómez-Raya. 2007. "Behaviour Influences Cholesterol Plasma Levels in a Pig Model." *Animal* 1 (6): 865–71. https://doi.org/10.1017/S1751731107000018.

Rechner, Andreas R, Gunter Kuhnle, Paul Bremner, Gary P Hubbard, Kevin P Moore, and Catherine A Rice-Evans. 2002. "The metabolic fate of dietary polyphenols in humans." *Free Radical Biology and Medicine* 33, (2): 220-235.

Rio, Daniele Del, Ana Rodriguez-Mateos, Jeremy P.E. Spencer, Massimiliano Tognolini, Gina Borges, and Alan Crozier. 2013. "Dietary (Poly)Phenolics in Human Health: Structures, Bioavailability, and Evidence of Protective Effects against Chronic Diseases." *Antioxidants and Redox Signaling*. 18, (14): 1818-1892. https://doi.org/10.1089/ars.2012.4581.

Rodriguez-Mateos, Ana, Rodrigo P. Feliciano, Albert Boeres, Timon Weber, Claudia Nunes dos Santos, M. Rita Ventura, and Christian Heiss. 2016. "Cranberry (Poly)Phenol Metabolites Correlate with Improvements in Vascular Function: A Double-Blind, Randomized, Controlled, Dose-Response, Crossover Study." *Molecular Nutrition and Food Research* 60 (10): 2130–40. https://doi.org/10.1002/mnfr.201600250.

Rodriguez-Mateos, Ana, Raquel del Pino-García, Trevor W. George, Alberto Vidal-Diez, Christian Heiss, and Jeremy P.E. Spencer. 2014. "Impact of Processing on the Bioavailability and Vascular Effects of Blueberry (Poly)Phenols." *Molecular Nutrition and Food Research* 58 (10): 1952–61. https://doi.org/10.1002/mnfr.201400231.

Rodríguez-Ramiro, Ildefonso, Sonia Ramos, Elvira López-Oliva, Angel Agis-Torres, Laura Bravo, Luis Goya, and Maria Angeles Martín. 2013. "Cocoa Polyphenols Prevent Inflammation in the Colon of Azoxymethane-Treated Rats and in TNF-α-Stimulated Caco-2 Cells." *British Journal of Nutrition* 110 (2): 206–15. https://doi.org/10.1017/S0007114512004862.

Rzeppa, Sebastian, Katharina Bittner, Susanne Döll, Sven Dänicke, and Hans Ulrich Humpf. 2012. "Urinary Excretion and Metabolism of Procyanidins in Pigs." *Molecular Nutrition and Food Research* 56 (4): 653–65. https://doi.org/10.1002/mnfr.201100471.

Santhakumar, Abishek B., Maurizio Battino, and José M. Alvarez-Suarez. 2018. "Dietary Polyphenols: Structures, Bioavailability and Protective Effects against Atherosclerosis." *Food and Chemical Toxicology*. Elsevier Ltd. https://doi.org/10.1016/j.fct.2018.01.022.

Selma, María V., Juan C. Espín, and Francisco A. Tomás-Barberán. 2009. "Interaction between Phenolics and Gut Microbiota: Role in Human Health." *Journal of Agricultural and Food Chemistry*. https://doi.org/10.1021/jf902107d.

Serra, Aida, Alba MacIà, Maria Paz Romero, Neus Anglès, José Ramón Morelló, and Maria José Motilva. 2011. "Distribution of Procyanidins and Their Metabolites in Rat Plasma and Tissues after an Acute Intake of Hazelnut Extract." *Food and Function* 2 (9): 562–68. https://doi.org/10.1039/c1fo10083a.

Sies, Helmut. 2010. "Polyphenols and Health: Update and Perspectives." *Archives of Biochemistry and Biophysics*. https://doi.org/10.1016/j.abb.2010.04.006.

Soobrattee, M. A., V. S. Neergheen, A. Luximon-Ramma, O. I. Aruoma, and T. Bahorun. 2005. "Phenolics as Potential Antioxidant Therapeutic Agents: Mechanism and Actions." *Mutation Research - Fundamental and Molecular Mechanisms of Mutagenesis* 579 (1–2): 200–213. https://doi.org/10.1016/j.mrfmmm.2005.03.023.

Stevens, Jan F., and Claudia S. Maier. 2016. "The Chemistry of Gut Microbial Metabolism of Polyphenols." *Phytochemistry Reviews*. Springer Netherlands. https://doi.org/10.1007/s11101-016-9459-z.

Terra, Ximena, Anna Ardevol, Mayte Blay, Montserrat Pinent, and Josepa Salvadó. 2017. "Flavonoids as Protective Agents Against Diet-Induced Oxidative Damage at Gastrointestinal Tract." In *Gastrointestinal Tissue: Oxidative Stress and Dietary Antioxidants*, 327–38. Elsevier Inc. https://doi.org/10.1016/B978-0-12-805377-5.00026-6.

Torres, Josep Lluís, Begoña Varela, Maria Teresa García, Josep Carilla, Cecilia Matito, Josep J. Centelles, Marta Cascante, Xavier Sort, and Raül Bobet. 2002. "Valorization of Grape (Vitis Vinifera) Byproducts. Antioxidant and Biological Properties of Polyphenolic Fractions Differing in Procyanidin Composition and Flavonol Content." *Journal of Agricultural and Food Chemistry* 50 (26): 7548–55. https://doi.org/10.1021/jf025868i.

Tsang, Catherine, Cyril Auger, William Mullen, Aurélie Bornet, Jean-Max Rouanet, Alan Crozier, and Pierre-Louis Teissedre. 2005. "The Absorption, Metabolism and Excretion of Flavan-3-Ols and Procyanidins Following the Ingestion of a Grape Seed Extract by Rats." *British Journal of Nutrition* 94 (2): 170–81. https://doi.org/10.1079/bjn20051480.

Williamson, G. 2017. "The Role of Polyphenols in Modern Nutrition." *Nutrition Bulletin*. Blackwell Publishing Ltd. https://doi.org/10.1111/nbu.12278.

Williamson, Gary, and Michael N. Clifford. 2017. "Role of the Small Intestine, Colon and Microbiota in Determining the Metabolic Fate of Polyphenols." *Biochemical Pharmacology*. Elsevier Inc. https://doi.org/10.1016/j.bcp.2017.03.012.

Xia, En Qin, Gui Fang Deng, Ya Jun Guo, and Hua Bin Li. 2010. "Biological Activities of Polyphenols from Grapes." *International Journal of Molecular Sciences*. https://doi.org/10.3390/ijms11020622.

Xiao, Jianbo. 2018. "Stability of Dietary Polyphenols: It's Never Too Late to Mend?" *Food and Chemical Toxicology* 119 (September): 3–5. https://doi.org/10.1016/j.fct.2018.03.051.

Zhang, Hua, and Rong Tsao. 2016. "Dietary Polyphenols, Oxidative Stress and Antioxidant and Anti-Inflammatory Effects." *Current Opinion in Food Science*. Elsevier Ltd. https://doi.org/10.1016/j.cofs.2016.02.002.

In: Grape Pomace in Health …
Editor: Veronica Sanda Chedea
ISBN: 978-1-68507-409-8


*Chapter 4*

# GRAPE POMACE AND GUT MICROBIOTA: A HEALTHY RELATIONSHIP

***Maria Adriana Neag[1,*], Adrian Catinean[2], Cristian Craciun[1] and Anca Dana Buzoianu[1]***
[1]Department of Pharmacology, Toxicology and Clinical Pharmacology, University Iuliu Hatieganu, Cluj-Napoca, Romania
[2]Department of Internal Medicine, University Iuliu Hatieganu, Cluj-Napoca, Romania

## ABSTRACT

Over the last decade, there has been a significant increase in research on the impact of many nutraceuticals on the composition of the intestinal microbiota and its relationship to various pharmacological effects. Grape pomace (GP) is a nutraceutical agent, rich in phenolic compounds, obtained during the production of wine from skins, seeds, and stalks. Many studies have examined the effect of GP and its active compounds on the intestinal microbiota and found that they can modulate the intestinal microbiota and thus prevent or treat various diseases. However, further studies are needed to better understand the

[*] Corresponding Author's E-mail: maria.neag@umfcluj.ro.

complex relationship between GP, its pharmacological effects, and the microbiota.

## INTRODUCTION

In the last decade, there was an increased number of studies on the microbiota role in general health and disease (Tojo et al. 2014). The role of microbiota in many conditions has been highlighted, from gastrointestinal (irritable bowel syndrome, inflammatory bowel disease) (Catinean et al. 2019; Morgan et al. 2012), cardiovascular (atherosclerosis, heart failure) (Li and Tang 2017; Org, Mehrabian, and Lusis 2015; Luedde et al. 2017) and neurological disorders (epilepsy) (Y. Zhang et al. 2018; Peng et al. 2018) to even cancer (W. Chen et al. 2012; Fernández et al. 2018).

The intestinal microbiota is constantly changing, but at the same time, it has a relatively stable profile (Gordon et al. 2012). There is a balance between beneficial bacteria and those associated with a negative impact on the organism (H. Wang et al. 2018). Several factors influence the stability of the gut microbiota: diet (Pareek et al. 2019), stress (Foster, Rinaman, and Cryan 2017), lifestyle (Rampelli et al. 2016), antibiotic treatment (Becattini, Taur, and Pamer 2016), etc. Several studies have looked at whether certain effects of some drugs or nutraceuticals are the consequences of microbiota modulation. For example, Wu et al. demonstrated that metformin can modify the gut microbiota of naïve type 2 diabetic patients and this may contribute to its therapeutic effect (Wu et al. 2017).

In the last 10 years, increasing researches have been focused on the beneficial effect of grape pomace (GP) obtained during wine production (Goula, Thymiatis, and Kaderides 2016; Oliveira et al. 2013; Pintać et al. 2018; Mitre et al. 2019). This product is made up of skins, seeds, and stalks and is rich in phenolic compounds. GP belongs to the nutraceutical class of substances. Agents in this class (herbal products, nutritional supplements, etc.) have physiological benefits and protect against certain chronic diseases (Das et al. 2012). Many polyphenolic compounds are isolated from GP: phenolic acids such as gallic, ellagic, and caftaric acid, flavanols such as catechin, epicatechin (procyanidins - PACs), flavonols such as quercetin, kaempferol, resveratrol (Wittenauer et al. 2015; Jara-Palacios et al. 2015; Cires et al. 2017). The GP's active compounds are known for their beneficial effects: antioxidant, antitumoral, antibacterial, anti-inflammatory, or anti-aging (Yu and Ahmedna 2013). In this chapter, we review studies that highlight the effects of GP, as a result of gut microbiota changes.

## The Relationship among GP, Microbiota and Some Pharmacological Effects

*Firmicutes* and *Bacteroidetes* phyla are known to be the dominant species of the intestinal microbiota. The *Bacteroides / Firmicutes* ratio is changed in several conditions, being lower in obese subjects compared to lean people (Qin et al. 2010) and in patients with type 2 diabetes (Koliada et al. 2017). *Roseburia* and *Faecalibacterium prausnitzii*, bacterial species belonging to *Firmicutes* phylum, are reduced in type 2 diabetes (La Rosa et al. 2019; Hartstra et al. 2015). These are two important butyrate-producing bacteria. Butyrate, along with acetate and propionate, is one of the most important short-chain fatty-acids (SCFAs). Butyrate is taken up by enterocytes and is used as an important source of cellular energy (Hartstra et al. 2015).

As mentioned before, butyrate has a major role in the host's metabolism homeostasis. Its low concentration is correlated with metabolic syndrome and cardiovascular diseases. Gao et al. showed in an experimental study in mice that the administration of sodium butyrate increased the levels of p-AMPK and GLUT4 in adipose tissue (Gao et al. 2019). Activation of AMPK has a positive effect on glucose metabolism disorders and atherosclerosis (increases glucose absorption, hepatic glucose production, and mitochondrial activity) (Kim et al. 2016).

GLUT4 is part of the family of glucose transporting proteins expressed mainly in adipose and skeletal muscle tissue. This transporter is a critical element in glucose homeostasis. AMPK activation stimulates GLUT4 translocation in the plasma membrane and thus increases glucose absorption (Yamaguchi et al. 2005). Butyrate, acetate, and propionate can activate G protein-coupled receptors (GPR): GPR41 and GPR43. Although angiotensin II is the key effector of the renin-angiotensin-aldosterone system that causes the downregulation of GPR41 and GPR43, butyrate can inhibit these changes. Butyrate supplementation may also reduce oxidative stress in atherosclerotic lesions. Moreover, butyrate and acetate, by activating GPR, increase the bioavailability of nitric oxide (NO) and improve endothelial dysfunction (Robles-vera et al. 2020).

Seo and collab. showed that flavonoids in chardonnay grape seed flour decrease the negative effects of high-fat diets in obese mice (body weight, adipose tissue, lipid profile – plasma LDL concentration), most likely through changes in the intestinal microbiota. Flavonoid from GP supplementation of the diet stimulated the growth of *Enterococcus, Blautia*, and *Roseburia* and inhibited the growth of *Clostridium* and *Lactobacillus* species (K. H. Seo et al. 2017). Another experimental study in mice demonstrated the beneficial effect of GP on the recovery of the intestinal microbiota after antibiotic therapy. Antibiotics have a negative impact on the overall composition of the intestinal microbiota with a decrease in gram-positive bacteria and an increase in gram-negative bacteria. A cocktail of antibiotics with vancomycin, ampicillin, neomycin sulfate, and metronidazole was administered to mice for 7 days. In the antibiotic-only group, *Firmicutes, Bacteroidetes*, and *Actinobacteria* decreased and *Proteobacteria* increased. In the group treated with GP, the improvement of the taxonomic diversity of the intestinal microbiota was observed. A significant increase in *Akkermansia* was observed, and based on this growth, *Verrucomicrobia* also grew (*Akkermansia* belongs to *Verrucomicrobia*) (Lu et al. 2019).

*Akkermansia muciniphila* is a mucin-degrading agent, a species of bacteria in healthy human feces that is found in the outer mucosal layer.

This bacterium strengthens the intestinal barrier, participating in reducing the grade of inflammation and metabolic disorders (T. Zhang et al. 2019). Regarding this bacterium, a study showed that the administration of pasteurized *Akkermansia muciniphila* for 3 months reduced the activity of dipeptidyl peptidase 4 (DPP4), which had a positive impact on lipid and carbohydrate metabolism and decreased lipo-poly-saccharides (LPS) (Depommier et al. 2019). DPP4 is a widely distributed enzyme in the body. It can exist in two forms: bound to the membrane in different tissues or soluble in the bloodstream. As an enzymatic activity, DPP4 can inactivate incretin hormones such as glucagon-like peptide (GLP) 1 or GLP-2 (Liu et al. 2014; Fujiwara et al. 2015). GLP-1 stimulates insulin secretion in pancreatic B cells, and GLP-2 promotes the integrity of the mucosal and gut barrier. Roopchand et al. showed that grape polyphenols increase, on the one hand, the abundance of *Akkermansia muciniphila*, and on the other hand increase the proglucagon, the precursor GLP-1, and GLP-2, in the ileum tissue. So, most likely, polyphenols through GLP-1 and GLP-2 proteins improve glucose tolerance and decrease serum LPS (Roopchand et al. 2015).

Because GP extract is a nutraceutical with a role in maintaining the body's physiological functions, there have been researchers who studied the effects of GP on intestinal microbiota diversity and molecular and biochemical biomarkers in healthy volunteers. In a clinical study, Gil-Sanchez et al. observed the effects of GP extract administration for 21 days in healthy volunteers. The results showed a significant reduction in blood glucose, a significant increase in total SCFA, and insignificant differences in lipid metabolism parameters, liver transaminases (ALT, AST) and the composition of the intestinal microbiota, and the content of phenolic metabolites in faeces and urine (Gil-Sánchez et al. 2018). The absence of statistically significant differences can be explained by the short duration of therapy or by the absence of pathological changes. Subjects included in the study were healthy, without cardiovascular, gastrointestinal, or metabolic disorders.

Some studies with GP have also been done on healthy young animals. For example, one category of animals on which GP effects were studied was young lambs. The 15-day-old animals were divided into two groups: the first group received the standard diet and the second group the standard diet supplemented with GP for 27 days. Blood, faecal, and tissue samples were taken at different ages: 15 days (before the start of the experiment), 42 days, or 70 days. Overall, GP had an antioxidant effect and lipid peroxidation and protein oxidation were inhibited. A particularity of this study was the evolution of the GSH level. This parameter increased in the spleen and quadriceps in the GP group in 70-day-old animals but decreased in liver tissue compared to the control group. But the GSH level at 42 days was more than 2 times higher than in the other tissues (Kafantaris et al. 2017). It may be because high levels of GSH can inhibit its synthesis by inhibiting the activity of γ-glutamate-cysteine ligase (GCL), a major enzyme that interferes with GSH synthesis (Figure 1). This feedback mechanism may explain the reduction in GSH levels after the previous increase (Z. H. Chen et al. 2008). Similar results were observed at GSH levels in piglets treated with GP-enriched feed. In the study on piglets, GSH decreased in the spleen and stomach 50 days after birth, compared to the control group (Kafantaris et al. 2018).

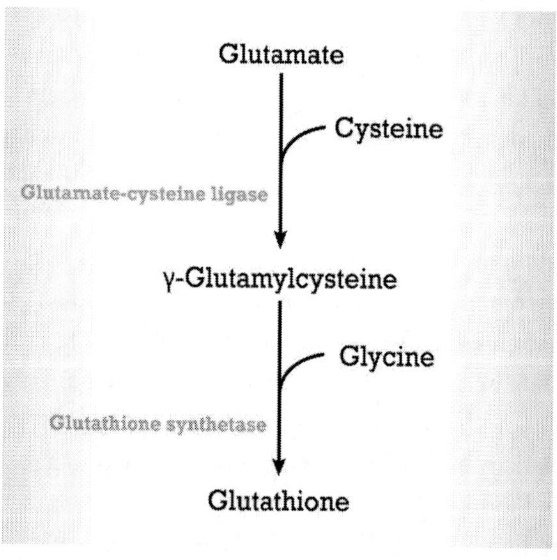


Figure 1. Glutathione synthesis pathway.

Regarding the microbiota, the administration of GP in young lambs promoted intestinal health by decreasing *Enterobacteriaceae* (especially *E. coli*) and increasing *Bifidobacterium* at 40 and 65 days. These effects on the microbiota could be explained by the presence of compounds such as polysaccharides, fructans (the polymer of fructose molecule), or polyphenols in GP (Kafantaris et al. 2017). The same microbiota changes were observed after the administration of GP to piglets: the population of Enterobacteriaceae decreased and the level of Bifidobacteria increased (Kafantaris et al. 2018). GP feed supplementation has also been studied in dairy calves. It was observed that the quantity of *Ruminiclostridium* and *Eubacterium* was increased in the rumen of GP supplementation calves (Biscarini et al. 2018).

## THE ACTIVE COMPOUNDS OF GP AND THEIR EFFECTS

*PACs* (proanthocyanidins) are known as condensed tannins and are flavan-3ol monomers. The degree of polymerization of the PACs influences their bioavailability. The monomers are absorbed in the small intestine, while the polymeric forms reach the colon and are transformed by the colonic bacteria into active metabolites (Cueva et al. 2013). However, it is important to note that, there is a two ways relationship between the PACs and the microbiota:

1. PACs have a prebiotic effect and cause the growth of *Lactobacillus spp* and *Bifidobacterium spp* or other bacteria have the ability to produce butyrate in the colon (Tzounis et al. 2011);
2. PACs could be metabolized into metabolites, such as aromatic acids or valerolactones, under the action of the intestinal microbiota and may have local (on the colonic epithelium) or systemic (extraintestinal tissue) effects. The effects are possible because some of the metabolites remain in the colon and others, due to their low molecular weight, can be absorbed into the

bloodstream (Appeldoorn et al. 2009). The effects of PACs are presented in Table 1.

**Table 1. Effects and mechanisms of PACs**

| **Sources of PACs** | **Effects of PACs** | **Mechanisms/ explications** | **References** |
|---|---|---|---|
| The fruit pulp of *Clausena lansium* (Lour.) | - strong inhibition of α-glucosidase activity | - numerous OH groups on (epi)gallocatechin rings | (Ou-Yang et al. 2020) |
| Grapeseed | - protected against nephrotoxicity induced by iron overload in rats<br>- reduced the level of iron in the blood and kidneys<br>- inhibited renal apoptosis | - increase in antioxidant mechanisms (decrease in glutathione peroxidase -GSH-Px, total antioxidant activity - T-AOC)<br>- down regulated the Fas and Bax genes | (Yun et al. 2020) |
| | - anti-arthritis effects on collagen-induced arthritis in mice | - reduction of cells that secrete proinflammatory cytokines (CD4 +, CD25 +)<br>- determined the upregulation of Foxp3 expression and decreasing of Il-1β, IL-6, TNF-α. | (Ahmad et al. 2013) |
| | - inhibited osteoclast formation and differentiation | - suppressed the NF-kB and JNK signaling pathway | (Zhu et al. 2019) |
| *Uncaria rhynchophylla* | - reduced viability and migration capacity of MDA-MB-231 breast cancer cell<br>- induced apoptosis<br>- synergistic cytotoxic effects with 5-FU on cells<br>The effects are dose-dependent. | - increased production of reactive oxygen species<br>- decreased mitochondrial membrane potential<br>- increased Bax/Bcl-2 ratio<br>- increased cleaved caspase-3 expression | (X. X. Chen, Leung, et al. 2017) |
| *Ficus virens* | | | (X. X. Chen, Lam, et al. 2017) |
| *Vaccinium macrocarpon* | - beneficial effect against diarrheagenic Escherichia coli<br>- antibacterial efficacy against Gram-negative diarrheagenic E. coli, enteropathogenic and enterotoxigenic strain | - inhibited the count of viable cell strains<br>- increased permeability of the outer membrane of enteropathogenic and enterotoxigenic strain | (Alshaibani, Zhang, and Wu 2017) |

**Table 2. Effects and mechanisms of quercetin**

| Effects of quercetin | Mechanisms/explications | References |
|---|---|---|
| - decreased liver fibrosis<br>- decreased liver cell apoptosis | - decreased the activation of nuclear NF-κB<br>- increased the expression of cytosolic NF-κB and IκBα<br>- inhibited the expression of p38 MAPK and p-p38 MAPK<br>- inhibited caspase-3 activation<br>- down-regulated Bax<br>- up-regulated Bcl-2 | (R. Wang et al. 2017) |
| - low dose – beneficial effect against the reproductive toxicity induced by Atrazine in adult male Albino rats | - relieved oxidative stress (increased TAC, reduced MDA)<br>- increased CYP17A1 mRNA expression | (Abdel Aziz et al. 2018) |
| - increased the hypotensive effect of bradykinin<br>- reduced the increase of blood pressure induced by angiotensin I in rats | - inhibited the angiotensin converting enzyme<br>- decreased bradykinin metabolism | (Häckl et al. 2002) |
| - improved endothelial function in spontaneously hypertensive rats | - increased NO bioactivity<br>- increased eNOS activity<br>- reduced activity of NADPH oxidase. | (Sánchez et al. 2006) |
| - inhibited lipid accumulation<br>- inhibited obesity-induced inflammation (in the cell and animal)<br>- improved insulin sensitivity | - inhibited MAPK signal expression<br>- suppressed activation of AP-1 and NF-κB in macrophages | (M. J. Seo et al. 2015) |
| - ameliorated DSS-induced colitis in mice | - decreased MPO, MDA and NO concentration, increased after the administration of DSS<br>- decreased the reduction of *Firmicutes* population and also the increasing of *Proteobacteria* | (Hong and Piao 2018) |

Another important active compound of the grape pomace is *quercetin.* The major glycosylated form of quercetin is rutin (quercetin-3-rhamno glucoside) (Carbonaro and Grant 2005). Several strains of intestinal bacteria (*Escherichia coli, Lactobacillus acidophilus, Clostridium perfringens, Bacteroides fragilis*) from human feces can degrade quercetin into other active/inactive compounds, but their ability to transform quercetin is different. *Clostridium perfringens* and *Bacteroides fragilis* have the highest quercetin metabolism capacity (Zhang et al. 2014). The pharmacological activity of quercetin metabolites has been studied in many pieces of research. Among the metabolites (3-hydroxyphenylacetic acid, 3,4 -dihydroxybenzoic acid, hippuric acid, benzoic acid), 3-hydroxyphenylacetic acid, 3,4 -dihydroxybenzoic acid have been the most studied and were demonstrated several effects. For example, 3,4 -dihydroxybenzoic acid metabolite decreased acetaminophen-induced hepatotoxicity and increased antioxidant capacity by increasing Nrf-2 translocation and increasing anti-oxidant enzymes or those involved in phase II of metabolism (Xue et al. 2016). Some effects of quercetin are shown in Table 2.

**Table 3. Relationship between resveratrol, microbiota and their pharmacological effects**

| Effects of resveratrol | Mechanism/ changes in microbiota composition | References |
|---|---|---|
| The effects were observed in high-fat diet (HFD)- fed mice treated with resveratrol:<br>- reduced the body weight gain<br>- reduced the liver oxidative stress<br>- decreased the liver inflammation<br>- decreased serum TG, TC, ALT, AST<br>- reversed fasting blood glucose and insulin levels<br>- improved gut permeability<br>- decreased plasma lipopolysaccharides | - increased mRNA expression of ZO-1 and occludin (tight junction proteins)<br>- increased junctional adhesion molecule A (JAM-A) in the ileum<br>- downregulated mRNA levels of goblet cell protein TFF3, the major mucin genes (Muc1 and Muc2)<br>- restored the *Bacteroidetes* population<br>- increased the abundance of *Allobaculum, Bacteroides*, and *Blautia*<br>- restored the *Desulfovibrio* population | (Wang et al. 2020) |
| - protected against atherosclerosis (ATS) (figure 2) | - decreased trimethylamine N-oxide (TMAO) - induced atherosclerosis<br>- increased *Bacteroidetes/Firmicutes* ratio<br>- increased *Lactobacillus, Bifidobacterium, and Akkermansia* population<br>- decreased trimethylamine (TMA) production<br>- decreased Trimethylamine N-oxide (TMAO) synthesis<br>- increased excretion of bile acid | (Chen et al. 2016) |
| - improved glucose homeostasis | - increased *Bacteroidetes/Firmicutes* ratio<br>- decreased the abundance of *Moryella* and *Akkermansia*<br>- increased *Bacteroides* and *Parabacteroides* population | (Sung et al. 2017) |

Along with PACs and quercetin, *resveratrol* is another active compound in GP. In the intestine, part of the resveratrol, under the action of the intestinal microbiota is metabolized and results in resveratrol metabolites. These compounds and free resveratrol are metabolized in the liver or intestine by glucuronidation and sulfation and result in circulating forms, conjugated metabolites. In the liver, resveratrol can be hydroxylated under the action of cytochrome P450 enzymes and results in piceatannol, a form that circulates in the bloodstream (Chaplin, Carpéné and Mercader 2018). The relationship between resveratrol, microbiota, and their pharmacological effects are presented in Table 3.

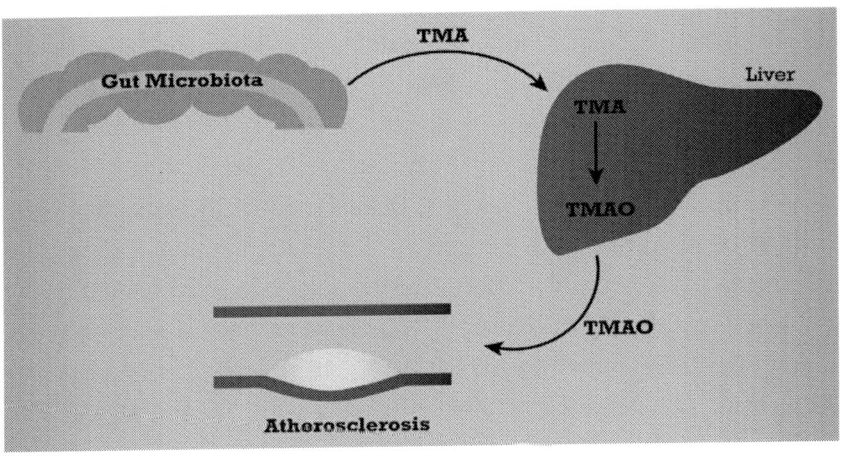


Figure 2. Gut microbiota influence on atherosclerosis (Abbreviations: TMA, trimethylamine; TMAO, Trimethylamine N-oxide).

## CONCLUSION

The microbiota is an important factor in maintaining the balance of host homeostasis. Some of the studies mentioned in this chapter have shown a close link between GP, its effects and the microbiota. GP and its active compounds could be considered as important and effective nutraceuticals in modulating the gut microbiota. However, further studies are needed to elucidate, from the mechanistic point of view, how modulation of the microbiota leads to certain beneficial effects. Human studies are also needed to establish the clear role of GP in the prevention and treatment of diseases.

## REFERENCES

Abdel Aziz, Rabie L., Ahmed Abdel-Wahab, Fatma I. Abo El-Ela, Nour El Houda Y. Hassan, El Shaymaa El-Nahass, Marwa A. Ibrahim, and Abdel Tawab A.Y. Khalil. 2018. "Dose-Dependent Ameliorative Effects of Quercetin and L-Carnitine against Atrazine- Induced Reproductive Toxicity in Adult Male Albino Rats." *Biomedicine and Pharmacotherapy* 102 (January): 855–64. https://doi.org/10.1016/j.biopha.2018.03.136.

Ahmad, Sheikh Fayaz, Khairy M.A. Zoheir, Hala E. Abdel-Hamied, Abdelkader E. Ashour, Saleh A. Bakheet, Sabry M. Attia, and Adel R.A. Abd-Allah. 2013. "Grape Seed Proanthocyanidin Extract Has Potent Anti-Arthritic Effects on Collagen-Induced Arthritis by Modifying the T Cell Balance." *International Immunopharmacology* 17 (1): 79–87. https://doi.org/10.1016/j.intimp.2013.05.026.

Alshaibani, Dhafer, Rong Zhang, and Vivian C.H. Wu. 2017. "Antibacterial Characteristics and Activity of Vaccinium Macrocarpon Proanthocyanidins against Diarrheagenic Escherichia Coli." *Journal of Functional Foods* 39: 133–38. https://doi.org/10.1016/j.jff.2017.10.003.

Appeldoorn, Maaike M., Jean Paul Vincken, Anna Marja Aura, Peter C.H. Hollman, and Harry Gruppen. 2009. "Procyanidin Dimers Are Metabolized by Human Microbiota with 2-(3,4-Dihydroxyphenyl)Acetic Acid and 5-(3,4-Dihydroxyphenyl)-γ-Valerolactone as the Major Metabolites." *Journal of Agricultural and Food Chemistry* 57 (3): 1084–92. https://doi.org/10.1021/jf803059z.

Becattini, Simone, Ying Taur, and Eric G. Pamer. 2016. "Antibiotic-Induced Changes in the Intestinal Microbiota and Disease." *Trends in Molecular Medicine* 22 (6): 458–78. https://doi.org/10.1016/j.molmed.2016.04.003.

Biscarini, Filippo, Fiorentina Palazzo, Federica Castellani, Giulia Masetti, Lisa Grotta, Angelo Cichelli, and Giuseppe Martino. 2018. "Rumen Microbiome in Dairy Calves Fed Copper and Grape-Pomace Dietary Supplementations: Composition and Predicted Functional Profile." *PLoS ONE* 13 (11): 1–20. https://doi.org/10.1371/journal.pone.0205670.

Carbonaro, Marina, and George Grant. 2005. "Absorption of Quercetin and Rutin in Rat Small Intestine." *Annals of Nutrition and Metabolism* 49 (3): 178–82. https://doi.org/10.1159/000086882.

Catinean, Adrian, Adriana Maria Neag, Andreea Nita, Mihaela Buzea, and Anca Dana Buzoianu. 2019. "*Bacillus* Spp. Spores-a Promising Treatment Option for Patients with Irritable Bowel Syndrome." *Nutrients* 11 (9): 1–10. https://doi.org/10.3390/nu11091968.

Chaplin, Alice, Christian Carpéné, and Josep Mercader. 2018. "Resveratrol, Metabolic Syndrome, and Gut Microbiota." *Nutrients* 10 (11): 1–29. https://doi.org/10.3390/nu10111651.

Chen, Ming-Liang, Long Yi, Yong Zhang, Xi Zhou, Li Ran, Jining Yang, Jun-dong Zhu, Qian-Yong Zhang, and Man-tian Mi. 2016. "Atherosclerosis by Regulating TMAO Synthesis and Bile Acid Metabolism via Remodeling of the Gut Microbiota." *MBio* 7 (2): 1–14. https://doi.org/10.1128/mBio.02210-15.Invited.

Chen, Weiguang, Fanlong Liu, Zongxin Ling, Xiaojuan Tong, and Charlie Xiang. 2012. "Human Intestinal Lumen and Mucosa-Associated Microbiota in Patients with Colorectal Cancer." *PLoS ONE* 7 (6). https://doi.org/10.1371/journal.pone.0039743.

Chen, Xiao Xin, Kar Ho Lam, Qing Xi Chen, George Pak Heng Leung, Sydney Chi Wai Tang, Stephen Cho Wing Sze, Jian Bo Xiao, et al. 2017. "Ficus Virens Proanthocyanidins Induced Apoptosis in Breast Cancer Cells Concomitantly Ameliorated 5-Fluorouracil Induced

Intestinal Mucositis in Rats." *Food and Chemical Toxicology* 110 (October): 49–61. https://doi.org/10.1016/j.fct.2017.10.017.

Chen, Xiao Xin, George Pak Heng Leung, Zhang Jin Zhang, Jian Bo Xiao, Li Xing Lao, Feng Feng, Judith Choi Wo Mak, Ying Wang, Stephen Cho Wing Sze, and Kalin Yan Bo Zhang. 2017. "Proanthocyanidins from Uncaria Rhynchophylla Induced Apoptosis in MDA-MB-231 Breast Cancer Cells While Enhancing Cytotoxic Effects of 5-Fluorouracil." *Food and Chemical Toxicology* 107: 248–60. https://doi.org/10.1016/j.fct.2017.07.012.

Chen, Zhi Hua, Yoshiro Saito, Yasukazu Yoshida, Noriko Noguchi, and Etsuo Niki. 2008. "Regulation of GCL Activity and Cellular Glutathione through Inhibition of ERK Phosphorylation." *BioFactors* 33 (1): 1–11. https://doi.org/10.1002/biof.5520330101.

Cueva, Carolina, Fernando Sánchez-Patán, María Monagas, Gemma E. Walton, Glenn R. Gibson, Pedro J. Martín-Álvarez, Begoña Bartolomé, and M. Victoria Moreno-Arribas. 2013. "In Vitro Fermentation of Grape Seed Flavan-3-Ol Fractions by Human Faecal Microbiota: Changes in Microbial Groups and Phenolic Metabolites." *FEMS Microbiology Ecology* 83 (3): 792–805. https://doi.org/10.1111/1574-6941.12037.

Das, Lipi, Eshani Bhaumik, Utpal Raychaudhuri, and Runu Chakraborty. 2012. "Role of Nutraceuticals in Human Health." *Journal of Food Science and Technology* 49 (2): 173–83. https://doi.org/10.1007/s13197-011-0269-4.

Depommier, Clara, Amandine Everard, Céline Druart, Hubert Plovier, Matthias Van Hul, Sara Vieira-Silva, Gwen Falony, et al. 2019. "Supplementation with Akkermansia Muciniphila in Overweight and Obese Human Volunteers: A Proof-of-Concept Exploratory Study." *Nature Medicine* 25 (7): 1096–1103. https://doi.org/10.1038/s41591-019-0495-2.

Fernández, Mariana F., Iris Reina-Pérez, Juan Manuel Astorga, Andrea Rodríguez-Carrillo, Julio Plaza-Díaz, and Luis Fontana. 2018. "Breast Cancer and Its Relationship with the Microbiota."

*International Journal of Environmental Research and Public Health* 15 (8): 1–20. https://doi.org/10.3390/ijerph15081747.

Foster, Jane A., Linda Rinaman, and John F. Cryan. 2017. "Stress & the Gut-Brain Axis: Regulation by the Microbiome." *Neurobiology of Stress* 7: 124–36. https://doi.org/10.1016/j.ynstr.2017.03.001.

Fujiwara, Kaori, Takuya Inoue, Naoki Yorifuji, Munetaka Iguchi, Taisuke Sakanaka, Ken Narabayashi, Kazuki Kakimoto, et al. 2015. "Combined Treatment with Dipeptidyl Peptidase 4 (DPP4) Inhibitor Sitagliptin and Elemental Diets Reduced Indomethacin-Induced Intestinal Injury in Rats via the Increase of Mucosal Glucagon-like Peptide-2 Concentration." *Journal of Clinical Biochemistry and Nutrition* 56 (2): 155–62. https://doi.org/10.3164/jcbn.14-111.

Gao, Feng, Yi Wei Lv, Jie Long, Jie Mei Chen, Jiu Ming He, Xiong Zhong Ruan, and Hai Bo Zhu. 2019. "Butyrate Improves the Metabolic Disorder and Gut Microbiome Dysbiosis in Mice Induced by a High-Fat Diet." *Frontiers in Pharmacology* 10 (September): 1–16. https://doi.org/10.3389/fphar.2019.01040.

Gil-Sánchez, Irene, Adelaida Esteban-Fernández, Dolores González de Llano, Marisa Sanz-Buenhombre, Alberto Guadarrana, Nuria Salazar, Miguel Gueimonde, et al. 2018. "Supplementation with Grape Pomace in Healthy Women: Changes in Biochemical Parameters, Gut Microbiota and Related Metabolic Biomarkers." *Journal of Functional Foods* 45 (March): 34–46. https://doi.org/10.1016/j.jff.2018.03.031.

Gordon, Jeffrey, T Yatsunenko, FE Rey, MJ Manary, I Trehan, MG Dominguez-Bello, M Contreras, et al. 2012. "F1000Prime Recommendations of Human Gut Microbiome Viewed across Age and Geography." *Nature* 486 (7402): 222–27. https://doi.org/10.1038/nature11053.Human.

Goula, Athanasia M., Konstantinos Thymiatis, and Kyriakos Kaderides. 2016. "Valorization of Grape Pomace: Drying Behavior and Ultrasound Extraction of Phenolics." *Food and Bioproducts Processing* 100: 132–44. https://doi.org/10.1016/j.fbp.2016.06.016.

Häckl, L. P.N., G. Cuttle, S. Sanches Dovichi, M. T. Lima-Landman, and M. Nicolau. 2002. “Inhibition of Angiotensin-Converting Enzyme by Quercetin Alters the Vascular Response to Bradykinin and Angiotensin I.” *Pharmacology* 65 (4): 182–86. https://doi.org/10.1159/000064341.

Hartstra, Annick V., Kristien E.C. Bouter, Fredrik Bäckhed, and Max Nieuwdorp. 2015. “Insights into the Role of the Microbiome in Obesity and Type 2 Diabetes.” *Diabetes Care* 38 (1): 159–65. https://doi.org/10.2337/dc14-0769.

Hong, Zhu, and Meiyu Piao. 2018. “Effect of Quercetin Monoglycosides on Oxidative Stress and Gut Microbiota Diversity in Mice with Dextran Sodium Sulphate-Induced Colitis.” *BioMed Research International* 2018. https://doi.org/10.1155/2018/8343052.

Kafantaris, I., B. Kotsampasi, V. Christodoulou, E. Kokka, P. Kouka, Z. Terzopoulou, K. Gerasopoulos, et al. 2017. “Grape Pomace Improves Antioxidant Capacity and Faecal Microflora of Lambs.” *Journal of Animal Physiology and Animal Nutrition* 101 (5): e108–21. https://doi.org/10.1111/jpn.12569.

Kafantaris, I., D. Stagos, B. Kotsampasi, A. Hatzis, A. Kypriotakis, K. Gerasopoulos, S. Makri, et al. 2018. “Grape Pomace Improves Performance, Antioxidant Status, Fecal Microbiota and Meat Quality of Piglets.” *Animal* 12 (2): 246–55. https://doi.org/10.1017/S1751731117001604.

Kim, Joungmok, Goowon Yang, Yeji Kim, Jin Kim, and Joohun Ha. 2016. “AMPK Activators: Mechanisms of Action and Physiological Activities.” *Experimental and Molecular Medicine* 48 (4): e224-12. https://doi.org/10.1038/emm.2016.16.

Koliada, Alexander, Ganna Syzenko, Vladislav Moseiko, Liudmyla Budovska, Kostiantyn Puchkov, Vyacheslav Perederiy, Yuriy Gavalko, et al. 2017. “Association between Body Mass Index and Firmicutes/Bacteroidetes Ratio in an Adult Ukrainian Population.” *BMC Microbiology* 17 (1): 4–9. https://doi.org/10.1186/s12 866-017-1027-1.

Li, Daniel Y., and W. H.Wilson Tang. 2017. "Gut Microbiota and Atherosclerosis." *Current Atherosclerosis Reports* 19 (10). https://doi.org/10.1007/s11883-017-0675-9.

Liu, Liehua, Bilal Omar, Piero Marchetti, and Bo Ahrén. 2014. "Dipeptidyl Peptidase-4 (DPP-4): Localization and Activity in Human and Rodent Islets." *Biochemical and Biophysical Research Communications* 453 (3): 398–404. https://doi.org/10.1016/j.bbrc.2014.09.096.

Lu, Feng, Fengjiao Liu, Qian Zhou, Xiaosong Hu, and Yan Zhang. 2019. "Effects of Grape Pomace and Seed Polyphenol Extracts on the Recovery of Gut Microbiota after Antibiotic Treatment in High-Fat Diet-Fed Mice." *Food Science and Nutrition* 7 (9): 2897–2906. https://doi.org/10.1002/fsn3.1141.

Luedde, Mark, Thorben Winkler, Femke Anouska Heinsen, Malte C. Rühlemann, Martina E. Spehlmann, Amer Bajrovic, Wolfgang Lieb, Andre Franke, Stephan J. Ott, and Norbert Frey. 2017. "Heart Failure Is Associated with Depletion of Core Intestinal Microbiota." *ESC Heart Failure* 4 (3): 282–90. https://doi.org/10.1002/ehf2.12155.

Mitre, Calin Iosif, Maria Adriana Neag, Andrei Otto Mitre, Vlad Morhan, Adrian Catinean, Emil Claudiu Botan, Carmen Stanca Melincovici, Dana Maria Muntean, and Anca Dana Buzoianu. 2019. "Paradoxical Effect of Grape Pomace Extract on Cisplatin-Induced Acute Kidney Injury in Rats." *Pharmaceutics* 11 (12): 1–12. https://doi.org/10.3390/pharmaceutics11120656.

Morgan, Xochitl C., Timothy L. Tickle, Harry Sokol, Dirk Gevers, Kathryn L. Devaney, Doyle V. Ward, Joshua A. Reyes, et al. 2012. "Dysfunction of the Intestinal Microbiome in Inflammatory Bowel Disease and Treatment." *Genome Biology* 13 (9). https://doi.org/10.1186/gb-2012-13-9-r79.

Oliveira, Daniela A., Ana Augusta Salvador, Artur Smânia, Elza F.A. Smânia, Marcelo Maraschin, and Sandra R.S. Ferreira. 2013. "Antimicrobial Activity and Composition Profile of Grape (Vitis Vinifera) Pomace Extracts Obtained by Supercritical Fluids." *Journal of Biotechnology* 164 (3): 423–32. https://doi.org/10.1016/j.jbiotec.2012.09.014.

Org, Elin, Margarete Mehrabian, and Aldons J. Lusis. 2015. "Unraveling the Environmental and Genetic Interactions in Atherosclerosis: Central Role of the Gut Microbiota." *Atherosclerosis* 241 (2): 387–99. https://doi.org/10.1016/j.atherosclerosis.2015.05.035.

Ou-Yang, Chong, Weiming Chai, Xiaohui Xu, Shuang Song, Qiming Wei, Qian Huang, and Zhengrong Zou. 2020. "Inhibitory Potential of Proanthocyanidins from the Fruit Pulp of Clausena Lansium (Lour.) Skeels against α-Glucosidase and Non-Enzymatic Glycation: Activity and Mechanism." *Process Biochemistry* 91 (December 2019): 364–73. https://doi.org/10.1016/j.procbio.2020.01.006.

Pareek, Siddhika, Takashi Kurakawa, Bhabatosh Das, Daisuke Motooka, Shuuichi Nakaya, Temsunaro Rongsen-Chandola, Nidhi Goyal, et al. 2019. "Comparison of Japanese and Indian Intestinal Microbiota Shows Diet-Dependent Interaction between Bacteria and Fungi." *Npj Biofilms and Microbiomes* 5 (1). https://doi.org/10.1038/s41522-019-0110-9.

Peng, Anjiao, Xiangmiao Qiu, Wanlin Lai, Wanling Li, Lin Zhang, Xi Zhu, Shixu He, Jianan Duan, and Lei Chen. 2018. "Altered Composition of the Gut Microbiome in Patients with Drug-Resistant Epilepsy." *Epilepsy Research* 147 (37): 102–7. https://doi.org/10.1016/j.eplepsyres.2018.09.013.

Pintać, Diandra, Tatjana Majkić, Ljilja Torović, Dejan Orčić, Ivana Beara, Nataša Simin, Neda Mimica–Dukić, and Marija Lesjak. 2018. "Solvent Selection for Efficient Extraction of Bioactive Compounds from Grape Pomace." *Industrial Crops and Products* 111 (March 2017): 379–90. https://doi.org/10.1016/j.indcrop.2017.10.038.

Qin, Junjie, Ruiqiang Li, Jeroen Raes, Manimozhiyan Arumugam, Kristoffer Solvsten Burgdorf, Chaysavanh Manichanh, Trine Nielsen, et al. 2010. "A Human Gut Microbial Gene Catalogue Established by Metagenomic Sequencing." *Nature* 464 (7285): 59–65. https://doi.org/10.1038/nature08821.

Rampelli, Simone, Marco Candela, Silvia Turroni, Elena Biagi, Maren Pflueger, Maike Wolters, Wolfgang Ahrens, and Patrizia Brigidi. 2016. "Microbiota and Lifestyle Interactions through the Lifespan." *Trends in Food Science and Technology* 57: 265–72. https://doi.org/10.1016/j.tifs.2016.03.003.

Robles-vera, Iñaki, Marta Toral, Néstor De Visitación, Nazaret Aguilera-sánchez, and Andrew Carley. 2020. "Protective Effects of Short-Chain Fatty Acids on Endothelial Dysfunction Induced by Angiotensin II" 11 (April). https://doi.org/10.3389/fphys.2020.00277.

Roopchand, Diana E., Rachel N. Carmody, Peter Kuhn, Kristin Moskal, Patricio Rojas-Silva, Peter J. Turnbaugh, and Ilya Raskin. 2015. "Dietary Polyphenols Promote Growth of the Gut Bacterium Akkermansia muciniphila and Attenuate High-Fat Diet-Induced Metabolic Syndrome." *Diabetes* 64 (8): 2847–58. https://doi.org/10.2337/db14-1916.

Rosa, Sabina Leanti La, Maria Louise Leth, Leszek Michalak, Morten Ejby Hansen, Nicholas A. Pudlo, Robert Glowacki, Gabriel Pereira, et al. 2019. "The Human Gut Firmicute Roseburia Intestinalis Is a Primary Degrader of Dietary β-Mannans." *Nature Communications* 10 (1): 1–14. https://doi.org/10.1038/s41467-019-08812-y.

Sánchez, Manuel, Milagros Galisteo, Rocío Vera, Inmaculada C. Villar, Antonio Zarzuelo, Juan Tamargo, Francisco Pérez-Vizcaíno, and Juan Duarte. 2006. "Quercetin Downregulates NADPH Oxidase, Increases ENOS Activity and Prevents Endothelial Dysfunction in Spontaneously Hypertensive Rats." *Journal of Hypertension* 24 (1): 75–84. https://doi.org/10.1097/01.hjh.0000198029.22472.d9.

Seo, Kun Ho, Dong Hyeon Kim, Dana Jeong, Wallace Yokoyama, and Hyunsook Kim. 2017. "Chardonnay Grape Seed Flour Supplemented Diets Alter Intestinal Microbiota in Diet-Induced Obese Mice." *Journal of Food Biochemistry* 41 (5): 1–9. https://doi.org/10.1111/jfbc.12396.

Seo, Min Jung, Yeon Joo Lee, Ji Hyun Hwang, Kui Jin Kim, and Boo Yong Lee. 2015. "The Inhibitory Effects of Quercetin on Obesity and Obesity-Induced Inflammation by Regulation of MAPK Signaling."

*Journal of Nutritional Biochemistry* 26 (11): 1308–16. https://doi.org/10.1016/j.jnutbio.2015.06.005.

Sung, Miranda M., Ty T. Kim, Emmanuel Denou, Carrie Lynn M. Soltys, Shereen M. Hamza, Nikole J. Byrne, Grant Masson, et al. 2017. "Improved Glucose Homeostasis in Obese Mice Treated with Resveratrol Is Associated with Alterations in the Gut Microbiome." *Diabetes* 66 (2): 418–25. https://doi.org/10.2337/db16-0680.

Tojo, Rafael, Adolfo Suárez, Marta G. Clemente, Clara G. De Los Reyes-Gavilán, Abelardo Margolles, Miguel Gueimonde, and Patricia Ruas-Madiedo. 2014. "Intestinal Microbiota in Health and Disease: Role of Bifidobacteria in Gut Homeostasis." *World Journal of Gastroenterology* 20 (41): 15163–76. https://doi.org/10.3748/wjg.v20.i41.15163.

Tzounis, Xenofon, Ana Rodriguez-Mateos, Jelena Vulevic, Glenn R. Gibson, Catherine Kwik-Uribe, and Jeremy P.E. Spencer. 2011. "Prebiotic Evaluation of Cocoa-Derived Flavanols in Healthy Humans by Using a Randomized, Controlled, Double-Blind, Crossover Intervention Study." *American Journal of Clinical Nutrition* 93 (1): 62–72. https://doi.org/10.3945/ajcn.110.000075.

Wang, Hao, Chuan Xian Wei, Lu Min, and Ling Yun Zhu. 2018. "Good or Bad: Gut Bacteria in Human Health and Diseases." *Biotechnology and Biotechnological Equipment* 32 (5): 1075–80. https://doi.org/10.1080/13102818.2018.1481350.

Wang, Pan, Jing Wang, Daotong Li, Weixin Ke, Fang Chen, and Xiaosong Hu. 2020. "Targeting the Gut Microbiota with Resveratrol: A Demonstration of Novel Evidence for the Management of Hepatic Steatosis." *The Journal of Nutritional Biochemistry*, 108363. https://doi.org/10.1016/j.jnutbio.2020.108363.

Wang, Rong, Hai Zhang, Yuanyuan Wang, Fuxing Song, and Yongfang Yuan. 2017. "Inhibitory Effects of Quercetin on the Progression of Liver Fibrosis through the Regulation of NF-KB/IκBα, P38 MAPK, and Bcl-2/Bax Signaling." *International Immunopharmacology* 47: 126–33. https://doi.org/10.1016/j.intimp.2017.03.029.

Wu, Hao, Eduardo Esteve, Valentina Tremaroli, Muhammad Tanweer Khan, Robert Caesar, Louise Mannerås-Holm, Marcus Ståhlman, et al. 2017. "Metformin Alters the Gut Microbiome of Individuals with Treatment-Naive Type 2 Diabetes, Contributing to the Therapeutic Effects of the Drug." *Nature Medicine* 23 (7): 850–58. https://doi.org/10.1038/nm.4345.

Xue, Huiting, Wenyan Xie, Zhihui Jiang, Meng Wang, Jian Wang, Hongqiong Zhao, and Xiaoying Zhang. 2016. "3,4-Dihydroxyphenylacetic Acid, a Microbiota-Derived Metabolite of Quercetin, Attenuates Acetaminophen (APAP)-Induced Liver Injury through Activation of Nrf-2." *Xenobiotica* 46 (10): 931–39. https://doi.org/10.3109/00498254.2016.1140847.

Yamaguchi, Shinya, Hiroshi Katahira, Sachihiko Ozawa, Yoko Nakamichi, Toshiaki Tanaka, Tatsuhiro Shimoyama, Kazuto Takahashi, et al. 2005. "Activators of AMP-Activated Protein Kinase Enhance GLUT4 Translocation and Its Glucose Transport Activity in 3T3-L1 Adipocytes." *American Journal of Physiology-Endocrinology and Metabolism* 289 (4 52-4): 643–49. https://doi.org/10.1152/ajpendo.00456.2004.

Yu, Jianmei, and Mohamed Ahmedna. 2013. "Functional Components of Grape Pomace: Their Composition, Biological Properties and Potential Applications." *International Journal of Food Science and Technology* 48 (2): 221–37. https://doi.org/10.1111/j.1365-2621.2012.03197.x.

Yun, Shaojun, Dongyang Chu, Xingshuai He, Wenfang Zhang, and Cuiping Feng. 2020. "Protective Effects of Grape Seed Proanthocyanidins against Iron Overload-Induced Renal Oxidative Damage in Rats." *Journal of Trace Elements in Medicine and Biology* 57 (April 2019): 126407. https://doi.org/10.1016/j.jtemb.2019.126407.

Zhang, Ting, Qianqian Li, Lei Cheng, Heena Buch, and Faming Zhang. 2019. "Akkermansia Muciniphila Is a Promising Probiotic." *Microbial Biotechnology* 12 (6): 1109–25. https://doi.org/10.1111/1751-7915.13410.

Zhang, Yunjian, Shuizhen Zhou, Yuanfeng Zhou, Lifei Yu, Linmei Zhang, and Yi Wang. 2018. "Altered Gut Microbiome Composition in Children with Refractory Epilepsy after Ketogenic Diet." *Epilepsy Research* 145 (June): 163–68. https://doi.org/10.1016/j.eplepsyres.2018.06.015.

Zhang, Zhichao, Xichun Peng, Shaoting Li, Ning Zhang, Yong Wang, and Hua Wei. 2014. "Isolation and Identification of Quercetin Degrading Bacteria from Human Fecal Microbes." *PLoS ONE* 9 (3): 1–5. https://doi.org/10.1371/journal.pone.0090531.

Zhu, Wei, Ziqing Yin, Qiang Zhang, Shuangfei Guo, Yi Shen, Tang Liu, Bo Liu, et al. 2019. "Proanthocyanidins Inhibit Osteoclast Formation and Function by Inhibiting the NF-KB and JNK Signaling Pathways during Osteoporosis Treatment." *Biochemical and Biophysical Research Communications* 509 (1): 294–300. https://doi.org/10.1016/j.bbrc.2018.12.125.

In: Grape Pomace in Health …
Editor: Veronica Sanda Chedea
ISBN: 978-1-68507-409-8


*Chapter 5*

# GRAPE POMACE – HEALTH BENEFITS IN OXIDATIVE STRESS AND INFLAMMATION

***Raluca Maria Pop[1,*], Dan Claudiu Măgureanu[2], Ștefan Octavian Macovei[2], Ioana Corina Bocșan[1] and Veronica Sanda Chedea[3]***

[1]Department of Pharmacology, Toxicology and Clinical Pharmacology, "Iuliu Hatieganu" University of Medicine and Pharmacy, Cluj-Napoca, Romania
[2]"Iuliu Hatieganu" University of Medicine and Pharmacy, Cluj-Napoca, Romania
[3]Research Station for Viticulture and Enology, Blaj, (SCDVV Blaj), Romania

## ABSTRACT

Recently the emphasis was placed on the role of oxidative stress and inflammation in different chronic diseases. Accordingly, there is a wide variety of diseases that are characterized by oxidative stress and inflammation such as diabetes, hypertension and cardiovascular diseases, alcoholic liver disease, chronic kidney disease,

* Corresponding Author's E-mail: raluca_parlog@yahoo.com.

neurodegenerative diseases, cancer, and aging. The classical medication used in the treatment of these diseases, besides their therapeutic effects, involves numerous side effects. Many studies have shown that numerous natural bioactive molecules have beneficial effects in counteracting these side effects. Therefore a lot of focus is directed toward the identification of these rich sources of natural compounds. Plants, fruits, food, and wine industry byproducts and their extracts are considered important alternative sources, being readily available. Among investigated resources, grape pomace (GP), the solid waste material obtained during wine production, is a very rich source of bioactive compounds, especially phenolics. In this context, this chapter aims to present the most recent studies that show the antioxidant and anti-inflammatory effects of GP, evidenced so far by the *in vitro* and *in vivo* studies. According to the most recent *in vitro* and *in vivo* animal studies, GP has shown promising results on inflammation and oxidative stress associated with various chronic diseases. The few *in vivo* studies on humans show that more research is needed to demonstrate its potential in chronic conditions prevention and/or treatment in humans.

**Keywords:** grape pomace, *in vitro*, *in vivo*, antioxidant activity, anti-inflammatory effect

## INTRODUCTION

Oxidative stress is the result of the imbalance between oxidants generation (e.g., free radicals reactive oxygen species (ROS) like hydroxyl radical (•OH), superoxide anion ($O_2^-$), hydrogen peroxide ($H_2O_2$), and reactive nitrogen species (RNS) (e.g., nitric oxide (NO•) peroxynitrite (ONOO•), nitrogen dioxide ($NO_2$)) and the existing endogenous antioxidants (e.g., enzymatic scavengers like Superoxide dismutase (SOD), Catalase (CAT), Glutathione peroxidase (GTPx), Glutathione transferase (GST) and non-enzymatic like A, C, E Vitamins, glutathione (GSH), carotenoids, phenolic compounds) used to scavenge the ROS and RNS production (Chatterjee 2016; Ozcan and Ogun 2015). The result of this imbalance is an excess in oxidants production generally termed "oxidative stress." When oxidative stress occurs, excessive ROS production is detrimental to the human organism since it can directly damage and alter the functions of nucleic acids, signal transduction, lipids, carbohydrates, and proteins (Chatterjee 2016).

As consequence, oxidative stress plays a pivotal role in various pathological conditions from cancer (Reuter et al. 2010) to neurological disorders (Patel 2016), cardiovascular diseases (Cervantes Gracia, Llanas-Cornejo, and Husi 2017) diabetes (Asmat, Abad, and Ismail 2016), acute and chronic respiratory diseases (Ramírez-Prieto, García-Río, and Villamor 2006; Birben et al. 2012). Overall, a significant role of oxidative stress was observed in several inflammatory conditions (glomerulonephritis arthritis, vasculitis, lupus erythematosus) (Lobo et al. 2010).

One explanation can be derived from the fact that ROS-regulated transcription factors (e.g., nuclear factor kappa B (NF-κB)) can be indirectly influenced via the modification of IκB proteins by oxidants. In its inactive form, NF-κB is bound to the IκB cytosolic proteins in the cell's cytoplasm (Chatterjee 2016). When IκB proteins are degraded by oxidants, the NF-κB is released. Further, NF-κB can be translocated to the nucleus where, single or with other transcription factors, can induce the expression of several inflammatory genes, thus influencing the production of inflammatory proteins (Chatterjee 2016). ROS production also affects the expression of specific genes like the activator protein-1 (AP-1), peroxisome proliferator activator receptor gamma (PPAR-γ), the hypoxia-inducible factor (HIF-1α), nuclear factor-like 2 (Nrf-2), and others (Espinosa-Diez et al. 2015; Chatterjee 2016). These can be translated into the alteration of several inflammatory genes, growth factors, cytokines, and chemokines which affect multiple inflammatory conditions.

On the other hand, inflammation is a defense mechanism response of the immune system to multiple factors like pathogens, toxic compounds, damaged cells or irradiation, to minimize their negative effects (Chen et al. 2018). This defense mechanism includes the initiation of immune responses (by innate and adaptive immune cells recruitment, proliferation, and differentiation) (Velazquez-Caldelas et al. 2019; Cronkite and Strutt 2018), of tissue components (e.g., stromal fibroblasts)

(Ball et al. 2016), of extracellular matrix (by its modulation effect on immune cell behavior) (Abudukelimu et al. 2018), of blood and lymphatic vasculature (by its influence on the drainage of extravasated fluid, leukocytes, and inflammatory mediators) (Schwager and Detmar 2019), of plasma proteins, cytokines, and chemokines (Abudukelimu et al. 2018). One of the links of inflammation with oxidative stress appears when proinflammatory cytokines and chemokines are produced by the innate immune system cells through ROS/RNS production (Khansari, Shakiba, and Mahmoudi 2009). This is possible because the elimination of the pathogens is mainly obtained by macrophages through ROS generation like $O_2^-$, NO•, $H_2O_2$, •OH, and others (Paiva and Bozza 2014). Further, the inflammation process continues until the pathogens will be eliminated and the tissue will be repaired (Khansari, Shakiba, and Mahmoudi 2009). However, a continued response to the acute inflammation process may lead to chronic inflammation. At this point, the inflammatory cells ROS overproduction is encountered. As known, ROS and RNS can have dual roles harmful and beneficial. The beneficial effects take place when low concentrations of ROS are produced and harmful when their overproduction takes place. Thus oxidative stress and inflammation can induce each other being strongly interrelated. That is why these two interconnected processes are impacting various physiological and pathological conditions (Pop et al. 2020).

Currently, there is a wide variety of diseases characterized by two components – oxidative stress and inflammation. Among diseases, we can mention type 2 diabetes and its complications, cardiovascular diseases and hypertension, alcoholic liver disease, neurodegenerative diseases, chronic kidney disease, cancer, and even aging (Ambade and Mandrekar 2012; Biswas et al. 2008; Biswas 2016). These are treated with classical medications which, unfortunately, besides their important therapeutic effects are also inducing numerous side effects. Therefore, it is crucial to identify alternative sources of bioactive compounds therapeutically potent, which, with no or minimal side effects could be able to improve the current treatments. Plants, fruits, food, and wine industry byproducts and their extracts are such sources, being readily available.

Grape pomace (GP) is a solid waste material obtained after grape pressing and fermentation and it accounts for 20 to 30% of the initial grape weight used in wine production (Dwyer, Hosseinian, and Rod 2014). Grape pomace contains unused skins, seeds, and stems, which have their chemical composition almost unaltered. The preservation of their chemical composition is possible because the main processes after which GP is obtained do not induce important chemical changes (Dwyer, Hosseinian, and Rod 2014). Thus, both white and red GP contains important quantities of bioactive compounds that can be exploited as an important source of bioactive compounds. For example, after wine production, GP contains approximately 70% of the total phenolic compounds in grapes (Ratnasooriya and Rupasinghe 2012). Therefore, GP is a rich source of phenolic compounds like phenolic acid (hydroxybenzoic acid and hydroxycinnamic acids), flavanols (epicatechin, epicatechin gallate), proanthocyanidins, flavonols (kaempferol quercetin, isorhamnetin 3-O-glucoside, kaempferol 3-O-glucoside, quercetin 3-O-glucoside, quercetin 3-O-galactoside, quercetin 3-O-rhamnoside), stilbenes (trans-resveratrol, trans-polydatin), anthocyanins (delphinidin 3-O-glucoside, delphinidin 3-O-acetylglucoside, malvidin, malvidin 3-O-p-coumaroylglucoside, peonidin, peonidin-3-O-p-coumaroylglucoside, peonidin 3-O-acetylglucoside, peonidin 3-O- p-coumaroylglucoside, petunidin, petunidin 3-O-glucoside, petunidin 3-O-acetylglucoside petunidin3-O- p-coumaroylglucoside) and tannins (Koutelidakis 2016). Besides phenolic compounds, GP contains high quantities of lipids (13–19% oil), proteins (11%), fibers, and minerals (Rasines-Perea et al. 2018; Ky, Lorrain, et al. 2014; Antoniolli et al. 2015; Fontana, Antoniolli, and Bottini 2013; González-Centeno et al. 2013; Ky, Crozier, et al. 2014; Deng, Penner, and Zhao 2011; Yu and Ahmedna 2013).

Also, taking into account that in 2018, the worldwide production of grapes exceeded 77 million tons, and that wine production (the principal source of GP production) represents one of the main ways of grapes usage with France as the world-leading country for wine production (41.4 million of hectoliters of wine), followed by Italy (40.1 million of hectoliters of wine) and Spain (30.4 million of hectoliters of wine) (OIV and International Organisation of Vine and Wine 2019; Zacharof 2017) it is compulsory to find viable alternative ways to reduce this waste production to our proper benefits.

In this light, this chapter aims to present the most recent studies that show the antioxidant and anti-inflammatory effects of using GP that could be further translated in the improvement of several disease conditions, evidenced so far by the existing *in vitro* and *in vivo* studies.

## Grape Pomace – A Promising Antioxidants Source

It is known that plants' bioactive compounds content, including the phenolics in grapes, varies strongly with grape varieties, degree of ripeness, environmental factors, and also winemaking technological processes. Because of this, numerous studies characterize the polyphenols' content and composition as they are affected by these factors (Ky, Lorrain, et al. 2014; Sousa et al. 2014; Kallithraka, Salacha, and Tzourou 2009; Correia, Cosme, and Jordão 2018; Lingua et al. 2016). These studies are extremely important since polyphenols' bioavailability differs considerably, thus having different *in vitro* and *in vivo* biological activities. Knowing these details can help the selection of optimum grape varieties, suitable for their further use as plant material for different applications (e.g., food, cosmetic, and pharmaceutical industries) (Nile et al. 2013).

Moreover, the phenolic compound composition can offer insight into the antioxidant capacity since it strongly depends on the number of hydroxyl groups existing in the phenolic molecules. Thus, phenolic compounds are important for their role as free radical scavengers, metal chelators, hydrogen donators, and singlet oxygen quenchers (Luchian et al. 2019). Accordingly, *in vitro* antioxidant activity evaluates phenolic antioxidant potential to eliminate free radicals. That is why most of the studies firstly analyze the total polyphenol content to further correlate the results with the antioxidant activities. In most situations, the antioxidant activities are reported as a synergistic effect of different bioactive substances that exist in the mixture. That is also the case for GP. The GP polyphenol extract profile determines its efficacy as compared to the individual activity of compounds which can widely vary (Maluf et al. 2018; Choueiri et al. 2012; Abou Samra et al. 2011). Therefore total polyphenol content (TPC) and antioxidant capacity measurement represent an important and useful strategy to offer preliminary results before the biological assays.

Currently, there are more than 19 methods for the *in vitro* evaluation of the antioxidant capacity of plant extracts (Alam, Bristi, and Rafiquzzaman 2013). These multiple assay strategies are strongly connected to the properties of the bioactive compounds to donate a hydrogen atom or to bind metal ions capable to catalyze oxidative processes, absorb UV radiation, inhibit enzymes of decomposing hydroperoxides (Kasote et al. 2015). Therefore, according to their inactivation mechanism, the antioxidant activity assays are classified in hydrogen atom transfer (HAT) assays and electron transfer (ET) reaction assays (Kasote et al. 2015). Because of this, there is a great discrepancy between thc tests used to evaluate the antioxidant activity and the corresponding results (Antoniolli et al. 2015). Consequently, it is recommended to use at least two different *in vitro* assay methods (Aruoma 2003; Schlesier et al. 2002; Ruberto et al. 2007).

Based on all aforementioned details, within this study, the GP characterization is presented considering its TPC and three different *in vitro* antioxidant activities. These are the 2,2-Diphenyl-1-picrylhydrazyl – (DPPH), the ({2,2' – azinobis-(3-ethyl-benzothiazoline-6-sulphonic acid)}- (ABTS) and ferric reducing antioxidant power assay – (FRAP). The choice was based on their frequent use (due to ease of use, simplicity, and instrumentation availability) and on their inactivation mechanism (DPPH, ABTS - both hydrogen atom and single electron transfer while FRAP- single electron transfer) (Kasote et al. 2015) (Table

1 and Table 2). At the same time, the GP origin was noted (Table 1 and Table 2). The main purpose was to offer in this way the possibility of having a broad overview of GP antioxidant capacity variability as determined by region, TPC, and compounds inactivation mechanism. As it can be observed in Table 1, at a first look, the TPC and antioxidant activity had higher values in seeds as compared with skins in all varieties, independent of the provenience region.

Xia et al., (2019) evaluated the TPC, phenolic composition, and *in vitro* antioxidant and antiproliferative activities of seeds and skins obtained from 31 different grape cultivars. Among investigated cultivars, they observed that seeds and skins belonging to the European cultivars had the highest TPC content as well as higher antioxidant activity. American and Oriental seeds had also high values, while the hybrids (Euro- Asian or Euro- American) were between parent varieties. Within their study, they had an important observation. They indicated a positive significant correlation among investigated antioxidant assays (ABTS, DPPH, and FRAP) in both seeds and skins. They also observed that a higher phenolic content will induce higher antioxidant activity (Xia et al. 2019). This study supports that TPC and antioxidant activities are higher in seeds as compared to skins (Xia et al. 2019).

Within their study, González-Centeno et al., (2013) characterized white GP in terms of polyphenol compounds and antioxidant activity. They also reported a positive correlation between TPC and antioxidant capacity (evaluated by ABTS and FRAP assays) (González-Centeno et al. 2013). The same positive correlation was observed when the GP was investigated as a mixture of bioactive compounds obtained after its extraction (Table 2). Moreover, Marchante et al., (2018) investigated GP, seed, and stems obtained from *Vitis vinifera* L. cv. Tempranillo, using a different approach. They have correlated the compounds identified in the GP extracts with their antioxidant capacity. As expected, a positive correlation between specific polyphenols (catechin, gallocatechin, epigallocatechin, catechin gallate, epicatechin gallate, procyanidin B1, and others) and the antioxidant activity (ABTS and DPPH) was observed (Marchante et al. 2018).

## Table 1. TPC and antioxidant activities of seeds and peels of grape pomace

| Source | TPC (mg GAE/g DM) | | Antioxidant activity | | | | | | References |
|---|---|---|---|---|---|---|---|---|---|
| | | | DPPH (µM TE/g DM) | | ABTS (µM TE/g DM) | | FRAP (µM TE/g DM) | | |
| | Seed | Skin | Seed | Skin | Seed | Skin | Seed | Skin | |
| *Vitis vinifera* L. (*V. vinifera*) American cultivars (7 cultivars –*cv.*) | 43 | 25 | 319 | 120 | 559 | 185 | 455 | 201 | (Xia et al. 2019) |
| Euro-American hybrids (5 *cv.*) | 50 | 27 | 308 | 129 | 570 | 206 | 455 | 184 | |
| *V. Vinifera* L (3 *cv.*) | 93 | 23 | 575 | 117 | 881 | 167 | 998 | 135 | |
| Euro-Asian hybrids (3 *cv.*) | 32 | 23 | 184 | 92 | 263 | 179 | 239 | 180 | |
| Oriental group (8 *cv.*) | 19 | 27 | 122 | 107 | 269 | 191 | 134 | 190 | |
| *V. vinifera* L. Muscadine (5 *cv.*) | 71 | 19 | 507 | 115 | 762 | 165 | 693 | 187 | |
| *V. vinifera* L. Italian Nero d'Avola *cv.* | 113 | 98 | 37 | 59 | - | - | - | - | (Messina et al. 2019) |
| *V. vinifera* L. cv. Grenache | 40.5 | 17.1 | 450.7 | 161.2 | 438.1 | 263.4 | 212.2* | 105.3* | (Ky, Lorrain, et al. 2014) |
| *V. vinifera* L. cv. Syrah | 35.6 | 24.3 | 322 | 190.6 | 486.3 | 299.3 | 232.7* | 190.8* | |
| *V. vinifera* L. cv. Carignan | 38.8 | 25.1 | 318.5 | 195.3 | 403.5 | 390.8 | 176.4* | 225.3* | |
| *V. vinifera* L. cv. Counois | 40.8 | 20.5 | 536.2 | 185 | 468.6 | 255.6 | 205.4* | 122.4* | |
| *V. vinifera* L. cv. Mourvèdre | 34.5 | 26.3 | 262.7 | 161.3 | 526.4 | 405.7 | 188.2* | 202.7* | |
| *V. vinifera* L. cv. Alicante Vallée du Rhône, France | 44.5 | 31.6 | 450.1 | 290.7 | 603.1 | 464.1 | 267.5* | 266.8* | |

* FRAP values are expressed as µM Fe2+/g DW.

Abbreviations: ABTS – 2,2-azino-bis(3-ethylbenzothiazoline -6-sulfonic acid); DPPH - 2,2-diphenyl-1-picryl -hydrazyl-hydrate; FRAP - Eric Reducing Antioxidant Power; TPC - Total Polyphenol Content.

**Table 2. TPC and antioxidant activities of some GPs**

| Source | TPC (mg GAE/g DM) | Antioxidant activity | | | References |
|---|---|---|---|---|---|
| | | DPPH (μM TE/g DM) | ABTS (μM TE/g DM) | FRAP (μM TE/g DM) | |
| | Region | | | | |
| | Brazil (Lagoa Grande, Pernambuco) | | | | |
| *V. vinifera* L. Alicante Bouschet grape pomace | 16 | 160 | 171 | 393 | (Costa et al. 2019) |
| | Brazil (Petrolina) | | | | |
| *V. vinifera* L. Chenin Blanc | 20.17 | 191 | 218 | - | (Melo et al. 2015) |
| *V. vinifera* L. Petit Verdo | 66.69 | 540 | 626 | - | |
| *V. vinifera* L. Syrah | 39.30 | 310 | 653 | - | |
| | Italy (Verona) | | | | |
| *V. vinifera* L. *(Corvina cv.)* | 34 | 171 | - | 393 | (Tolve et al. 2020) |
| | USA (Virginia) | | | | |
| *V. vinifera* L. Cabernet Franc | 153.8 | 11.2 | 1013 | - | (Xu et al. 2016) |
| Hybrid grape Chambourcin | 92 | 28.2 | 378 | - | |
| Hybrid grape Vidal Blanc | 55.5 | 7.71 | 334 | - | |
| *V. vinifera* L. Viognier | 99.1 | 3.54 | 951 | - | |
| *V. vinifera* L. Cabernet Franc | 153.8 | 11.2 | 1013 | - | |
| | Spain (Castilla y León) | | | | |
| *V. vinifera* L. Tempranillo | 71.3 | - | 840 | 530 | (Ayuda-Durán et al. 2019) |
| | Spain (Mallorca, Balearic Islands) | | | | |
| *V. vinifera* L. Chardonnay | 38.91 | - | 92.4 | 76.1 | (González-Centeno et al. 2013) |
| *V. vinifera* L. Macabeu | 30.93 | - | 71.6 | 49 | |
| *V. vinifera* L. Parellada | 46.54 | - | 134 | 124.8 | |
| *V. vinifera* L. Premsal Blanc | 36.39 | - | 93.8 | 68.3 | |
| | Spain, Cordoba | | | | |
| *V. vinifera* L. Zalema | 25.13 | - | 567.7 | - | (José Jara-Palacios et al. 2014) |
| *V. vinifera* L. Pedro Ximénez | 7.14 | - | 266.9 | - | |
| *V. vinifera* L. Moscatel | 21.93 | - | 314.2 | - | |
| *V. vinifera* L. Baladí | 4.54 | - | 286.2 | - | |
| *V. vinifera* L. Parellada | 31.13 | - | 594.2 | - | |
| *V. vinifera* L. Sauvignon blanc | 23.04 | - | 538.5 | - | |

| Source | TPC (mg GAE/g DM) | Antioxidant activity | | | References |
|---|---|---|---|---|---|
| | | DPPH (μM TE/g DM) | ABTS (μM TE/g DM) | FRAP (μM TE/g DM) | |
| *V. vinifera* L. Montepila | 5.39 | - | 296.6 | - | |
| *V. vinifera* L. Airén | 11.53 | - | 253 | - | |
| *V. vinifera* L. Verdejo | 12.77 | - | 225 | - | |
| | Spain (Ciudad Real) | | | | |
| *V. vinifera* L. Cv. Tempranillo | 39.5 | 273 | 156 | - | (Marchante et al. 2018) |

Abbreviations: ABTS – 2,2-azino-bis(3-ethylbenzothiazoline -6-sulfonic acid); DPPH - 2,2-diphenyl-1-picryl -hydrazyl-hydrate; FRAP - Feric Reducing Antioxidant Power; TPC - Total Polyphenol Content.

So far, the existing studies have shown that GP can be considered a strong candidate to be further tested in the *in vivo* studies for its potential antioxidant effect.

## Grape Pomace – *In Vivo* Antioxidant Activity

Another aim of this study was to analyze the *in vitro* GP antioxidant activity in the light of a possible correspondence with the *in vivo* antioxidant activity further detailed in this chapter. As previously described, most of the studies have shown that GPs are strong *in vitro* antioxidants (Table 1 and Table 2).

Knowing that, under *in vivo* conditions, the antioxidant potential of phytochemicals is influenced by several factors (e.g., absorption, distribution, metabolism, transportation and excretion, co-antioxidants presence, drug interactions) only a few of them further confirm their antioxidant activities in the *in vivo* experiments (Kasote et al. 2015) (Veskoukis et al. 2012). Consequently, the results of the *in vivo* antioxidant assays are often inconsistent and controversial. Generally, the *in vivo* methods used to test the antioxidant capacity includes the administration of different samples (e.g., bioactive compounds, single or in combinations, antioxidant-rich plant, fruits, or vegetable extracts) in different experimental settings to experimental animals (mice, rats, pigs, and so on) in known dosage. Blood antioxidant capacity can be performed during and at the end of the experiments, while organs' antioxidant capacity is determined at the end after the experimental animals are euthanatized.

There is a large variety of assays suitable to measure the plant's antioxidant activity or reducing potential. These methods evaluate the antioxidant effect of plants to see whether the host is capable to handle the free radical stress as induced in the experimental settings (Wood, Gibson, and Garg 2006; Chedea and Pop 2018). Generally, there are two approaches in the *in vivo* antioxidant activity assessment. The first one is the direct measurement of antioxidant activity through the analysis of antioxidant concentrations, while the second one is the indirect measurement of oxidative stress markers. The direct approach includes the analysis of dietary antioxidants (e.g., vitamins A, E, C, carotenoids, and flavonoids concentrations), endogenous antioxidants (GSH, GSHPx, SOD, CAT), and total antioxidant capacity (ORAC, TRAP, FRAP, TEAC). The indirect approach consists in assessing the markers of lipid damage (e.g., 8-isoprostane, TBARS/MDA, 4-HNE, lipid hydroperoxides, hydrocarbons –ethane, pentane and antibodies against LDL), of protein damage (e.g., protein carbonyls nitrotyrosine), of DNA damage (e.g., 8-ohdG) and free radical measurement (ESR, $H_2O_2$) (Wood, Gibson, and Garg 2006). Furthermore, the use of direct and indirect methods is extremely important when antioxidant supplementation needs to be monitored. Firstly, with the help of the direct methods by antioxidant levels measurement, it can be demonstrated if the tested samples were absorbed in the host systemic circulation. Secondly, with the help of indirect methods, it can be demonstrated if sample administration produces an antioxidant effect as indicated by the host oxidative stress markers levels (Wood, Gibson, and Garg 2006). However, because the highly available methods are rarely standardized, data comparison between studies is hampered.

For example, Chedea et al., (2019) used both directly and indirectly assay methods to evaluate the influence of the red GP diet (5% red GP incorporated in the conventional compound piglets feed) on the antioxidant status in piglet's organs. They determined TPC in both feed and organs (liver, spleen, kidney, heart, brain, mesenteric lymph nodes, and Longissimus Dorsi muscle). It was observed that the GP diet significantly influenced plasma TPC. After 36 days, at the end of the experiment, TPC was higher in the group feed with GP as compared with the control group. Regarding the organs, GP pomace determined significantly higher levels of TPC only in kidneys. Concerning antiradical activity, as determined by DPPH, the liver of piglets belonging to the GP feed group was the single organ (among the studied ones) which had significantly higher activity (144 μM Trolox equivalents) as compared with the control group (109 μM Trolox equivalents) (Chedea, Palade, et al. 2019). The total antioxidant status (TAS) and antioxidant enzyme activity (CAT, SOD, and -GPx) completed the direct analysis methods assays. It was observed that GP diet significantly increased TAS in the liver, spleen, and kidneys with 21, 20, and 11% respectively, towards the control group. Increased CAT activity was also observed in the spleen and kidneys, with 13 and 18% respectively, as compared with control. Regarding SOD activity significantly higher levels were identified in the liver, kidneys, and spleen, with increments of 13, 11, and 21%, respectively. Further, an increased GPx activity was observed in the kidneys (33%) and a decreased lipid peroxidation in the liver (-34%) and kidneys (-30%). The authors of this study showed that GP was absorbed in the pigs' plasma and further had antioxidant activity (Chedea et al. 2019).

Within Veskoukis et al., (2012) study, the antioxidant effects of GP extract were also studied to check if the *in vitro* activity corresponds with the *in vivo* one, using a swimming protocol in rats as an oxidant stimulus. Within this study, the authors used again both direct and indirect methods for antioxidant capacity determination. Firstly, they characterized the GP in terms of TPC, radical scavenging capacity (DPPH and ABTS), and DNA prevention damage as induced by ROO• and OH• radicals. Next, they investigated the potent GP *in vivo* activity by examining TAC and GSH in rats' blood and tissue samples. Last, they evaluated the oxidative stress markers like xanthine oxidase, TBARS (lipid damage), and protein carbonyls (protein damage) in blood and tissues. GP was found to have high quantities of TPC (648 mg GAE/ g extract), with potent antioxidant activities (IC 50 values for DPPH and ABTS being of 25 and 5.5 mg/mL) and potent effect against free radical-induced damage (ROO• and OH• radicals having IC50 of 1.5 and 500 mg/ml, respectively) (Veskoukis et al. 2012). The GP extract effect, administered before exhaustive swimming, was investigated in rat's plasma, erythrocytes, gastrocnemius muscle, heart, and liver. Interestingly, they observed that, at rest and after exercise, GP administration induced oxidative stress and did not affect exercise performance (Veskoukis et al. 2012). As we discussed before, these findings suggest that GP extract can have different effects *in vitro* than *in vivo*.

## GRAPE POMACE –*IN VITRO* AND *IN VIVO* OXIDATIVE STRESS AND INFLAMMATION EVIDENCE

The information provided so far will further enable an overview of the antioxidant and anti-inflammatory effects of GP in both *in vitro* and *in vivo* assays. Following, the next section of the chapter will analyze the effect of GP on oxidative stress and inflammation biomarkers in different experimental settings, trying to identify the mechanism of action responsible for these effects (Table 3, 4, and 5).

### *In Vitro* Studies

According to Table 3, we can observe that GP has great potential in controlling oxidative stress and inflammation processes encountered in cancer or different inflammatory diseases. In their study, Pistol et al., (2019) investigated the effect of a symbiotic combination (grape pomace extract as prebiotic and Lactobacillus sp. as probiotic) using an *in vitro* experiment. Markers of the intestinal inflammatory condition were investigated in lipopolysaccharide-treated Caco-2 cells with a focus on the intracellular signaling routes (Pistol et al. 2019). The TPC of GP extract used in this study was 6710 mg with high epicatechin and procyanidin dimer concentrations (52 and 23 mg/100 g, respectively). The lipopolysaccharide (LPS) stimulated Caco-2 cells were treated with the above-mentioned extract (50 μg/ml GAE) and Lactobacillus strains (3 $\times 10^8$ colony-forming units/ml). According to the PCR array results, the identified inflammatory markers were the cytokines, chemokines, receptors of cytokine soluble forms, adhesion molecules, growth factors, and matrix metalloproteinases inhibitors (Pistol et al. 2019). Under the symbiotic treatment, more than 50% of the investigated genes and proteins were down-regulated (with 57 and 60%, respectively). The following pro-inflammatory cytokines and chemokines IFN-γ, TNF-α, IL-7, IL-12p40, GCSF, and GM-CSF had the values restored under the positive control (LPS) cells towards the unstimulated cells. The NF-κB and mitogen-activated protein kinase pathways were involved in their reduction. The authors of this study observed that LPS activated signaling molecules were decreased when cells were treated with the GP extract and Lb mix (Pistol et al. 2019). This study is very important since it provides promising results to be further used in nutraceuticals and pharmaceutical industries, especially in the development of adjunctive therapies specific for inflammatory bowel diseases.

The *in vitro* antioxidant capacity was also investigated by de Sales et al., (2018). In their study, the effect of GP extract was investigated on the metabolism and redox status using human hepatocarcinoma HepG2 cells. The GP used in this study was very rich in polyphenols (34.000 mg GAE/100g DM). The main phenolic classes were represented by flavonoids (2146 catechin equivalents/100g DM), anthocyanins (1582 cyanidin 3-glucoside equivalents/100g DM), and monomeric anthocyanins (1441 cyanidin 3-glucoside equivalents/100g DM). As expected, the GP extract had high antioxidant capacity as determined by ABTS (1014 μmol TE/g DM), FRAP (3220 Fe(II) sulfate equivalents/L), and ORAC (167 μmol TE/g DM) assays (de Sales et al. 2018).

**Table 3. *In vitro* evidence-based use of grape pomace**

| Source | Models | Methods | Mechanism of action | References |
|---|---|---|---|---|
| *V. Vinifera* L. Cagnulari cv. (Santa Maria La Palma, Alghero, Italy) | Human umbilical vein endothelial cells (HUVECs) culture in the presence of the $H_2O_2$ | MTT assay and ROS fluorescent sensor H2DCF-DA | • antioxidant and protective vascular effect effects due to polyphenolic substances in its composition: malvidin, peonidin-3-O-glucoside, malvidin-3-(6-acetyl)-glucoside | (Posadino et al. 2018) |
| *V. Vinifera* L Batiki Tyrnavou cv. (Greece) | Muscle cells (C2C12) and endothelial cells (EA.hy926) cultures | • XTT assay kit<br>• flow cytometry using mercury orange and DCF-DA for ROS and GSH<br>• spectrophoto metrically for protein carbonyls and TBARS<br>• Cytotoxic activity for C2C12 (>10 mg/mL) and for EA.hy926 (>0.675 mg/mL) | • Treatment with GP extract C2C12 cells<br>• significantly reduced ROS, TBARS, and protein carbonyls levels<br>• increased GSH levelsEA.hy926<br>• significantly increased GSH levels<br>• significantly decreased protein carbonyls levels<br>• no difference in ROS and TBARS levels<br>• Treatment with GP extract + tBHPC2C12<br>• significantly inhibited the tBHP-induced increase in protein carbonyls and TBARS<br>• neutralized free radicals produced by tBHP (radicals reacted with GSH and lipids)<br>EA.hy926<br>• significantly inhibited the tBHP-induced decrease in GSH levels<br>• significantly inhibited the tBHP-induced increase in protein carbonyls and TBARS | (Goutzourelas et al. 2014) |

| Source | Models | Methods | Mechanism of action | References |
|---|---|---|---|---|
| - | N13 microglia cells culture stimulated with LPS | SDS-polyacrylamide gel electrophoresis | • reduced the expression of the mRNA of the pro-inflammatory factors: TNF-α, TLR-4, IL-1β, Iba-1, and iNOS | (Rodríguez-Morgado et al. 2015) |
| *V. Vinifera* L. Red varieties GP (Valea Calugareasca, Romania) | Caco-2 cells (model for intestinal inflammation) stimulated with LPS and cultured with GP extract and Lactobacillus sp. Mixture | MTT assay qPCR array Qiagen GmbH Abcam array | • decreased chemokine and cytokines genes expression and proteins levels(pro-inflammatory molecules)<br>• decreased MMP-2 and MMP-9 mRNA expression (pro-inflammatory effect)<br>• increased TIMP1, TIMP2 expression (anti-inflammatory effect)<br>• decreased MAPK, Akt/P70S6K/ mTOR, NF-κB, Nrf2 (inflammation signaling pathways) | (Pistol et al. 2019) |
| *V. Vinifera* L. | Caco-2 cells (model for colon adenocarcinoma) | tBPH assay | • antioxidant activity (reduced ROS induced by tBPH) | (Lazze et al. 2009) |
| *V. Vinifera* L. Negroamaro – Southern Italy fermented with *Lactobacillus plantarum* | RBL-2H3 (leukemia basophilic cells) – a model for type I allergic reactions | β-Hexosaminidase assay Western blot | • inhibited β-Hexosaminidase release (reduced degranulation)<br>• suppressed Syk phosphorylation (degranulation role) | (Kaneko et al. 2010) |

Abbreviations: Abcam - Inflammation Human Membrane Antibody Array; DCF-DA - 2,7-dichlorofluorescein diacetate; GSH - glutathione; H2DCF-DA – 2',7'-dichlorodihydrofluorescein diacetate; $H_2O_2$ - hydrogen peroxide (oxidative stress-inducing substance); Iba-1 - Ionized calcium binding adaptor molecule-1; IL-1β - Interleukin 1β; iNOS - Inducible nitric oxide synthase; LPS - Lipopolysaccharide; MAPK - Mitogen-activated protein kinases; MMP2 - matrix metalloproteinase-2; MMP9 - matrix metalloproteinase-9; MTT - 3-(4,5-dimethylthiazol-2-yl)-2,5-diphenyltetrazolium bromide (colorimetric assay used in cell metabolic activity); NF-kB - nuclear factor - kappa-light-chain-enhancer of activated B cells; PBMC- Peripheral Blood Mononuclear cells; Qiagen GmbH - Qiagen RNeasy mini kit; qPCR - quantitative PCR; ROS- reactive oxygen species; Syk - spleen tyrosine kinase (transmitting signals to Fc receptor - lymphocytes, mast cells, basophils cells, neutrophils cells); TBARS - thiobarbituric reactive substances; tBHP- tert-butyl hydroperoxide (oxidative stress-inducing substance); TIMP1 - tissue inhibitor of metalloproteinases 1; TIMP2 - tissue inhibitor of metalloproteinases 2; TLR-4 - Toll-like receptor 4; TNF-α - Tumor necrosis factor alpha; XTT - Cell proliferation kit II.

Thus, the GP treatment induced an increment of mitochondrial respiration as well as antioxidant capacity enhancement in HepG2 cells. Antioxidant capacity was tested concerning mitochondrial function because the authors of this study observed that HepG2 cells treatment with GP extract induced an increased mitochondrial function that could induce an altered redox state. For this purpose, the cells were stimulated with antimycin A, known for its capacity to increase ROS intracellular production. They observed that incubation for 1h with GP extracts in different concentrations promotes a significant decrease (85–90%) in maximal oxidation of the chloromethyl derivative (H2DCFDA -indicator for ROS in cells). This decrease shows a reduced accumulation of ROS in HepG2 cells (de Sales et al. 2018). Metabolic effects seemed somehow targeted to mitochondria and preceded the observed decrease in cell proliferation and viability. The results indicated that GPE possessed important pharmacological properties, with increased potential to be used as functional or nutraceutical food ingredients.

## *In Vivo* - Animal Studies

Antioxidant activity or anti-inflammatory effects of GP, taken individually or associated with various *in vivo* experimental pathological conditions were largely studied (Rho and Kim 2006; Bralley et al. 2007; Denny et al. 2014; Nishiumi et al. 2012; Souza et al. 2019). The simultaneous effect of GP on these parameters was also investigated, but in a lower percent (Table 4). As observed in Table 4, most of these studies investigated the effect of GP on inflammation and oxidative stress, encountered in various models of metabolic diseases like obesity, diabetes, or cardiovascular diseases. Others refer to oxidative stress and inflammation in different inflammatory conditions.

For example, Rivera et al., (2019) investigated the effect of red GP on atherosclerosis, myocardial damage, and survival rates, using a lethal ischemic heart disease murine model.

The lethal ischemic heart disease model was obtained using atherogenic SR-B1 KO/ApoER61h/h mice fed with an enriched diet in fat, cholesterol, and cholic acid. These mice were additionally fed (for 7 or 14 days) with a 20% high-fat diet (control group), with 20% GP flour (GP group), or with a combination of 10% chow and 10% oat fiber (fiber group). Afterward, the survival rate, inflammation, oxidative stress, and antioxidant activity markers were measured (Rivera et al. 2019). Plasma total antioxidant capacity, oxidative stress status (MDA quantification), and systemic inflammation (circulating levels of TNF-α and IL-10) were investigated. The results indicated that GP flour supplementation significantly increased the lifespan of the atherogenic feed mice, their median survival being of 31 days as compared to the control group (23.5 days) or fiber group (21 days). The antioxidant plasma activity was investigated using HDL-containing plasma with a dihydrorhodamine based fluorescent assay after non-HDL lipoprotein was removed. They observed that after 14 days, the GP feed group had the HDL containing plasma antioxidant activity increased as compared to the control group, indicating that GP might modulate lipid peroxidation. The other parameters used to investigate the oxidation status (MDA) had no significant changes in values after 14 days of GP administration, compared to the control group. Regarding the inflammatory status, as expressed by TNF- α and IL-10 cytokines, after 7 days of a high-fat diet, significantly lower plasma levels in the mice's feed with GP were identified as compared to the control group. Interestingly, after 14 days of GP supplementation, these markers had a non-significant trend to reduce their levels as compared to the control group (Rivera et al. 2019). Even though GP had a positive influence on systemic inflammation and on plasma HDL-containing antioxidant activity that is associated with significantly reduced atherosclerotic lesions, further studies need to be performed to check more specific biomarkers for oxidative stress and inflammation and to see why the investigated (MDA, IL-10, and TNF-α) did not keep their significance over a longer period.

**Table 4. *In vivo* evidence-based use of grape pomace in animal models**

| Source | Models | Mechanism of action | References |
|---|---|---|---|
| *Vitis aestivalis* hybrid-Norton GP extract- Blackstone, Virginia | Obese C57BLK/6J mice (high-fat diet) supplementation | • suppressed inflammation (reduced C-reactive protein)<br>• no significant anti-oxidative effects | (Hogan et al. 2010) |
| Grape pomace (GP) mixture and Omija (*Schisandra chinensis*) | Type 2 diabetes mice into 3 groups: control group; high dose GP + omija (HGO); low dose GP + omija (LGO) | • LGO is more efficient than HGO against oxidative stress<br>• LGO significantly decreased $H_2O_2$, TBARS, erythrocyte peroxides<br>• LGO significantly decreased erythrocyte oxidation by increasing the levels of the antioxidant enzyme: SOD, CAT, GSH-Px<br>• LGO and HGO significantly decreased liver oxidation | (Cho et al. 2017) |
| *Vitis vinifera* L. GP Cabernet Sauvignon | Mice (atherogenic diet) | • reduced atherosclerosis lesion<br>• suppressed inflammatory status by reducing TNF-α and IL-10 levels<br>• increased plasma antioxidant status | (Rivera et al. 2019) |
| *V. vinifera* L.- Garibaldi, Rio Grande do Sul state, Brazil | Grass carps (*Pseudomonas aeruginosa* infection)- a model for hepatic oxidative lesion | • significantly reduced the increase of NOx, ROS, TBARS levels<br>• reduced CAT, SOD levels*<br>• ACAP levels stopped increasing | (Souza et al. 2019) |
| *V. vinifera L.*- Mures county, Târnavelor Plateau, Romania | Induced myocardial infarction in male rats (albino Wistar) orally fed with Fetească neagră fresh GP (FNFs) or Fetească neagră fermented GP (FNFr) | • FNFs decreased ST segments elevation, reduced increasing of RR, QT interval; FNFr only decreased ST segments and reduced RR interval (EGC parameters) | Balea et al. 2018) |

| Source | Models | Mechanism of action | References |
|---|---|---|---|
| | | • FNFs, FNFr decreased CK-MB, AST, ALT (Cardiac enzymes)<br>• antioxidant activity: FNFs, FNFr significantly decreased TOS, OSI, MDA, and increased TAR | (Balea et al. 2018) |
| *V. vinifera* -red and white GP-Kobe City (Japan) | I[st] experiment: mice (red and white GP extracts) injected after one-hour LPS and galactosamine (hepatoxic) (pro-inflammatory substance) | • Red GP diet more potent than white GP diet to suppress NF-kB (inflammation signaling pathway); decreased pro-inflammatory cytokines | (Nishiumi et al. 2012) |
| | II[nd] experiment: rats fed with red GP diet for 7 days and injected after with lipopolysaccharide and galactosamine | • suppressed the expression of the protein of COX-2 (pro-inflammatory) and iNOS (mutagenesis and carcinogenesis) | |
| *Vitis vinifera* L. Red varieties GP, Valea Calugareasca Romania | Dissected organs (liver, spleen, kidneys) of pigs with a 5% GP diet | • antioxidant activity had the highest values in the liver<br>• decreased lipid peroxidation levels in all organs<br>• TAS increased in all organs<br>• increased CAT activity in spleen and kidney;<br>• increased SOD activity in all organs | (Chedea, Palade, et al. 2019) |
| *Vitis vinifera* L. Alicante red wine-Rhone valley, France | Mice fed with dextran sodium sulfate (model for inflammatory bowel disease) | • decreased PMN cell infiltration<br>• increased SOD | (Boussenna et al. 2016) |
| *Vitis vinifera* L. *GP and GPE* | Male rats (high-fat fructose diet-model for metabolic syndrome) | • reduced NADPH oxidase activity<br>• prevented the increase of altered adipocytokine expression (pro-inflammatory) | (Rodriguez Lanzi et al. 2016) |

**Table 4. (Continued)**

| Source | Models | Mechanism of action | References |
|---|---|---|---|
| *Vitis vinifera* L. Red varieties GP from a Romanian distillery | Longissimus Dorsi muscle from 24 hybrid pigs | • increased by 1.27 times the concentration of n-3 PUFA (significantly increased, by 1.35 times, the concentration of alpha-linolenic FA)<br>• increased by 1.14 times the concentration of n-6 PUFA (increased the concentration of linoleic FA by 1.17 times)<br>• decreased by 1.40 times the concentration of arachidonic FA<br>• no significant effects on the MUFA<br>• no statistically significant decrease in the ration-6:n-3<br>• no statistically significant increase in the predisposition to peroxidation by 1.11 times (p=0.24) | (Habeanu et al. 2015) |
| *Vitis vinifera L.* Red grape varieties GP -Valea Calugareasca, Romania | Dairy cows (GP diet) | • increased β-lactoglobulin (exhibit antiviral, hypocholesterolemic, anti-pathogen adhesion, and anticarcinogenic effects) | (Chedea, Pelmus, et al. 2019) |
| *Vitis vinifera* L. Red grape varieties GP-Valea Calugareasca, Romania | Piglets duodenum and colon(5% GP diet) | • decreased lipid peroxidation<br>• increased TAS<br>• increased CAT and GPx activity<br>• increased SOD (duodenum) | (Chedea et al. 2018) |
| *V. vinifera* L.- Yllera Wineries, Spain-GP enzymatic extract | Arterial vessels (male rats) | • prevented contraction (inhibited ET-1 and DETCA to produce Superoxide anion-antioxidant effect) | (Rodriguez-Rodriguez et al. 2012) |

| Source | Models | Mechanism of action | References |
|---|---|---|---|
| *V. vinifera* L. *Koshu* (Katsunuma, Japan) – fermented with *Lactobacillus plantarum* | Female rats (asthma induced – a model for type I allergic reaction) | • suppressed IgE response<br>• reduced eosinophils in BALF<br>• reduced anaphylaxis reaction after intradermal injection | (Tominaga et al. 2010) |
| *V. vinifera* L.– La Mancha, Spain | Raw and cooked chicken patties stored up to 20 days and 6 months (0, 30, 60mg/kg GPC diet for 6 weeks) | • reduced TBARS levels (the lowest value after 20 days; the lowest value in cooked chicken with the highest dose of GPC after 6 months) (antioxidant effect) | (Sáyago-Ayerdi et al. 2009) |
| *V. vinifera* L. *Petit Verdot* - Pernambuco, Brazil | Male mice (orally fed with PVE) injected with Carrageenan (pro-inflammatory agent) in paw | • reduced paw edema after 2, 3 and respectively 5h (dose: 30, 100, 300, 1000 mg $kg^{-1}$) reduced neutrophils migration to the intraperitoneal cavity (dose: 300 mg $kg^{-1}$)<br>• reduced levels of TNF-α and IL1-β (dose: 300 mg $kg^{-1}$) (anti-inflammatory effect) | (Denny et al. 2014) |
| Korean *Vitis labruscana* | 120 male rats were evaluated at 16, 18, and 20 months. (experimental diet with 2% GP and 0.02% CdCl2-P+; experimental diet with 2% GP – P-; Control diet – C-; control diet with 0.02% CdCl2 – C+) | • TBARS plasma levels: P+ lower than C+ and similar with C-;<br>• TBARS liver levels: P+ similar with C- at 16months, P+ similar with P- at 20 months<br>• SOD, CAT, GSH Px erythrocytes levels: lower in P+ than in P- but similar with C-;<br>• SOD liver levels: no significant changes;<br>• CAT liver levels: P+/- higher than C+/- groups at 16 mo; | (Rho and Kim 2006) |

**Table 4. (Continued)**

| Source | Models | Mechanism of action | References |
|---|---|---|---|
| | | • GSH Px liver levels: P+/- higher than C+/- groups at 18months; P+ higher than C+ but lower than P- and C- at 20 months;<br>• 8-Hydroxy-2¢-deoxyguanosine (oxidative stress levels) similar between P+ and P- but lower than C+/- at 16and 18 months; | |

*due to its antioxidant effect, grape pomace impaired oxidative response of the liver due to infection with *Pseudomonas aeruginosa* and reduced antioxidant response of CAT and SOD.

Abbreviations: ACAP - antioxidant capacity against peroxyl radicals; ALT - alanine transaminase; AST - aspartate transaminase; BALF - bronchial alveolar lavage fluids; CAT - catalase; CK-MB - creatine kinase myocardial band; COX-2 - cyclooxygenases-2; DETCA - diethyldithiocarbamic acid; ET-1 - endothelin-1; FA - fatty acid; GP - grape pomace; GPC – grape pomace concentrate; GPE- grape pomace extract; GPx- Glutathione Peroxidase; GSH-Px - glutathione-paraoxonase; H2O2 - hydrogen peroxide (oxidative stress-inducing substance); IgE - Immunoglobulin E - antibody for allergic reactions; IL-10 - interleukin-10; MDA - malondialdehyde; MUFA – monounsaturated fatty acid; NADPH - nicotinamide adenine dinucleotide phosphate; NF-kB – nuclear factor - kappa-light-chain-enhancer of activated B cells; NOx -nitrate oxide; OSI - oxidative stress index; PMN - polymorphonuclear; PUFA - polyunsaturated fatty acid; PVE- Petit Verdot Extract; QT interval - the duration between the beginning of the Q wave and the end of the T wave on an ECG; ROS- reactive oxygen species; RR interval - the interval of time between two successive R waves on an ECG; SOD - superoxide dismutase; TAR - total antioxidant response; TAS - total antioxidant status; TBARS - thiobarbituric reactive substances; TNF-α - Tumor necrosis factor alpha; TOS - total oxidative status.

A different approach was observed in the research performed by Gonçalves et al., (2017) which investigated the effect of GP hydroalcoholic extract using an adjuvant-induced arthritic model in rats. The total phenolics level as determined by mass spectrometry was approximately 74 mg (non-anthocyanin and anthocyanin compounds)/g. Using this extract, the dose administered during the experiment (23 days) was 250 mg/kg body weight (Gonçalves et al. 2017). The oxidative stress indicators were analyzed in plasma samples, liver, or brain homogenates.

Total ROS, total protein carbonyl groups, reduced (GSH), oxidized glutathione (GSSG), antioxidant capacity (FRAP method), CAT, SOD, MPO were used to evaluate the oxidative stress process. The inflammation process was evaluated clinically by the measurement of posterior paw edema formation and leukocyte migration in the knee cartilages (a known phenomenon encountered in both patients and arthritic rats). The results showed that GP treatment positively influenced the oxidative stress parameter, most of them being normal or close to normal levels as compared to the control group. The same positive effect was observed in the inflammation process. The GP extract reduced or delayed the paw edema as compared to control arthritic rats. Also, the GP administration in arthritic rats reduced the polymorphonuclear leukocytes infiltration in the femorotibial joint cavities, in a similar way to the effect produced by ibuprofen administration (Gonçalves et al. 2017).

## *In Vivo* – Human Studies

Although several studies are trying to elucidate the antioxidant and anti-inflammatory effect of GP in various methods, most of them have inconclusive results that need further studies. This might be the reason why *in vivo* human studies are very rare. In total 6 studies were identified, out of which three included patients involving metabolic syndrome while two included healthy volunteers (Table 5).

The study conducted by Annunziata et al., (2019) investigated the effect of GP extract of a commercial product (Taurisolo®) in reducing the serum level of Trimethylamine N-oxide (TMAO) in humans. Considering that TMAO is a key factor for oxidative stress and CVD, they have investigated the effect of GP administration on TMAO levels in a cross-over, randomized, placebo-controlled study. After 4 weeks of administration (300 mg Taurisolo® containing 136 µg/g resveratrol), the TMAO serum level was significantly lower in the GP group as compared to the placebo group (63,6% vs. 0,54%, respectively, p <0,0001) (Annunziata et al. 2019). Because Resveratrol was the major compound in the GP extract, the bioavailability and pharmacokinetic studies were performed in relationship with Resveratrol. Knowing that TMAO is produced after trimethylamine (TMA) hepatic oxidation by Flavin-containing monooxygenase-3 (FMO3) (7.8) (Annunziata et al. 2019) and is involved in redox reaction (electron acceptor in bacteria), the authors of this study considered that polyphenols identified in GP extract can directly reduce TMAO to TMA. This study is also important because the authors gavc ideas of GP incorporation into a nutraceutical product. They showed that encapsulation in an acid-resistant matrix may improve intestinal bioavailability. Although improvement of TMAO levels was achieved within this study, more investigation is needed with a larger sample size and a longer period of administration on patients with different diseases.

The study conducted by Urquiaga et al., (2015) investigated the effect of GP flour on blood pressure, protein damage, and fasting glucose level in a randomized controlled clinical trial. They started with the hypothesis that red GP flour intake can reduce metabolic syndrome in humans. The study included 38 patients having at least one component of metabolic syndrome and they received red GP flour for 16 weeks. The GP flour had the TPC of 41 mg GAE/ g, total anthocyanin of 1.49 mg cyaniding 3-glucoside/ g, and antioxidant capacity of 363 μmoles TE/g as determined by ORAC assay. Out of this extract, the patients received 20g, summing 822 mg polyphenols with an ORAC of 7258 μmoles TE/g (Urquiaga et al. 2015). Besides the effect of GP on different metabolic factors, glucose tolerance test, glycosylated hemoglobin, the antioxidant capacity (total radical trapping potential - TRAP and DPPH), and proteins oxidative damage (carbonyl proteins groups) were also investigated. GP flour had a positive effect on systolic and diastolic blood pressure and fasting glucose levels. Also, the group fed with GP had the γ-tocopherol and δ-tocopherol plasma levels significantly increased while the carbonyl group, significantly decreased. Still, there was no significant difference for HDL cholesterol, triglycerides waist circumference, vitamin C, and total antioxidant capacity in and between groups

(Urquiaga et al. 2015). It would be interesting to see the effect of GP administration on a longer period.

More recently, the same author Urquiaga et al., (2018) investigated the effect of red GP flour, included in the preparation of beef burgers, on plasma antioxidant levels, oxidative damage, and fasting glucose. This time, the study took place over three months, including 27 male patients. As in the previous study, the patients had different metabolic syndrome components. The GP supplementation was made via a beef burger containing 7% GP flour. In this way, a daily constant administration of 3.5% fiber and 1.2 mg GAE/g of polyphenols was assured for the first month (Urquiaga et al. 2018). Again, metabolic syndrome components, oxidative stress damage (MDA, advanced oxidation protein products - AOPPs and oxidized low-density lipoproteins - oxLDLs), and plasma antioxidant activity (DPPH, vitamin E, and vitamin C) were investigated. As expected, GP supplementation significantly reduced glycemia but did not affect high blood pressure, triglycerides, low HDL cholesterol, or metabolic syndrome. This time Vitamin C content was increased, but Vitamin E, $\alpha$, and $\gamma$ tocopherols which are important antioxidants, did not change in a significant matter during the study. Still, GP-burger consumption had a positive effect in significantly decreasing AOPP and oxLDL levels. Vitamin E and MDA levels showed no significant changes. Also, a significant decrease was observed for DPPH radical scavenging activity and uric acid level. The authors assumed that these parameters were diminished during the period of GP enriched burger consumption because of its ability to reduce oxidative injury as expressed by the AOPP and oxLDL analyses (Urquiaga et al. 2018).

Although the consumption of GP as such, as ingredients in different foods or as nutraceuticals seems to have promising results on positive modulation of the pathophysiological processes like inflammation and oxidative stress associated with various chronic diseases, more studies are needed.

**Table 5. *In vivo* evidence-based use of grape pomace in human**

| Source | Models | Mechanism of action | References |
|---|---|---|---|
| *V. vinifera* L.<br>GP Cabernet sauvignon | 27 subjects in a clinical, placebo-controlled trial | • antioxidant effects demonstrated by:<br>• increased serum Vitamin C levels<br>• decreased serum uric acid levels<br>• significantly decreased DPPH radical activity<br>• decreased oxidative damage markers: AOPP and oxLDL | (Urquiaga et al. 2018) |
| Korean GP<br>*V. vinifera* L. + Omija fruits (*S. chinensis* Baillon) | 76 obese subjects in a randomized, double-blind, placebo-controlled trial | • antioxidant effects demonstrated by:<br>• significant increase of SOD activity in erythrocytes<br>• significant elevated GSH-Px and GR activities<br>• significant decrease of erythrocytic TBARS and $H_2O_2$ concentrations<br>• anti-inflammatory effects by decreasing serum IL-1β, IL-6, and TNF-α | (Han et al. 2016) |
| *V. vinifera L.*GP *Cabernet Sauvignon-* Maipo Valley, Chile | 29 male participants (at least one metabolic syndrome component) in a prospective, controlled, randomized, parallel-group trial | • decreased the damages of the proteins due to oxidative stress<br>• decreased DPPH radical activity | (Urquiaga et al. 2015) |
| *V. vinifera L.*GP *Aglianico-* Italy | 20 healthy subjects in a randomized, placebo-controlled, cross-over trial | • significantly reduced TMAO (a risk factor for cardiovascular disease, atherosclerosis) levels | (Annunziata et al. 2019) |
| Lyophilized grape powder | 44 women (pre-and postmenopausal) in a crossover, single-blind study | • decreased LDL-C and TG, apoB, apoE<br>• decreased TNF-α (anti-inflammatory effect)<br>• decreased urinary isoprostane (anti-oxidative effect) | (Zern et al. 2005) |

| Source | Models | Mechanism of action | References |
|---|---|---|---|
| Grape polyphenol powder | 24 men (MetS) in a randomized, double-blind, crossover study | • reduced sICAM-1 (anti-inflammatory effect)<br>• a low positive association between changes of sVCAM-1 (pro-inflammatory) and decreased SBP<br>• a low negative association between changes of SPB and NOx | (Barona et al. 2012) |

Abbreviations: AOPP - advanced oxidation protein product; apoB – Apolipoprotein B (main component of LDL-C); apoE – apolipoprotein E (involved in metabolism of fats); DPPH - 2,2-diphenyl-1-picryl - hydrazyl-hydrate; GR - glutathione reductase; GSH-Px - glutathione-paraoxonase; H2O2 - hydrogen peroxide (oxidative stress-inducing substance); IL-10 – interleukin-10; IL-1β – interleukin-1β; LDL – low-density lipoprotein; LDL-C - Low-density lipoprotein Cholesterol; MetS – Metabolic Syndrome; NOx - The total plasma nitrite + nitrate; oxLDL - oxidized low-density lipoprotein; SBP- systolic blood pressure; sICAM-1 - Soluble intercellular adhesion molecule-1; SOD - superoxide dismutase; sVCAM-1 - soluble vascular cell adhesion molecule-1; TBARS - thiobarbituric reactive substances; TG – triglyceride; TMAO – trimethylamine N-oxide; TNF-α – Tumor necrosis factor alpha.

## CONCLUSION

GP proved so far, in the *in vitro* and on the animal *in vivo* studies that it is a promising candidate to fight against oxidative stress and inflammation. Still, because there are also several contradictory studies, more research is needed to elucidate GP's molecular mechanism and to provide more scientific evidence. These can lead towards its safe and efficient use in developing different formulations, like nutraceuticals designed for disease prevention. Because the few existing *in vivo* human studies showed promising results, they should be continued, broadening their research spectrum. Besides GP's effect on different diseases, studies should also be oriented towards its safety, pharmacokinetics, pharmacodynamics, toxicity, and drug interaction effects.

## References

Abou Samra, Mario, Veronica Sanda Chedea, Anastasios Economou, Antony Calokerinos, and Panagiotis Kefalas. 2011. "Antioxidant/ Prooxidant Properties of Model Phenolic Compounds: Part I. Studies on Equimolar Mixtures by Chemiluminescence and Cyclic Voltammetry." *Food Chemistry* 125 (2): 622–29. https://doi.org/ 10.1016/j.foodchem.2010.08.076.

Abudukelimu, Abulikemu, Matteo Barberis, Frank A. Redegeld, Nilgun Sahin, and Hans V. Westerhoff. 2018. "Predictable Irreversible Switching between Acute and Chronic Inflammation." *Frontiers in Immunology* 9 (AUG): 1596. https://doi.org/10.3389/fimmu.2018. 01596.

Alam, Md Nur, Nusrat Jahan Bristi, and Md Rafiquzzaman. 2013. "Review on in Vivo and in Vitro Methods Evaluation of Antioxidant Activity." *Saudi Pharmaceutical Journal*. Elsevier. https://doi.org/10.1016/j.jsps.2012.05.002.

Ambade, Aditya, and Pranoti Mandrekar. 2012. "Oxidative Stress and Inflammation: Essential Partners in Alcoholic Liver Disease." *International Journal of Hepatology* 2012: 1–9. https://doi.org/10. 1155/2012/853175.

Annunziata, Giuseppe, Maria Maisto, Connie Schisano, Roberto Ciampaglia, Viviana Narciso, Gian Carlo Tenore, and Ettore Novellino. 2019. "Effects of Grape Pomace Polyphenolic Extract (Taurisolo ®) in Reducing Tmao Serum Levels in Humans: Preliminary Results from a Randomized, Placebo-Controlled, Cross-over Study." *Nutrients* 11 (1): 139. https://doi.org/10.3390/ nu11010139.

Antoniolli, Andrea, Ariel R. Fontana, Patricia Piccoli, and Rubén Bottini. 2015. "Characterization of Polyphenols and Evaluation of Antioxidant Capacity in Grape Pomace of the Cv. Malbec." *Food Chemistry* 178: 172–78. https://doi.org/10.1016/j.foodchem. 2015.01.082.

Aruoma, Okezie I. 2003. "Methodological Considerations for Characterizing Potential Antioxidant Actions of Bioactive Components in Plant Foods." In *Mutation Research - Fundamental and Molecular Mechanisms of Mutagenesis*, 523–524:9–20. https://doi.org/10.1016/S0027-5107(02)00317-2.

Asmat, Ullah, Khan Abad, and Khan Ismail. 2016. "Diabetes Mellitus and Oxidative Stress—A Concise Review." *Saudi Pharmaceutical Journal*. Elsevier B. V. https://doi.org/10.1016/j.jsps.2015.03.013.

Ayuda-Durán, Begoña, Susana González-Manzano, Irene Gil-Sánchez, M. Victoria Moreno-Arribas, Begoña Bartolomé, Marisa Sanz-Buenhombre, Alberto Guadarrama, Celestino Santos-Buelga, and Ana M. González-Paramás. 2019. "Antioxidant Characterization and Biological Effects of Grape Pomace Extracts Supplementation in Caenorhabditis Elegans." *Foods* 8 (2). https://doi.org/10.3390/foods8020075.

Balea, Ştefania Silvia, Alina Elena Pârvu, Nastasia Pop, Fernando Zamora Marín, and Marcel Pârvu. 2018. "Polyphenolic Compounds, Antioxidant, and Cardioprotective Effects of Pomace Extracts from Fetească Neagră Cultivar." *Oxidative Medicine and Cellular Longevity* 2018 (March): 1–11. https://doi.org/10.1155/2018/8194721.

Ball, Stephen L., Derek A. Mann, Janet A. Wilson, and Andrew J. Fisher. 2016. "The Role of the Fibroblast in Inflammatory Upper Airway Conditions." *American Journal of Pathology*. Elsevier Inc. https://doi.org/10.1016/j.ajpath.2015.09.020.

Barona, Jacqueline, Juan C. Aristizabal, Christopher N. Blesso, Jeff S. Volek, and Maria Luz Fernandez. 2012. "Grape Polyphenols Reduce Blood Pressure and Increase Flow-Mediated Vasodilation in Men with Metabolic Syndrome." *The Journal of Nutrition* 142 (9): 1626–32. https://doi.org/10.3945/jn.112.162743.

Birben, E., Umit Murat Sahiner, Cansin Sackesen, Serpil Erzurum, and Omer Kalayci. 2012. "Oxidative Stress and Antioxidant Defense." *World Allergy Organization Journal*. BioMed Central Ltd. https://doi.org/10.1097/WOX.0b013e3182439613.

Biswas, Subrata K., Elisa B. Peixoto, Denise S. Souza, and Jose B. Lopes de Faria. 2008. "Hypertension Increases Pro-Oxidant Generation and Decreases Antioxidant Defense in the Kidney in Early Diabetes." *American Journal of Nephrology* 28 (1): 133–42. https://doi.org/10.1159/000109993.

Biswas, Subrata Kumar. 2016. "Does the Interdependence between Oxidative Stress and Inflammation Explain the Antioxidant Paradox?" *Oxidative Medicine and Cellular Longevity* 2016 (January): 1–9. https://doi.org/10.1155/2016/5698931.

Boussenna, Ahlem, Juliette Joubert-Zakeyh, Didier Fraisse, Bruno Pereira, Marie Paule Vasson, Odile Texier, and Catherine Felgines. 2016. "Dietary Supplementation with a Low Dose of Polyphenol-Rich Grape Pomace Extract Prevents Dextran Sulfate Sodium-Induced Colitis in Rats." *Journal of Medicinal Food* 19 (8): 755–58. https://doi.org/10.1089/jmf.2015.0124.

Bralley, Eve E., James L. Hargrove, Phillip Greenspan, and Diane K. Hartle. 2007. "Topical Anti-Inflammatory Activities of Vitis Rotundifolia (Muscadine Grape) Extracts in the Tetradecanoylphorbol Acetate Model of Ear Inflammation." *Journal of Medicinal Food* 10 (4): 636–42. https://doi.org/10.1089/jmf.2006.244.

Cervantes Gracia, Karla, Daniel Llanas-Cornejo, and Holger Husi. 2017. "CVD and Oxidative Stress." *Journal of Clinical Medicine* 6 (2): 22. https://doi.org/10.3390/jcm6020022.

Chatterjee, Shampa. 2016. *Oxidative Stress, Inflammation, and Disease. Oxidative Stress and Biomaterials*. Elsevier Inc. https://doi.org/10.1016/B978-0-12-803269-5.00002-4.

Chedea, Veronica Sanda, Laurentiu Mihai Palade, Daniela Eliza Marin, Rodica Stefania Pelmus, Mihaela Habeanu, Mircea Catalin Rotar, Mihail Alexandru Gras, Gina Cecilia Pistol, and Ionelia Taranu. 2018. "Intestinal Absorption and Antioxidant Activity of Grape Pomace Polyphenols." *Nutrients* 10 (5). https://doi.org/10.3390/nu10050588.

Chedea, Veronica Sanda, Laurentiu Mihai Palade, Rodica Stefania Pelmus, Catalin Dragomir, and Ionelia Taranu. 2019. "Red Grape Pomace Rich in Polyphenols Diet Increases the Antioxidant Status in Key Organs— Kidneys, Liver, and Spleen of Piglets." *Animals* 9 (4): 149. https://doi.org/10.3390/ani9040149.

Chedea, Veronica Sanda, Rodica Stefania Pelmus, Cristina Lazar, Gina Cecilia Pistol, Loredana Georgeta Calin, Smaranda Mariana Toma, Catalin Dragomir, and Ionelia Taranu. 2019. "Effects of a Diet Containing Dried Grape Pomace on Blood Metabolites and Milk Composition of Dairy Cows." *Statistical Field Theor* 53 (9): 1689–99.

Chedea, Veronica Sanda, and Raluca Maria Pop. 2018. "Total Polyphenols Content and Antioxidant DPPH Assays on Biological Samples." In *Polyphenols in Plants: Isolation, Purification and Extract Preparation*, 169–84.

Chen, Linlin, Huidan Deng, Hengmin Cui, Jing Fang, Zhicai Zuo, Junliang Deng, Yinglun Li, Xun Wang, and Ling Zhao. 2018. "Inflammatory Responses and Inflammation-Associated Diseases in Organs." *Oncotarget. Impact Journals LLC.* https://doi.org/10.18632/oncotarget.23208.

Cho, Su Jung, Hye Jin Kim, Ji Young Choi, Eun Young Kwon, Ye Jin Kim, Ri Ryu, Myung Sook Choi, and Yong Bok Park. 2017. "Low-Dose Grape Pomace and Omija Fruit Extract Is More Effective than High-Dose in Lowering Oxidative Stress and Fat-Pad Mass in Db/Db Mice." *Food Science and Biotechnology* 26 (6): 1709–14. https://doi.org/10.1007/s10068-017-0227-7.

Choueiri, Lamis, Veronica Sanda Chedea, Antony Calokerinos, and Panagiotis Kefalas. 2012. "Antioxidant/pro-Oxidant Properties of Model Phenolic Compounds. Part II: Studies on Mixtures of Polyphenols at Different Molar Ratios by Chemiluminescence and LC-MS." *Food Chemistry* 133 (3): 1039–44. https://doi.org/10.1016/j.foodchem.2012.01.057.

Correia, Ana C., Fernanda Cosme, and António M. Jordão. 2018. "The Impact of Modern Winemaking Technologies on Phenolic

Composition of Red Wines." *A Closer Look at Grapes, Wines, and Winemaking*, no. January: 129–72.

Costa, Gislaine N. S., Renata V. Tonon, Caroline Mellinger-Silva, Melicia C. Galdeano, Marcello Iacomini, Manuela C. P. A. Santiago, Eveline L. Almeida, and Suely P. Freitas. 2019. "Grape Seed Pomace as a Valuable Source of Antioxidant Fibers." *Journal of the Science of Food and Agriculture* 99 (10): 4593–4601. https://doi.org/10.1002/jsfa.9698.

Cronkite, David Alex, and Tara M. Strutt. 2018. "The Regulation of Inflammation by Innate and Adaptive Lymphocytes." *Journal of Immunology Research* 2018: 1–14. https://doi.org/10.1155/2018/1467538.

Deng, Qian, Michael H. Penner, and Yanyun Zhao. 2011. "Chemical Composition of Dietary Fiber and Polyphenols of Five Different Varieties of Wine Grape Pomace Skins." *Food Research International* 44 (9): 2712–20. https://doi.org/10.1016/J.FOODRES.2011.05.026.

Denny, C., J. G. Lazarini, M. Franchin, P. S. Melo, G. E. Pereira, A. P. Massarioli, I. A.M. Moreno, J. A.R. Paschoal, S. M. Alencar, and P. L. Rosalen. 2014. "Bioprospection of Petit Verdot Grape Pomace as a Source of Anti-Inflammatory Compounds." *Journal of Functional Foods* 8 (1): 292–300. https://doi.org/10.1016/j.jff.2014.03.016.

Dwyer, Kyle, Farah Hosseinian, and Michel Rod. 2014. "The Market Potential of Grape Waste Alternatives." *Journal of Food Research* 3 (2). https://doi.org/10.5539/jfr.v3n2p91.

Espinosa-Diez, Cristina, Verónica Miguel, Daniela Mennerich, Thomas Kietzmann, Patricia Sánchez-Pérez, Susana Cadenas, and Santiago Lamas. 2015. "Antioxidant Responses and Cellular Adjustments to Oxidative Stress." *Redox Biology*. Elsevier B. V. https://doi.org/10.1016/j.redox.2015.07.008.

Fontana, Ariel R., Andrea Antoniolli, and Rubén Bottini. 2013. "Grape Pomace as a Sustainable Source of Bioactive Compounds: Extraction, Characterization, and Biotechnological Applications of

Phenolics." *Journal of Agricultural and Food Chemistry* 61 (38): 8987–9003. https://doi.org/10.1021/jf402586f.

Gonçalves, Geferson A., Andréia A. Soares, Rúbia C. G. Correa, Lillian Barros, Charles W. I. Haminiuk, Rosane M. Peralta, Isabel C. F. R. Ferreira, and Adelar Bracht. 2017. "Merlot Grape Pomace Hydroalcoholic Extract Improves the Oxidative and Inflammatory States of Rats with Adjuvant-Induced Arthritis." *Journal of Functional Foods* 33: 408–18. https://doi.org/10.1016/j.jff.2017.04.009.

González-Centeno, María Reyes, Michael Jourdes, Antoni Femenia, Susana Simal, Carmen Rosselló, and Pierre Louis Teissedre. 2013. "Characterization of Polyphenols and Antioxidant Potential of White Grape Pomace Byproducts (Vitis Vinifera L.)." *Journal of Agricultural and Food Chemistry* 61 (47): 11579–87. https://doi.org/10.1021/jf403168k.

Goutzourelas, N., D. Stagos, N. Demertzis, P. Mavridou, H. Karterolioti, S. Georgadakis, E. Kerasioti, et al. 2014. "Effects of Polyphenolic Grape Extract on the Oxidative Status of Muscle and Endothelial Cells." *Human and Experimental Toxicology* 33 (11): 1099–1112. https://doi.org/10.1177/0960327114533575.

Habeanu, Mihaela, Nicoleta A. Lefter, Mariana Ropota, Veronica S. Chedea, Anca Gheorghe, Smaranda M. Toma, Georgeta Ciurescu, and Cătălin Dragomir. 2015. "Dried Grape Pomace Influenced Fatty Acids Composition of Longissimus Dorsi Muscle and Plasma Polyphenols Spectrum in Finishing Pigs." *Indian Journal of Animal Sciences* 85 (7): 786–89.

Han, Hye Jin, Un Ju Jung, Hye Jin Kim, Su Jung Cho, Ae Hyang Kim, Youngji Han, and Myung Sook Choi. 2016. "Combined Supplementation with Grape Pomace and Omija Fruit Ethanol Extracts Dose-Dependently Improves Body Composition, Plasma Lipid Profiles, Inflammatory Status, and Antioxidant Capacity in Overweight and Obese Subjects." *Journal of Medicinal Food* 19 (2): 170–80. https://doi.org/10.1089/jmf.2015.3488.

Hogan, Shelly, Corene Canning, Shi Sun, Xiuxiu Sun, and Kequan Zhou. 2010. "Effects of Grape Pomace Antioxidant Extract on Oxidative Stress and Inflammation in Diet Induced Obese Mice." *Journal of Agricultural and Food Chemistry* 58 (21): 11250–56. https://doi.org/10.1021/jf102759e.

José Jara-Palacios, M., Dolores Hernanz, M. Luisa Escudero-Gilete, and Francisco J. Heredia. 2014. "Antioxidant Potential of White Grape Pomaces: Phenolic Composition and Antioxidant Capacity Measured by Spectrophotometric and Cyclic Voltammetry Methods." *Food Research International* 66: 150–57. https://doi.org/10.1016/j.foodres.2014.09.009.

Kallithraka, S., M. I. Salacha, and I. Tzourou. 2009. "Changes in Phenolic Composition and Antioxidant Activity of White Wine during Bottle Storage: Accelerated Browning Test versus Bottle Storage." *Food Chemistry* 113 (2): 500–505. https://doi.org/10.1016/j.foodchem.2008.07.083.

Kaneko, Masahiro, Manabu Kanesaka, Miho Yoneyama, Takanari Tominaga, Emilio Jirillo, and Yoshio Kumazawa. 2010. "Inhibitory Effects of Fermented Grape Marc from Vitis Vinifera Negroamaro on Antigen-Induced Degranulation." *Immunopharmacology and Immunotoxicology* 32 (3): 454–61. https://doi.org/10.3109/08923970903513139.

Kasote, Deepak M., Surendra S. Katyare, Mahabaleshwar V. Hegde, and Hanhong Bae. 2015. "Significance of Antioxidant Potential of Plants and Its Relevance to Therapeutic Applications." *International Journal of Biological Sciences*. Ivyspring International Publisher. https://doi.org/10.7150/ijbs.12096.

Khansari, Nemat, Yadollah Shakiba, and Mahdi Mahmoudi. 2009. "Chronic Inflammation and Oxidative Stress as a Major Cause of Age-Related Diseases and Cancer." *Recent Patents on Inflammation & Allergy Drug Discovery* 3 (1): 73–80. https://doi.org/10.2174/187221309787158371.

Koutelidakis, Antonios. 2016. "Grape Pomace: A Challenging Renewable Resource of Bioactive Phenolic Compounds with

Diversified Health Benefits." *MOJ Food Processing & Technology* 3 (1). https://doi.org/10.15406/mojfpt.2016.03.00065.

Ky, Isabelle, Alan Crozier, Gérard Cros, and Pierre-Louis Teissedre. 2014. "Polyphenols Composition of Wine and Grape Sub-Products and Potential Effects on Chronic Diseases." *Nutrition and Aging* 2: 165–77. https://doi.org/10.3233/NUA-130027.

Ky, Isabelle, Bénédicte Lorrain, Natallia Kolbas, Alan Crozier, and Pierre Louis Teissedre. 2014. "Wine By-Products: Phenolic Characterization and Antioxidant Activity Evaluation of Grapes and Grape Pomaces from Six Different French Grape Varieties." *Molecules* 19 (1): 482–506. https://doi.org/10.3390/molecules19010482.

Lazze, M. C., R. Pizzala, P. Gutiérrez Pecharromán, F. J. Gatón Garnica, J. M. Antolín Rodríguez, N. Fabris, and L. Bianchi. 2009. "Grape Waste Extract Obtained by Supercritical Fluid Extraction Contains Bioactive Antioxidant Molecules and Induces Antiproliferative Effects in Human Colon Adenocarcinoma Cells." *Journal of Medicinal Food* 12 (3): 561–68.

Lingua, Mariana S., María P. Fabani, Daniel A. Wunderlin, and María V. Baroni. 2016. "In Vivo Antioxidant Activity of Grape, Pomace and Wine from Three Red Varieties Grown in Argentina: Its Relationship to Phenolic Profile." *Journal of Functional Foods* 20: 332–45. https://doi.org/10.1016/j.jff.2015.10.034.

Lobo, V., A. Patil, A. Phatak, and N. Chandra. 2010. "Free Radicals, Antioxidants and Functional Foods: Impact on Human Health." *Pharmacognosy Reviews*. Wolters Kluwer -- Medknow Publications. https://doi.org/10.4103/0973-7847.70902.

Luchian, C. E., V. V. Cotea, L. Vlase, A. M. Toiu, L. C. Colibaba, I. E. Răschip, G. Nadăş, A.M. Gheldiu, C. Tuchiluş, and L. Rotaru. 2019. "Antioxidant and Antimicrobial Effects of Grape Pomace Extracts." *BIO Web of Conferences* 15: 04006. https://doi.org/10.1051/bioconf/20191504006.

Maluf, Daniela F., Melissa M. Gonçalves, Rebeca W. O. D. Angelo, Ana B. Girassol, Ana P. Tulio, Yasmine M. Pupo, and Paulo V. Farago.

2018. "Cytoprotection of Antioxidant Biocompounds from Grape Pomace: Further Exfoliant Phytoactive Ingredients for Cosmetic Products." *Cosmetics* 5 (46): 1–11. https://doi.org/10.3390/cosmetics 5030046.

Marchante, Lourdes, Sergio Gómez Alonso, María Elena Alañón, María Soledad Pérez-Coello, and María Consuelo Díaz-Maroto. 2018. "Natural Extracts from Fresh and Oven-Dried Winemaking by-Products as Valuable Source of Antioxidant Compounds." *Food Science and Nutrition* 6 (6): 1564–74. https://doi.org/10. 1002/fsn3.697.

Melo, Priscilla Siqueira, Adna Prado Massarioli, Carina Denny, Luciana Ferracini Dos Santos, Marcelo Franchin, Giuliano Elias Pereira, Thais Maria Ferreira De Souza Vieira, Pedro Luiz Rosalen, and Severino Matias De Alencar. 2015. "Winery By-Products: Extraction Optimization, Phenolic Composition, and Cytotoxic Evaluation to Act as a New Source of Scavenging of Reactive Oxygen Species." *Food Chemistry* 181: 160–69. https://doi.org/10.1016/j.foodchem. 2015.02.087.

Messina, Concetta Maria, Simona Manuguerra, Giuseppe Catalano, Rosaria Arena, Massimo Cocchi, Maria Morghese, Lucia Montenegro, and Andrea Santulli. 2019. "Green Biotechnology for Valorisation of Residual Biomasses in Nutraceutic Sector: Characterization and Extraction of Bioactive Compounds from Grape Pomace and Evaluation of the Protective Effects in Vitro." *Natural Product Research*, June, 1–6. https://doi.org/10.1080/14786419. 2019.1619727.

Nile, Shivraj Hariram, S. H. Kim, Eun Young Ko, and Se Won Park. 2013. "Polyphenolic Contents and Antioxidant Properties of Different Grape (V. Vinifera, V. Labrusca, and V. Hybrid) Cultivars." *BioMed Research International* 2013. https://doi.org/10. 1155/2013/718065.

Nishiumi, Shin, Rie Mukai, Takashi Ichiyanagi, and Hitoshi Ashida. 2012. "Suppression of Lipopolysaccharide and Galactosamine-Induced Hepatic Inflammation by Red Grape Pomace." In *Journal of*

*Agricultural and Food Chemistry*, 60:9315–20. https://doi.org/10.1021/jf302298n.

OIV, and International Organisation of Vine and Wine. 2019. “2019 Statistical Report on World Vitiviniculture.” *2019 Statistical Report on World Vitiviniculture*, 23. https://doi.org/64/19/6835 [pii]\n 10.1158/ =0008-5472.CAN-04-1678.

Ozcan, Ayla, and Metin Ogun. 2015. “Biochemistry of Reactive Oxygen and Nitrogen Species.” In *Basic Principles and Clinical Significance of Oxidative Stress*. InTech. https://doi.org/10.5772/61193.

Paiva, Claudia N., and Marcelo T. Bozza. 2014. “Are Reactive Oxygen Species Always Detrimental to Pathogens?” *Antioxidants and Redox Signaling*. Mary Ann Liebert, Inc. https://doi.org/10.1089/ars.2013.5447.

Patel, Manisha. 2016. “Targeting Oxidative Stress in Central Nervous System Disorders.” *Trends in Pharmacological Sciences*. Elsevier Ltd. https://doi.org/10.1016/j.tips.2016.06.007.

Pistol, Gina Cecilia, Daniela Eliza Marin, Catalin Dragomir, and Ionelia Taranu. 2019. “Synbiotic Combination of Prebiotic Grape Pomace Extract and Probiotic Lactobacillus Sp. Reduced Important Intestinal Inflammatory Markers and in-Depth Signalling Mediators in Lipopolysaccharide-Treated Caco-2 Cells.” *British Journal of Nutrition* 121 (3): 291–305. https://doi.org/10.1017/S0007114518003410.

Pop, Raluca Maria, Adrian Pavel Trifa, Ada Popolo, Veronica Sanda Chedea, Claudia Militaru, Ioana Corina Bocsan, and Anca Dana Buzoianu. 2020. “Nigella Sativa : Valuable Perspective in the Management of Chronic Diseases.” *Iran J Basic Med Sci* 23 (2): 1–15.

Posadino, Anna Maria, Grazia Biosa, Hatem Zayed, Haissam Abou-Saleh, Annalisa Cossu, Gheyath K. Nasrallah, Roberta Giordo, et al. 2018. “Protective Effect of Cyclically Pressurized Solid-Liquid Extraction Polyphenols from Cagnulari Grape Pomace on Oxidative Endothelial Cell Death.” *Molecules* 23 (9). https://doi.org/10.3390/molecules23092105.

Ramírez-Prieto, María Teresa, Francisco García-Río, and José Villamor. 2006. "Role of Oxidative Stress in Respiratory Diseases and Its Monitoring." *Medicina Clinica* 127 (10): 386–96. https://doi.org/10.1157/13092440.

Rasines-Perea, Zuriñe, Isabelle Ky, Gérard Cros, Alan Crozier, Pierre-Louis Teissedre, Zuriñe Rasines-Perea, Isabelle Ky, Gérard Cros, Alan Crozier, and Pierre-Louis Teissedre. 2018. "Grape Pomace: Antioxidant Activity, Potential Effect against Hypertension and Metabolites Characterization after Intake." *Diseases* 6 (3): 60. https://doi.org/10.3390/diseases6030060.

Ratnasooriya, Charmila C., and H. P.Vasantha Rupasinghe. 2012. "Extraction of Phenolic Compounds from Grapes and Their Pomace Using β-Cyclodextrin." *Food Chemistry* 134 (2): 625–31. https://doi.org/10.1016/j.foodchem.2012.02.014.

Reuter, Simone, Subash C. Gupta, Madan M. Chaturvedi, and Bharat B. Aggarwal. 2010. "Oxidative Stress, Inflammation, and Cancer: How Are They Linked?" *Free Radical Biology and Medicine*. NIH Public Access. https://doi.org/10.1016/j.freeradbiomed.2010.09.006.

Rho, Kyoung Ah, and Mi Kyung Kim. 2006. "Effects of Different Grape Formulations on Antioxidative Capacity, Lipid Peroxidation and Oxidative DNA Damage in Aged Rats." *Journal of Nutritional Science and Vitaminology* 52 (1): 33–46. https://doi.org/10.3177/jnsv.52.33.

Rivera, Katherine, Francisca Salas-Pérez, Guadalupe Echeverría, Inés Urquiaga, Sara Dicenta, Druso Pérez, Paula de la Cerda, et al. 2019. "Red Wine Grape Pomace Attenuates Atherosclerosis and Myocardial Damage and Increases Survival in Association with Improved Plasma Antioxidant Activity in a Murine Model of Lethal Ischemic Heart Disease." *Nutrients* 11 (9): 2135. https://doi.org/10.3390/nu11092135.

Rodríguez-Morgado, B., M. Candiracci, C. Santa-María, E. Revilla, B. Gordillo, J. Parrado, and A. Castaño. 2015. "Obtaining from Grape Pomace an Enzymatic Extract with Anti-Inflammatory Properties."

*Plant Foods for Human Nutrition* 70 (1): 42–49. https://doi.org/10.1007/s11130-014-0459-0.

Rodriguez-Rodriguez, Rosalia, Maria Luisa Justo, Carmen Maria Claro, Elisabet Vila, Juan Parrado, Maria Dolores Herrera, and Maria Alvarez De Sotomayor. 2012. "Endothelium-Dependent Vasodilator and Antioxidant Properties of a Novel Enzymatic Extract of Grape Pomace from Wine Industrial Waste." *Food Chemistry* 135 (3): 1044–51. https://doi.org/10.1016/j.foodchem.2012.05.089.

Rodriguez Lanzi, Cecilia, Diahann Jeanette Perdicaro, Andrea Antoniolli, Ariel Ramón Fontana, Roberto Miguel Miatello, Rubén Bottini, and Marcela Alejandra Vazquez Prieto. 2016. "Grape Pomace and Grape Pomace Extract Improve Insulin Signaling in High-Fat-Fructose Fed Rat-Induced Metabolic Syndrome." *Food and Function* 7 (3): 1544–53. https://doi.org/10.1039/c5fo01065a.

Ruberto, Giuseppe, Agatino Renda, Carmelo Daquino, Vincenzo Amico, Carmela Spatafora, Corrado Tringali, and Nunziatina De Tommasi. 2007. "Polyphenol Constituents and Antioxidant Activity of Grape Pomace Extracts from Five Sicilian Red Grape Cultivars." *Food Chemistry* 100 (1): 203–10. https://doi.org/10.1016/J.FOODCHEM.2005.09.041.

Sales, Nathalia F. F. de, Leandro Silva da Costa, Talita I. A. Carneiro, Daniela A. Minuzzo, Felipe L. Oliveira, Lourdes M. C. Cabral, Alexandre G. Torres, and Tatiana El-Bacha. 2018. "Molecules Anthocyanin-Rich Grape Pomace Extract (*Vitis Vinifera* L.) from Wine Industry Affects Mitochondrial Bioenergetics and Glucose Metabolism in Human Hepatocarcinoma HepG2 Cells." *Molecules* 23 (611): 1–17. https://doi.org/10.3390/molecules23030611.

Sáyago-Ayerdi, S. G., A. Brenes, A. Viveros, and I. Goñi. 2009. "Antioxidative Effect of Dietary Grape Pomace Concentrate on Lipid Oxidation of Chilled and Long-Term Frozen Stored Chicken Patties." *Meat Science* 83 (3): 528–33. https://doi.org/10.1016/j.meatsci.2009.06.038.

Schlesier, K., M. Harwat, V. Böhm, and R. Bitsch. 2002. "Assessment of Antioxidant Activity by Using Different in Vitro Methods." *Free*

*Radical Research* 36 (2): 177–87. https://doi.org/10.1080/10715760290006411.

Schwager, Simon, and Michael Detmar. 2019. "Inflammation and Lymphatic Function." *Frontiers in Immunology*. Frontiers Media S.A. https://doi.org/10.3389/fimmu.2019.00308.

Sousa, Eldina Castro, Ana Maria Athayde Uchôa-Thomaz, José Osvaldo Beserra Carioca, Selene Maia de Morais, Alessandro de Lima, Clécio Galvão Martins, Cristiane Duarte Alexandrino, et al. 2014. "Chemical Composition and Bioactive Compounds of Grape Pomace (Vitis Vinifera L.), Benitaka Variety, Grown in the Semiarid Region of Northeast Brazil." *Food Science and Technology* 34 (1): 135–42. https://doi.org/10.1590/S0101-20612014000100020.

Souza, Carine F., Matheus D. Baldissera, Sharine N. Descovi, Carla C. Zeppenfeld, Camila M. Verdi, Roberto C. V. Santos, Aleksandro S. da Silva, and Bernardo Baldisserotto. 2019. "Grape Pomace Flour Alleviates Pseudomonas Aeruginosa-Induced Hepatic Oxidative Stress in Grass Carp by Improving Antioxidant Defense." *Microbial Pathogenesis* 129 (April): 271–76. https://doi.org/10.1016/j.micpath.2019.02.024.

Tolve, Roberta, Gabriella Pasini, Fabiola Vignale, Fabio Favati, and Barbara Simonato. 2020. "Effect of Grape Pomace Addition on the Technological, Sensory, and Nutritional Properties of Durum Wheat Pasta." *Foods* 9 (3): 354. https://doi.org/10.3390/foods9030354.

Tominaga, Takanari, Kiichiro Kawaguchi, Manabu Kanesaka, Hideyuki Kawauchi, Emilio Jirillo, and Yoshio Kumazawa. 2010. "Suppression of Type-I Allergic Responses by Oral Administration of Grape Marc Fermented with Lactobacillus Plantarum." *Immunopharmacology and Immunotoxicology* 32 (4): 593–99. https://doi.org/10.3109/08923971003604786.

Urquiaga, Inés, Sonia D'Acuña, Druso Pérez, Sara Dicenta, Guadalupe Echeverría, Attilio Rigotti, and Federico Leighton. 2015. "Wine Grape Pomace Flour Improves Blood Pressure, Fasting Glucose and Protein Damage in Humans: A Randomized Controlled Trial."

*Biological Research* 48: 49. https://doi.org/10.1186/s40659-015-0040-9.

Urquiaga, Inés, Danitza Troncoso, Maria José Mackenna, Catalina Urzúa, Druso Pérez, Sara Dicenta, Paula María de la Cerda, et al. 2018. "The Consumption of Beef Burgers Prepared with Wine Grape Pomace Flour Improves Fasting Glucose, Plasma Antioxidant Levels, and Oxidative Damage Markers in Humans: A Controlled Trial." *Nutrients* 10 (10). https://doi.org/10.3390/nu10101388.

Velazquez-Caldelas, Tadeo Enrique, Sergio Antonio Alcalá-Corona, Jesús Espinal-Enríquez, and Enrique Hernandez-Lemus. 2019. "Unveiling the Link Between Inflammation and Adaptive Immunity in Breast Cancer." *Frontiers in Immunology* 10 (JAN): 56. https://doi.org/10.3389/fimmu.2019.00056.

Veskoukis, Aristidis S., Antonios Kyparos, Michalis G. Nikolaidis, Dimitrios Stagos, Nektarios Aligiannis, Maria Halabalaki, Konstantinos Chronis, Nikolaos Goutzourelas, Leandros Skaltsounis, and Dimitrios Kouretas. 2012. "The Antioxidant Effects of a Polyphenol-Rich Grape Pomace Extract in Vitro Do Not Correspond in Vivo Using Exercise as an Oxidant Stimulus." *Oxidative Medicine and Cellular Longevity* 2012. https://doi.org/10.1155/2012/185867.

Wood, Lisa G., Peter G. Gibson, and Manohar L. Garg. 2006. "A Review of the Methodology for Assessing in Vivo Antioxidant Capacity." *Journal of the Science of Food and Agriculture* 86 2057–66. https://doi.org/10.1002/jsfa.

Xia, Lanlan, Changmou Xu, Kunlun Huang, Jiang Lu, and Yali Zhang. 2019. "Evaluation of Phenolic Compounds, Antioxidant and Antiproliferative Activities of 31 Grape Cultivars with Different Genotypes." *Journal of Food Biochemistry* 43 (6): 1–13. https://doi.org/10.1111/jfbc.12626.

Xu, Yixiang, Sheanell Burton, Chyer Kim, and Edward Sismour. 2016. "Phenolic Compounds, Antioxidant, and Antibacterial Properties of Pomace Extracts from Four Virginia-Grown Grape Varieties." *Food Science and Nutrition* 4 (1): 125–33. https://doi.org/10.1002/fsn3.264.

Yu, Jianmei, and Mohamed Ahmedna. 2013. "Functional Components of Grape Pomace: Their Composition, Biological Properties and Potential Applications." *International Journal of Food Science and Technology* 48 (2): 221–37. https://doi.org/10.1111/j.1365-2621.2012.03197.x.

Zacharof, Myrto Panagiota. 2017. "Grape Winery Waste as Feedstock for Bioconversions: Applying the Biorefinery Concept." *Waste and Biomass Valorization*. Springer Netherlands. https://doi.org/10.1007/s12649-016-9674-2.

Zern, Tosca L., Richard J. Wood, Christine Greene, Kristy L. West, Yanzhu Liu, Dimple Aggarwal, Neil S. Shachter, and Maria Luz Fernandez. 2005. "Grape Polyphenols Exert a Cardioprotective Effect in Pre- and Postmenopausal Women by Lowering Plasma Lipids and Reducing Oxidative Stress." *The Journal of Nutrition* 135 (8): 1911–17. https://doi.org/10.1093/jn/135.8.1911.

In: Grape Pomace in Health …
Editor: Veronica Sanda Chedea ISBN: 978-1-68507-409-8


*Chapter 6*

# GRAPE POMACE AND CARDIOVASCULAR RISK FACTORS

***Octavia Sabin****
Department of Pharmacology, Toxicology and Clinical Pharmacology, "Iuliu Haţieganu" University of Medicine and Pharmacy, Cluj-Napoca, Romania

## ABSTRACT

Current studies show that nutrition can be considered a two-way road towards reducing or increasing the risk factors for several chronic conditions such as metabolic diseases, cardiovascular disease (CVD), and certain types of cancer. Worldwide, at the forefront, CVD remains the leading cause of mortality, with 26% out of total deaths. It was already demonstrated that diets low in saturated fat, salt, and cholesterol, with high intakes of fruit, vegetables and fish are protective factors against CVD. Grapes are a rich source of bioactive phenolic compounds and some of them have been associated with a reduction in CVD risk. Therefore, the chapter aims to review grape pomace effects on cardiovascular risk factors in both *in vivo* and *in vitro* studies. The

* Corresponding Author's E-mail: octaviasabin@gmail.com.

effects will be discussed starting from the molecular mechanisms of action of the main polyphenols found in the composition, focusing on the cellular effects that could influence the CVD risk factors: lipid profile, anti-atherosclerotic effect, antioxidant status, effects on blood pressure. The second part of the chapter discusses epidemiological and interventional studies in humans, comparing the results obtained on resveratrol, the most studied component, and different grape products, to highlight the idea that the observed beneficial effects are not due to a single component, but that it is a accumulation of effects of the grape as a whole.

## ABBREVIATIONS

| | |
|---|---|
| BP | Blood pressure |
| CRP | C reactive protein |
| CVD | Cardiovascular disease |
| DBP | diastolic blood pressure |
| ERR | estrogen-related receptor |
| eNOS | endothelial nitric oxide synthase |
| MAPK | mitogen-activated protein kinases |
| NF-κB | nuclear factor κB |
| NOS | NO synthase |
| NOX | NADPH oxidase |
| PGC-1 | peroxisome proliferator-activated receptor gamma coactivator-1 |
| RCT | randomized clinical trial |
| ROS | reactive oxygen species |
| SBP | systolic blood pressure |
| SIRT | sirtuin |
| TC | total cholesterol |
| TNF | tumour necrosis factor |
| UCP2 | Mitochondrial uncoupling protein 2 |

## INTRODUCTION

Cardiovascular disease (CVD) is the leading cause of morbidity and mortality, despite improvements in prevention and treatment over the last three decades. Types of CVD that involve atherosclerosis are characteristic of older adults and include coronary artery diseases (CAD), such as angina and myocardial infarction, stroke, heart failure, peripheral artery disease. Modifiable risk factors such as hypertension, smoking, diabetes mellitus, sedentary behavior, excessive weight, dyslipidemia, poor diet, high alcohol consumption, are involved in atherosclerosis progression and development of complications (WHO 2014) (Figure 1).

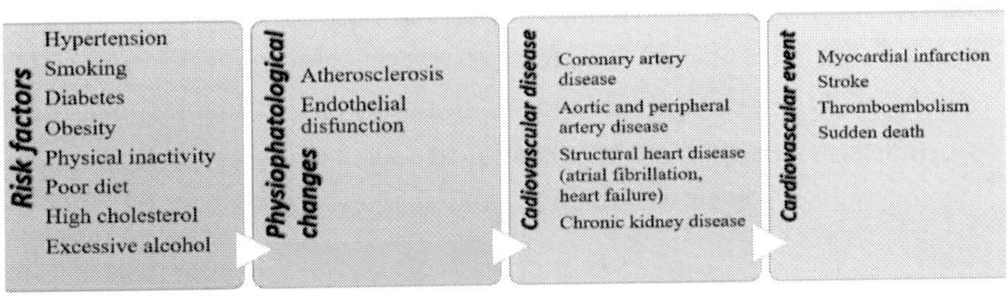


Figure 1. The spectrum of cardiovascular disease from risk factors to cardiovascular events.

Prevention is extremely effective. It is estimated that, by reducing modifiable risk factors, it is possible to reduce by at least 80% the incidence of CVDs, thus the burden of complications and poor outcomes (Piepoli 2016). CVD prevention is defined as a set of measures and recommendations to reduce the impact of CVDs, limiting the disabilities, and improving the outcomes. Some recommendations (e.g., lowering high blood pressure or stopping smoking) have strong evidence from multiple studies to be not only effective but also cost-efficient, while for others the indisputable evidence is still being built. Dietary factors play an important role in the development of CVD and its risk factors and may contribute to the geographic differences in CVD morbidity and mortality (Piepoli 2016). These measures are taken at the population level by promoting healthy lifestyle behaviors or at an individual level, targeting individual risk factors.

The epidemiological research in the 1980s and early 1990s began to evaluate the so-called French paradox, a lower cardiovascular risk observed in the French population compared to other Western developed countries, despite their traditional consumption of foods that are rich in animal fats (butter, cheese, red meat). There was a time when the main culprit for the high prevalence of CVD was considered to be the "bad" cholesterol originated from animal fats. We now know that there are also other dietary factors, such as a trans-fat, low-fiber, or high-sugar diet that influence CVD risk (Piepoli 2016). Moderate red wine intake was correlated with decreased incidence of obesity and heart disease. The initial hypothesis at that moment was that wine consumption not only was correlated but had a direct effect on protection against CVD (Streppel 2009). The questions raised from this observation led to a series of studies to identify the component of wine that confers this effect and to demonstrate its positive benefits. And the resveratrol was the first in front.

The first studies on resveratrol appeared in the 1990s and continue even today, reaching over 200 clinical studies published both in cardiovascular prevention and in other pathologies. There are more resveratrol studies published in the last ten years than in the mid-1990s. The increased interest is understandable because resveratrol can be produced by cheap chemical synthesis and is easier to standardize and use. For these obvious practical reasons and due to the growing commercial interest from nutritional supplement manufacturers, research in this area has flourished. Fifteen years ago, David Sinclair, a biologist, and professor at Harvard University publicly declared that resveratrol is

> "as close to a miraculous molecule as you can find... One hundred years from now, people will maybe be taking these molecules on a daily basis to prevent heart disease, stroke, and cancer."

This optimistic view was not endorsed by the scientific community, who casually argued that large clinical trials are needed, not only animal studies and small-scale human studies (KHN 2019). Moreover, serious allegations of scientific misconduct and fraud were made against Dr. Das, who had resveratrol in cardiovascular disease as one of his areas of interest and who published several dozen articles, which were later retracted (Retraction Watch 2012). Of course, many researchers were working on resveratrol, but the hype around it, combined with commercial interest and misconduct accusations have cast a shadow over the whole scientific community's work on this subject.

Resveratrol was initially thought to have anti-aging and cardiovascular protective benefits through its powerful antioxidant effect. We now know that there are several molecular mechanisms: antioxidant, anti-proliferative, anti-inflammatory, and anti-angiogenesis, but also low bioavailability, which may reduce or cancel *in vivo* effects. The original claim that the protective effects of wine and grape products were due to the direct antioxidant property of resveratrol was overcome by detailed studies on other polyphenols' molecular mechanisms of action (Cheng 2020). Other bioactive components of grapes and wine may have additive effects to those shown for resveratrol.

Meanwhile, enthusiasm for resveratrol has declined due to several inconclusive clinical trials. New epidemiological and interventional studies have shown that more plant-originated foods high in polyphenols may provide a cardiovascular protective effect and that resveratrol is only one of the multiple bioactive components with a potential cardioprotective effect (Mink 2007). Polyphenols represent a large and diverse group of secondary plant metabolites that are present virtually in all plant foods: fruit, vegetables, legumes, dark chocolate, tea, and wine. Several epidemiological studies indicate a positive correlation between polyphenol-rich food intake and several cardiovascular endpoints, such as reduction of myocardial infarction, chronic heart disease, heart failure, and overall, in cardiovascular mortality.

As a consequence of these observations, the paradigm of searching for that "miracle" molecule responsible for all observed positive effects has changed. Now, the objectives of studies in preventive medicine and nutraceuticals focus on assessing the global effects of polyphenols in food, as well as the effect of non-digestible carbohydrates on the human body and microbiota in reducing the risk of CVD. This chapter summarizes the molecular, pre-clinical, and clinical basis of the effects observed for both resveratrol and other grape pomace components.

## Molecular Basis of Cardiovascular Effects of Grape Pomace and Derivates

Grape pomace (GP) is a residue of *Vitis vinifera* obtained during the production of wine and consisting of skin, seeds, and stems. As discussed in previous chapters, GP has a complex structure and composition. GP is rich in polyphenols originated mainly from grape seed such as resveratrol, phenolic acid, flavonoids, procyanidins, and the derivatives of grape skins, anthocyanins. GP also has an important amount of non-extractable polyphenols such as proanthocyanidins and dietary fibers that are not present in wine. This section summarizes the molecular and cellular mechanisms of the various bioactive molecules present in GP.

The proposed mechanisms for the cardiovascular protection of GP derivates are based on modulation of oxidative processes, energy metabolism regulation, stress resistance, exercise and fasting mimetics, and modulation of microbiota composition, often involving binding to specific proteins and effects on cell signaling. Not all polyphenols act in the same way, the mechanisms are different, some of them intensively studied, especially for resveratrol (Cheng 2020).

A key mechanism of polyphenols that can provide protective effects against CVD is the increase in nitric oxide (NO) at the endothelial level. In blood vessels, NO is a powerful vasodilator, reduces vasoconstrictor influences, but also reduces platelet aggregation and adherence of platelets and leukocytes to endothelium, inhibits oxidation of low-density lipoproteins (LDL) and diminishes vascular smooth muscle cell proliferation. Thus, polyphenols inhibit endothelial dysfunction and induce vascular endothelium-dependent vascular relaxation by redox regulation and NO production.

## Stilbenes

The main 2 stilbenes that are found in grape pomace, resveratrol, and piceatannol, are natural phytoalexins, produced by grapevine in response to injury or when it is under attack by pathogens, such as bacteria or fungi. Other stilbenes (desoxyrhapontigenin, rhapontigenin, piceid, rhaponticin, and epsilon-viniferin) are present in small quantities in grape products.

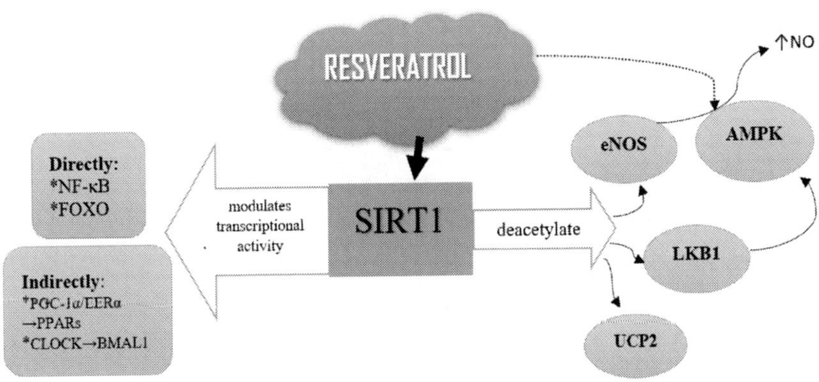


- Molecular level: activator of SIRT1, the NAD+-dependent protein deacetylase
- Cellular level:
  - Endothelial cells: reduced inflammation, increased endothelial function, reduced oxidative stress, reduced apoptosis, reduced eNOS uncoupling, reduced angiogenesis
  - Vascular smooth muscle: reduced hyperplasia, reduce fibrosis
  - Cardiac myocytes: reduced hypertrophy, reduced apoptosis, inflammation, reduced cardiac remodeling, and fibrosis
  - Monocyte/macrophage: Reduced monocyte-to-macrophage differentiation, macrophage infiltration, and foam cell formation
  - Platelets: reduced aggregation

Figure 2. Resveratrol schematic mechanism of action.

*Resveratrol* (3,4′,5-trans-trihydroxystilbene), a stilbene molecule belonging to the polyphenol family, is commonly found in other foods aside from grape, such as berries, peanuts, and cocoa. Although certain amount of resveratrol in grape transfers into wine during grape maceration, a significant amount of resveratrol remains in the pomace. Following reports on a cardioprotective effect of red wine, studies aiming to unravel the intimate mechanisms of resveratrol began to be published. Initially, the protective effect was explained by its free-radical scavenging capacity, so a direct antioxidant effect. We now know that this effect is secondary. At the molecular level, the cardioprotective effect of resveratrol is based on activating SIRT1 that regulates aging, transcription, proliferation, apoptosis, inflammation, and may mimic calorie restriction through further detailed mechanisms (Cheng 2020).

SIRT1 or Sirtuin 1 or NAD-dependent deacetylase sirtuin-1 is an enzyme that deacetylates proteins that are essential to the metabolic process involved in cellular regulation as a response to stress and aging. Human SIRT1 is probably one of the intracellular regulatory proteins involved in epigenetic gene silencing.

SIRT1 deacetylates and enhances the activity of eNOS, which also undergoes phosphorylation by AMPK for NO production. SIRT1 up-regulates endothelial NOS (eNOS) expression and controls the activity of the NO/ROS balance to prevent endothelial dysfunction. SIRT1 deacetylates LKB1 to promote AMPK phosphorylation for downstream eNOS activation contributing to NO production. LKB1 is an essential element in cell metabolism that is required for maintaining energy homeostasis. Activation of AMPK by LKB1 suppresses growth and proliferation when energy and nutrient levels are scarce. SIRT1 directly and indirectly through AMPK activates UCP2 (mitochondrial uncoupling protein 2) to reduce oxidative stress. SIRT1 modulates transcriptional activity by directly deacetylating the transcription factors themselves (NF-κB, FOXOs, KLF2). SIRT1 deacetylates and affects the activity of the PGC1-alpha/ERR-alpha complex, which are essential mitochondrial transcriptional regulators. Mitochondria is essential for obtaining ATP, the cellular energy battery, by oxidative phosphorylation. Decreased mitochondrial activity and progressive build-up of mitochondrial oxidative stress are biological consequences of aging. Evidence of alterations at the mitochondrial level by accumulating ROS accounts for oxidative damage, potentially increasing the risk of CVDs. One study correlated alterations in PGC-1alpha and ERRalpha target gene sets with the severity of left ventricular ejection fraction in heart failure in humans (Sihag 2009) while in animal studies, resveratrol induced mitochondrial biogenesis in cardiomyocytes to attenuate angiotensin II-induced cardiac remodeling (Biala 2010). In endothelial cells, triggering SIRT1 upregulation reduces levels of reactive oxygen species (ROS) and, as a consequence, induces inhibition of monocyte recruitment, increased autophagy, endothelial elongation, and an improved re-endothelialisation. Resveratrol also acts independently of SIRT1 to modulate several other molecular targets such as a direct free-radical scavenger to reduce oxidative stress and as a direct AMPK or PPARδ activator. Resveratrol was found to largely inhibit platelet aggregation induced by collagen and arachidonic acid, but isorhapontigenin, the methoxylated analogue of resveratrol, with better bioavailability, acts by selectively inhibiting ADP-induced platelet activation at reduced concentrations ($IC_{50}$ of around 1.85 μM). Isorhapontigenin may interfere with cAMP and PI3K signaling pathways that are associated with the $P2Y_{12}$ receptor (Ravishankar 2019).

Due to its chemical characteristics (e.g., poor water-solubility, instability, susceptibility to degradation during food processing, and low bioavailability), the benefits of resveratrol have been questioned. However, favorable results from animal studies have encouraged researchers to seek explanations. Most resveratrol administered orally is rapidly metabolized in the enterocytes (Rotches-Ribalta 2012) and in the liver, so it has low bioavailability and an extended first-pass metabolism (Wenzel 2005). This pharmacokinetics contradiction between poor bioavailability and observed *in vivo* effects of resveratrol raises the question as to whether these metabolites are partially responsible for the beneficial effects. Resveratrol is metabolized to piceatannol in hepatocyte hydroxylation by the action of CYP1B1, and both are extensively glucuronidated in a second phase. In this way, other metabolites result at the intestinal level.

GP polyphenols and other bioactive molecules interact with the gut microbiota in the large intestine. First, polyphenols and non-digestible fibers may regulate the composition of the gut microbiota and second, the gut microbiota can metabolize polyphenols to active bioavailable metabolites (Espin 2017). Therefore, the intestinal microbiota may be a decisive factor in polyphenols pharmacokinetics, resveratrol included, as discussed further.

*Trans-piceatannol* (3,3′,4,5′-trans-trihydroxystilbene), the less-known stilbene, shadowed by the famous resveratrol, possesses a similarly broad spectrum of biological activity, as antioxidant and anti-inflammatory. Piceatannol is abundant in red wine, more than resveratrol in some varieties and it has an even higher free-radical scavenging capacity than resveratrol due to an extra OH group to the phenol ring.

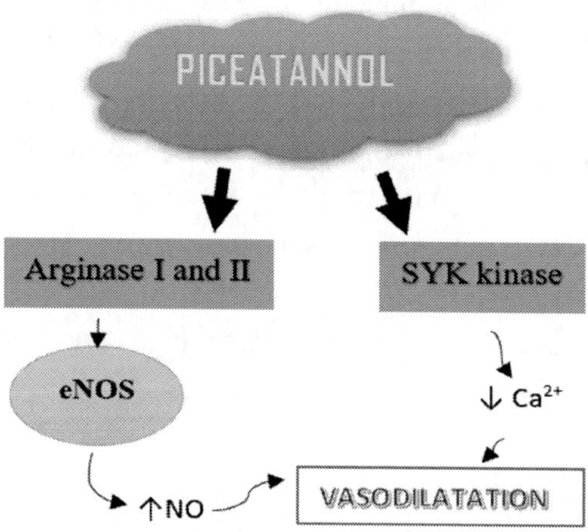


- Molecular level: inhibits the activity of arginase I and II; Syk kinase inhibitor; activate PPAR-α
- Cellular level:
  - Endothelial cells: reduced endothelial dysfunction, reduced oxidative stress by increased eNOS protein expression (via arginase inhibition) and increased NO,
  - Vascular smooth muscle: relaxation due to reduced $Ca^{2+}$ mobilization (via Syk kinase inhibition), reduced hyperplasia and proliferation, reduced angiogenesis
  - Cardiac myocytes: membrane-stabilizing (class Ia antiarrhythmic), reduced hypertrophy, reduced oxidative stress

Figure 3. Piceatannol mechanism of action.

The cardioprotective effect of piceatannol is based on inhibiting arginase I and II. Arginase II is co-expressed with NOS in smooth muscle and endothelium and competes for the same substrate (L-arginine). An over-expressed arginase can affect eNOS activity; therefore, inhibiting arginase will maintain normal cellular levels of arginine thus allowing for normal NO production. It also inhibits Syk kinase and has a membrane-stabilizing effect. SYK inhibition modulates transcriptional activity of NF-κB, PPAR-α, and partly regulates NO production via activating the MAPK cascade. The activation of Syk and NF-κB is an important factor in inflammation and atherosclerosis. Inhibiting Syk may reduce expressions of cell adhesion molecules, resulting in a reduction of monocyte-
endothelial cell adhesion and prevention of early development of atherosclerotic plaque (Tang 2014).

Piceatannol has an acute vasodilator effect demonstrated in the animal model study. Piceatannol is the most potent vascular relaxant in rat-isolated aortic rings among different stilbene compounds including resveratrol. The mechanism may be dual, direct action on vascular muscle by Syk kinase inhibition and reduced intracellular $Ca^{2+}$ mobilization, via $Ca^{2+}$-activated $K^+$ channels and indirect action by eNOS activation responsible for long term effects. Pineatannol has a membrane-stabilizing effect in ischemic-reperfusion rats' aorta by a prolonged action potential duration through delaying sodium ion current ($I_{Na}$) inactivation to increase the effective refractory period (Yoo 2007). Possible side effects for this compound should also be considered given that Syk has important roles in cellular immunity, that the effects on Na and K channels on myocyte may prove proarrhythmogenic.

## Monomeric Flavonols

Monomeric flavan-3-ols (catechin, epicatechin, and gallic acid) found in grape seeds and skins have antioxidant activity. Their total antioxidant capacity was additive to each component (Iacopini 2008).

Some monomeric flavan-3-ols (especially epigallocatechin gallate), have an inhibitory α-amylase and α-glucosidase activity. These enzymes are needed to digest carbohydrates and their inhibition reduces the rate of digestion of complex carbohydrates, thus reducing glycemia in diabetic patients (Ylmazer-Musa 2012)

Quercetin has an anti-inflammatory effect by inhibiting lipopolysaccharide (LPS)-induced tumor necrosis factor α (TNF-α) production in macrophages (Manjeet 1999)

## Procyanidins (Condensed Tannins)

Procyanidins are a group of condensed flavan-3-ols that can be found in grape seed, grape skin, red wine, and many plants, most notably apples and aronia fruit. Procyanidins have antioxidant, anti-inflammatory, and serum lipid-lowering effects. These effects may contribute to the cardiovascular protective effect.

GP procyanidins inhibit human endothelial NADPH oxidase, the enzyme responsible for the increased production of ROS. The procyanidin fractions are inhibiting ROS production at both extra- and intracellular levels (Alvarez et al., 2012). They also enhance endothelial NO-synthase–mediated relaxation. Procyanidins are effective *in vitro* inhibitors of human platelet aggregation and low-density lipoprotein oxidation.

Procyanidin anti-inflammatory molecular mechanisms include modulation of the arachidonic acid pathway, inhibition of gene transcription, protein expression and enzymatic activity of eicosanoid pathway, production and secretion of inflammatory mediators (such as cytokines and nitric oxide), inhibition of mitogen-activated protein kinase (MAPK) pathway activation, and modulation of the NF-κB pathway. The NF-κB pathway can be regulated by procyanidins at several levels. Furthermore, procyanidins have a strong anti-inflammatory effect, directly by inhibiting cyclo-oxygenase activity. They are selective inhibitors; procyanidins B2 and C1 are more COX 2 selective and procyanidin B1 is more COX 1 selective (Martinez-Micaelo 2012). This raises the issue of possible cardiovascular side effects through selective inhibition of COX2 and a possible prothrombotic effect. This is probably offset by the other effects but needs further evaluation.

GP's procyanidins regulate intestinal *Fxr*-target gene expression *in vivo,* a critical regulatory point of biliary acids absorption and transport. This partly explains the triglyceride reductions observed in studies (Heidker 2016)

## Other Bioactive Components

### *Anthocyanidins*

Anthocyanins are polyphenolic compounds produced by plants, that give the red-violet color to many fruits and vegetables such as red grapes, berries, and red cabbages. In plants, they exist exclusively as glycosides compounds.

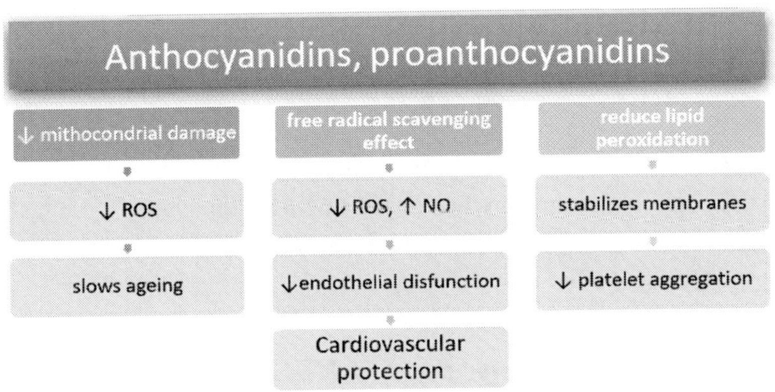


Figure 4. Anthocyanins and proanthocyanidins can limit oxidative stress and, as result, have cardiovascular protection. ROS, reactive oxygen species; NO, nitric oxide (adapted after Kruger 2014).

Anthocyanins have a strong free radical scavenging effect, thus antioxidant activity due to increased activity of antioxidant enzymes such as superoxide dismutase (SOD) and catalase (CAT). They also block the NF-κB signaling pathway involved in the inhibition of COX-2 gene expression. Cyclooxygenase inhibitory activity of cyanidin glycosides increased with a decreasing number of sugar units (Kruger 2014)

### *Phenolic Acids*

Hydroxycinnamates, hydroxybenzoic and hydroxycinnamic acids (tartaric esters of caftaric acid and coumaric acid) and their conjugates are components of GP. Starting from epidemiological data that have suggested an inverse association between consumption of whole grains that are rich in hydroxycinnamates and the incidence of atherosclerosis, *in vitro* studies have demonstrated potent antioxidant activity, which might be correlated with the beneficial health impact *in vivo*. The proposed mechanism of action is assumed to be a free radical scavenging property against hydroxyl radical, peroxynitrite, and oxidation of LDL. One study demonstrated that the phenolic acid metabolites isolated from the serum of animals fed with blueberries were able to reduce foam-cell formation *in vitro* by inhibiting CD36 expression and increased the expression of ABCA1, possibly contributing to the removal of excess cholesterol from macrophages (Xie 2011).

### *Lignans*

Lignans are diphenolic compounds such as matairesinol, found in grape. These compounds are converted to enterolignans by the intestinal microflora and possess estrogen-like activities and antioxidant effect (Milder 2006).

### *Non-Digestible or Very-Low Bioavailable Compounds*

GP is rich in non-digestible dietary fiber, mainly cell wall polysaccharides and lignin, and non-absorbable polyphenols. A major part of polyphenols is not absorbed or poorly absorbed and can interact with intestinal microbiota acting as prebiotics, promoters of bacterial growth.

The human digestive system is host to a diverse selection of microorganisms, up to a thousand different species. Research has proved that gut microbiota composition is highly influenced by the diet. The type and quantity of food derivatives passing thru intestines have an important impact on microbiota composition and activity. GP polyphenols can promote intestinal growth of *Lactobacillus* sp. (Hervert-Hernandez 2009). Large studies have demonstrated that a high fiber diet that promotes colonic fermentation by a different type of microorganisms is positively correlated with protection against CVD, type 2 diabetes, obesity, and other high prevalence diseases. Fiber and other plant-originating compounds are the main energy source for the gut microbiota and the source of secondary metabolites that have multiple functions in the host: energy source, immune system, lipid metabolism, gut motility, and permeability, thus affecting the risk of gastrointestinal disorders, cancers, and CVD. Complex polyphenols and dietary fiber can also have a chelating effect on biliary acids in the intestine or facilitate changes in the microbiota composition and their capacity to deconjugate and hydrolyze bile acids into secondary bile acids. Thus, they modify bile acid's enterohepatic circulation.

As discussed above, some polyphenols can be metabolized by the colonic bacterial flora and transformed into active compounds with higher bioavailability. Microorganisms transform polyphenols into simple aromatic metabolites while polyphenols can modulate the gut microbiota composition, inhibiting some bacterial populations while stimulating others. This dual interaction may be an essential key to explaining the positive influence of foods high in polyphenols on the prevention of CVD. After oral administration, GP does not alter normal gut bacteria but has a modulatory action on gut microbiota to a healthier phenotype. The concentration of acetic, propionic, and butyric acids, markers of microbiota fermentative activity, increased, as well as ammonium concentration, a marker of the proteolytic activity of the microbiota. Bacteria groups like *Lactobacillus* and *Bacteroides* increased, while non-beneficial bacteria like *Clostidioides* decreased (Gil-Sánchez 2017).

**Table 1. Grape pomace components and molecular/cellular mechanisms of action in cardiovascular protection**

| **Phenolic components** | Stilbenes | **Resveratrol** and its glycosides | activator of SIRT1<br>AMPK activation (direct and indirect by SIRT1)<br>PPARδ activator |
|---|---|---|---|
| | | **Trans-piceatannol** | Syk kinase inhibitor<br>inhibit the activity of arginase I and II |
| | Phenolic acids: Hydroxycinnamic ac.<br>Hydroxybenzoic ac. | | antioxidant activity |
| | Flavonoids | Flavan-3-ols (catechin) | antioxidant activity<br>inhibit α-amilase |
| | | Flavonol (quercitin) | Inhibit TNF α |
| | Procyanidins | | Inhibit NADPH oxidase<br>Inhibit COX |
| | Lignans | | antioxidant activity by microbiota transformation, estrogen-like effect |
| **Other components** | Essential fatty acids – linoleic acid | | ↓ LDL cholesterol |
| | tocopherols | | Antioxidant |
| | Non-digestible carbohydrates | | Secondary antioxidant activity by microbiota transformation |
| | Dietary fiber (lignin) | | Secondary antioxidant activity by microbiota transformation |
| | Beta-carotenes | | Antioxidant |

The recommended intake of dietary fiber according to guidelines is 25–30 grams per day. Since this amount is not easily reachable, alternative sources of fiber should be sought, and GP can be one such source. The positive effects of GP-based fiber are supporting the research, development, and marketing of GP-based fiber-rich products.

## Pharmacokinetics Considerations

This subchapter summarizes the main ideas related to the pharmacokinetics components, without going into detail on the characteristics and metabolic transformations for each component, which can be found in other chapters but focusing instead on the relevant points in terms of cardiovascular prevention.

The effects of polyphenols are dependent on the ingested quantity and their pharmacokinetics properties. To have cardiovascular effects, at the endothelial or cardiac level, active molecules must reach the systemic circulation. But it is possible to have a favorable effect as antiaggregant on platelets on portal circulation of some molecules that are circulating in the enterohepatic circuit before they are reaching hepatic metabolization, by a mechanism similar to aspirin.

Bioavailability is influenced by absorption and metabolization at the intestinal level and by the hepatic first pass. The absorption of polyphenols is influenced by various factors such as their physicochemical properties (e.g., molecular size, degree of polymerization, solubility, pKa), biological factors (through their passage in the gastrointestinal tract), food matrix, interaction with other dietary components, and gut microbiota composition. For some polyphenols is not surprising that the concentration in human plasma is lower than the concentration observed to have potential health effects *in vitro* due to their low bioavailability. After oral administration, there are several possible pathways of absorption and metabolism of bioactive molecules in GP, depending on the chemical structure and nature of attached moieties. The gut microbiota is responsible for the breakdown of the original polyphenolic structures into many low-molecular-weight compounds, which could be more absorbable than their original counterparts found in plants. This metabolization may have multiple steps of ester and glycoside hydrolysis, demethylation, dehydroxylation, and decarboxylation by different bacteria.

Some of the metabolized and conjugated forms of different polyphenols could have higher biological activity than their parent compounds. Metabolization by microbiota is a rich source of highly absorbable active molecules. For instance, in a study of healthy volunteers consuming berries rich in polyphenols, the sulfa-metabolites reached high serum concentrations up to 20 μM and no detectable concentration of parent compounds (Pimpao 2015). At this level of metabolite concentration, and *in vivo* positive effect might occur. Anthocyanins and procyanidins are also poorly absorbed in their intact form, but microbial and chemical breakdown metabolites are well absorbed and appear in plasma and urine.

Resveratrol is quickly absorbed, but rapidly metabolized at an intestinal and hepatic level resulting in low bioavailability of the parent compound, but one of the metabolites is piceatannol, an active molecule with proven effects. The use of resveratrol as a nutraceutical ingredient is limited due to its chemical characteristics (e.g., instability and low bioavailability). Therefore, attempts have been made to produce pharmaceutical forms of delivery systems that would increase its bioavailability, such as nanoemulsions, nanocrystals, liposomes, solid dispersion, and micelles. These pharmaceutical forms are known to improve bioavailability, but it is not known if they also increase efficiency.

It is not known for every bioactive molecule in grape's composition whether an active concentration of polyphenols or their metabolites is achieved by consumption of wine or grapes seed extract or other supplemented sources, but there is indirect evidence that they, indeed, increase to pharmacologically relevant levels.

Evaluating single compounds *in vitro* does not consider the complex mixture of plasma metabolites that could have additive, synergistic or antagonistic effects. Also, the tested molecules are those that are found in foods or in raw plant material, at high doses, ranging from low micromolar to millimolar concentrations. We need to consider pharmacokinetic processes after oral administration, because these compounds are extensively modified by human and microbial enzymes, and their appearance in the internal compartments of the human body rarely exceeds nanomolar concentrations. Individual and population variability of metabolic pathways should also be considered. In conclusion, studying the effects at the molecular and cellular level gives us a suitable direction to investigate the individual clinical effects of these bioactive compounds.

## EPIDEMIOLOGICAL STUDIES WITH GRAPE DERIVATES

Over time, several epidemiological longitudinal studies have evaluated the influence of some foods on cardiovascular risk factors, on the progression of atherosclerosis and its manifestations, cardiovascular diseases, and their complications.

The Seven Countries Study, launched in the 1960s, was the first major cross-cultural prospective study to link diet and serum cholesterol to coronary heart disease. It showed that populations in the Mediterranean region experienced lower coronary heart disease mortality probably due to different dietary patterns. Later observational studies have confirmed the benefits of adherence to a Mediterranean dietary pattern on CVD risk factors, not because of the low cholesterol content, but because of the association of several dietary factors.

Pieces of evidence for modifiable diet factors were gathered from a part of this large study, the so-called Zutphen cohort. On the one hand, information on alcoholic drinks consumed was collected by questionnaires seven times between 1960 and 2000. Wine drinkers in the Zutphen study who consumed less than 20 g alcohol from wine per day, the equivalent of two glasses, had a 39% lower risk of coronary death and a 32% lower risk of overall cardiovascular mortality. Initially, the reduced risk was attributed to its ethanol content, but this study demonstrated that the consumption of beer and spirits was related to neither long-term coronary nor cardiovascular mortality. These results are compatible with the idea that a low intake of wine may protect against CVD. Statistically, light wine consumption was associated with 5 years longer life expectancy (Streppel 2009).

On the other hand, epidemiological data suggest that dietary flavonoids may have beneficial cardiovascular effects in human populations, and wine and grape products are a rich source of both flavan-3-ols and flavonols. An extension of Zutphen, called Zutphen Elderly Study showed a beneficial effect of food polyphenols over the 15-year incidence of stroke, in men with an average flavonol intake of 33 mg/d, compared to 14 mg/d, had a 73% lower risk of stroke (Hertog

1993). In the same cohort, an average intake of monomeric flavan-3-ols of 124 mg/d, compared to an average intake of 25 mg/d, was associated with a 51% lower 10-year cardiovascular associated mortality (Arts 2001). These are the results for men, as for women, a large prospective study of postmenopausal women, with 16 y of follow-up, reported on total flavonoids and on 7 subclasses of flavonoids and found that dietary intakes of flavanones and anthocyanidins were associated with a decreased risk of death due to coronary heart disease, CVD, and all causes combined (Mink 2007). These observational studies do not allow the identification of specific phenolic compounds or polyphenol-rich foods that effectively improve cardio-metabolic risk factors.

Epidemiological studies have suggested an inverse association between flavonoids and CVD. However, the results might be biased due to the methods of dietary assessment. A systematic review of observational studies on associations between polyphenol biomarkers and CVD and mortality risk identified 16 different polyphenol biomarkers in association with CVD and mortality. A reduction in all-cause and CVD mortality risk by 30% and 45% respectively were revealed at higher enterolactone concentrations, a lignan metabolite. Protective associations were demonstrated for polyphenol biomarkers and all-cause mortality, kaempferol, and acute coronary syndrome. This underlines the important role of microbiota in disease prevention (Rienks 2017). Let us not forget that these results were not specifically for grape products and that the epidemiological studies were mainly based on dietary assessments without independent validation by objective methods that do not depend on one individual's memory. However, it is exceedingly difficult to find those markers, those metabolites that can be measured on a large scale, in large studies.

More recent epidemiological studies provide further support for a beneficial effect of wine, indicating that wine might confer benefits above and beyond those of other alcoholic beverages, and suggesting that nonalcoholic factors in wine may also play a protective role. For instance, wine consumption was found to be cardioprotective, whereas beer intake was not, in a meta-analysis of 13 studies and 209,418 participants (Di Castelnuovo 2002).

Other studies approached this question differently, measuring urinary metabolites of some bioactive components to estimate total consumption and to associate those with CVD protection. A large cross-sectional study (PREDIMED) evaluated 1000 participants measuring total urinary resveratrol metabolites as biomarkers of wine and resveratrol consumption and the associations with CVD risk factors. Both resveratrol and wine intake were associated with beneficial changes in blood lipid profiles and heart rate, fasting blood glucose only for resveratrol, suggesting that resveratrol intake via wine consumption might help decrease CVD risk factors (Zamora 2012).

A prospective cohort study, the InCHIANTI Study, conducted in two villages in Italy in a population-based sample of 783 community-dwelling men and women 65 years or older, with a primary outcome the all-cause mortality, measured total urinary resveratrol metabolite concentration during 9 years of follow-up. In this study, total urinary resveratrol metabolite did not have a substantial influence on health status and mortality risk of the population and was not associated with secondary outcome measurements, serum CRP, IL-6, IL-1β, TNF, prevalent or incident cardiovascular disease, or cancer (Semba 2014).

Like all observational studies it is hard to point out a cause, it is more about making a correlation. However, these studies are essential to establish directions for interventional clinical trials.

## Interventional Studies with Grape Derivates on CVD Risk Factors

### Arterial Hypertension

High blood pressure is a major risk factor for developing atherosclerosis, endothelial dysfunction, and their consequences, CVD.

High blood pressure can be caused by an increased cardiac output or by a higher systemic vascular resistance. Lower vascular elasticity and/or an excess of vasoconstriction stimuli can result in arterial hypertension.

Mechanisms associated with blood pressure regulation, for different GP products or wine:

1. Polyphenols demonstrated an effect of increasing the endothelial-derived nitric oxide (NO), via modulation of endothelial NO synthase (eNOS) expression and activity. NO is one of the major vasodilator factors at endothelium level. NO causes vascular smooth muscle relaxation following activation of soluble guanylate cyclase, which in turn increases cGMP, followed by blockage of the release of intracellular calcium, preventing it from causing vascular smooth muscle contraction.
2. Reducing reactive oxygen species (ROS) damage at endothelial level inducing vasoconstriction and hypertension. Due to their strong antioxidant activity, some of the grape polyphenols act to prevent NO oxidative damage and radical-induced NO conversion, such as the reaction caused by NADPH oxidase.
3. Some polyphenols, especially stilbenes (piceatannol) have been shown to have a direct vasodilator effect by reducing the $Ca^{2+}$ intracellular mobilization.

## Dyslipidemia, Metabolic Syndrome, and Diabetes

Dyslipidemia, particularly elevated plasma low-density lipoprotein (LDL) cholesterol levels, is the most important risk factor for CVD. In animal models, dietary grape seed significantly increased fecal excretion of cholesterol and reduced total cholesterol (TC), LDL cholesterol, very-low-density lipoprotein VLDL cholesterol, triglycerides, and increased HDL cholesterol (Tebib 1994). Beneficial effects of grape may be due to enhanced expression of insulin signaling pathway-related proteins, decrease of plasma lipoproteins concentrations, scavenging of hydroxyl and peroxyl radicals, antioxidant activities, suppressing of the oxidation of LDL, and also inhibiting intestinal cholesterol absorption.

Metabolic syndrome, an association between disturbed glucose and insulin metabolism, overweight and abdominal fat distribution, dyslipidemia, and hypertension, is associated with subsequent development of type 2 diabetes mellitus and CVD.

## Platelet Activation

Platelets are involved in atherosclerotic coronary heart disease development and thrombosis processes. Following vascular damage, the endothelium releases pro-aggregate factors, allowing the adhesion of subendothelium to platelets. Several flavonoids have shown preclinical antiplatelet effects through various mechanisms. The inhibition of platelet aggregation is a mechanism largely used in cardioprotection.

Nowadays, the number of studies with grape derivatives or resveratrol is constantly increasing, there is an abundance of interventional clinical trials, but not all are of a quality that allows relevant conclusions. Therefore, in this section of the chapter, we chose to present results from meta-analyses or systematic reviews that evaluate the effects on CVD risk factors.

*Grape products* A 2019 meta-analysis evaluating grape products (whole grape extract, grape juice, raisin, and grape seed extract) supplementation in improving the lipid profiles in adults on TC, LDL-cholesterol, HDL-cholesterol. A significant heterogeneity across the studies was observed. Combined results from 56 randomized clinical trials (RCT) including a total of 2373 participants revealed that grape supplementation significantly decreases LDL serum level with grape supplementation and had no significant effect on HDL-cholesterol. Also, the meta-analysis significantly decreased TC serum level in 57 RCTs including a total of 2352 participants (Ghaedi 2019). However, the available evidence from these RCTs does not allow the identification of specific phenolic compounds in the grape that effectively improve cardio-metabolic risk factors.

The amount of grape polyphenols administered may influence the final result. This quantity depends on the type of grape product. A meta-analysis of 10 studies assessing the total amount and effect on BP showed that daily grape polyphenol intake could modestly reduce systolic blood pressure (by 1.48 mmHg) when compared to control subjects. Subgroup analyses indicated that greater reductions were identified in patients with metabolic syndrome. Contrarily, diastolic blood pressure was not significantly decreased in the grape polyphenols group as compared to controls (Li 2015). A 2020 meta-analysis on 9 studies found no beneficial effects of grape polyphenols on the selected inflammatory mediators (Haghighatdoost 2020).

Still, more studies with higher doses of polyphenols, longer treatment durations, different sources of grape polyphenols, and larger numbers of participants are required.

## Grape Seed Extract

Grape seed has high flavonoid content as previously discussed. The antioxidant properties of grape seed polyphenols are central to their mechanisms of action, which also include cellular signaling mechanisms and interactions at the genomic level. Multiple clinical studies have reported that grape seed polyphenols had a beneficial effect on lipid metabolism and other metabolic abnormalities in patients with metabolic syndrome by antioxidant properties, improved lipoprotein metabolism, and reduced inflammation. A first meta-analysis published in 2011, in which nine RCTs were included, showed that grape seed extract administration did not have any effect on total cholesterol (TC), LDL cholesterol, HDL cholesterol, triglycerides, and C-reactive protein (CRP) levels (Feringa 2011).

Meanwhile, new evidence was gathered, such as the study by Argani (2016), showing that taking grape seed extract for 8 weeks by patients with mild to moderate hyperlipidemia led to a significant decrease in TC, triglycerides, and LDL cholesterol levels. In 2020, a new meta-analysis taking into account fifteen RCT showed that grape seed extract intake significantly reduced fasting plasma glucose, TC, LDL cholesterol, and triglycerides levels, but did not have any significant effect on HbA1c and HDL cholesterol levels (Asbaghi 2020).

Sixteen clinical trials (810 subjects) on blood pressure effects after grape seed extract treatment were analyzed and found significant reductions for SBP and DBP. This impact was more obvious in younger or obese subjects, as well as in patients with metabolic disorders (Zhang 2016).

*Resveratrol* A meta-analysis of 31 RCT demonstrated that resveratrol supplementation among patients with metabolic syndrome and related disorders significantly reduced total cholesterol, but did not affect triglycerides, LDL-, HDL-cholesterol, ALT, and AST concentrations (Akbari 2020). A meta-analysis of data from 12 RCTs did not support significant effects of resveratrol supplementation on circulating levels of some markers of oxidative stress: superoxide dismutase, catalase, and glutathione peroxidase, although resveratrol significantly increased circulating total antioxidant capacity (Koushki 2020). Another meta-analysis on the effects of resveratrol supplementation on biomarkers of inflammation and oxidative stress among patients with metabolic syndrome and related disorders showed that resveratrol supplementation significantly decreased C-reactive protein (CRP) and tumor necrosis factor-α (TNF-α), but concentrations of Interleukin 6 (IL-6) and superoxide dismutase (SOD) did not significantly change following resveratrol supplementation (Tabrizi 2018). A meta-analysis of 9 RCTs with resveratrol intervention in patients with type 2 diabetes involving 283 participants showed that resveratrol significantly improved fasting plasma glucose in a dose-dependent manner and reduced systolic blood pressure and diastolic blood pressure.

Changes in HbA1c, LDL cholesterol, and HDL cholesterol were negligible in diabetics (Zhu 2017). Data from 10 RCTs showed no beneficial effect of resveratrol on blood pressure (Sahebkar 2015). Resveratrol supplementation did not bring benefits on the metabolic modulation and anti-inflammatory effects as evaluated in a 12 trials meta-analysis (455 patients with high cardiovascular risk). No significant effect was found on the secretion of leptin, adiponectin, and fasting glucose (Rui 2014).

A 2019 Meta-analysis of 17 RCTs (782 participants) confirmed that resveratrol has a blood pressure-lowering effect only in type 2 diabetic patients and that high dosages are needed, which however implies high cost, and efficacy is limited to insulin-resistant individuals (Fogacci 2019). A marked reduction in BP was found only in studies testing doses of resveratrol greater than 300 mg/day and depending on the bioavailability of the resveratrol pharmaceutical formulation tested in the different trials.

Because of this difference in resveratrol effect on blood pressure, the European Society of Hypertension issued in 2020 a position document, "Nutraceuticals and blood pressure control" stating that

> "several possible nutraceutical compounds that might contribute to the improvement of BP control in the general population" and that "among nonnutrient-nutraceuticals, [...], resveratrol in insulin-resistant patients"

may be recommended (Borghi 2020).

Many studies have shown the antihypertensive effects of resveratrol in different preclinical models of hypertension that did not entirely validate on humans.

The favorable effects observed in those who consume an increased amount of polyphenols through a balanced diet, rich in fruit and vegetables, have only been partially confirmed in resveratrol studies (Table 2).

**Table 2. The most recent meta-analysis on grape and cardiovascular risk factors**

| CVD risk factors | Grape products/grape polyphenols | Grape seed extract | Resveratrol | Wine/grape juice* |
|---|---|---|---|---|
| High blood pressure | ↓SBP (in metabolic syndrome)<br>NS: DBP (Li 2015) | ↓SBP<br>↓DBP<br>(Zhang 2016) | ↓SBP (in D2M)<br>↓DBP (in D2M)<br>(Zhu 2017, Foggaci 2019)<br>NS: BP (Sahebkar 2015) | ↓BP (Barbalho 2020) |
| Dyslipidemia | ↓LDL, ↓TC,<br>NS: HDL, TG<br>(Ghaedi 2019)<br>↓LDL↓oxLDL<br>(Lupoli 2020) | ↓LDL, ↓TC,<br>↓TG<br>NS: HDL<br>(Asbaghi 2020) | ↓TC<br>NS: LDL, HDL, TG<br>(Akbari 2020)<br>NS: LDL, HDL (in D2M) (Zhu 2017) | ↓LDL, ↓TC,<br>↓TG (Barbalho 2020) |
| Metabolic syndrome /Obesity | * | ↓FPG<br>NS: HbA1c, BMI, BW<br>(Asbaghi 2020) | NS: HbA1c (Zhu 2017)<br>NS: leptin, adiponectin, HbA1c, FPG (Rui 2014)<br>↓BW (Asgary 2019) | ↓ BMI, BW (Barbalho 2020) |
| Biomarkers of inflammation and oxidative stress | NS: TNF-α, IL-6, CRP (Haghighatdoost 2020) | NS: CRP (Asbaghi 2020) | ↑TAC<br>NS: CAT, SOD, GPx (Koushki 2020)<br>↓CRP, ↓ TNF-α<br>NS: IL-6, SOD (Tabrizi 2018) | ↓Homocysteine (Barbalho 2020) |

* no meta-analysis, only systematic review; BMI-body mass index, BW-Body weight superoxide dismutase, CAT-catalase, CRP C reactive protein D2M type 2 diabetes, FPG fasting plasma glucose, GPx-glutathione peroxidase NE-no effect, SOD-superoxide dismutase, TAC-total antioxidant capacity.

# Conclusion

GP is a residual, cheap product that could be used in the food industry to fortify certain foods to increase the amount of polyphenols. But the overall picture regarding the properties of substances found in GP and their metabolites is far from complete.

The compounds that are now tested *in vitro* are those that occur in foods or in raw plant material, at doses ranging from low micromolar to millimolar concentrations although, following ingestion, these substances are largely metabolized. These transformations are carried out by human and microbial enzymes, at the intestinal or hepatic level and the quantity of parent substance rarely reaches nanomolar concentrations in tissues. It is more likely that the metabolites have the beneficial effects observed in epidemiological studies, so they should be the focus of further study. Because colonic microbiota is involved in these transformations and leads to a plethora of metabolites, it is just as important to study the influence of bacteria types on different metabolic pathways.

Therefore, a different approach than the classic drug research and development is necessary for evaluating nutraceuticals or food with CVD protective potential. From a pharmacological perspective, research begins at the molecular level, with the screening of a novel substance that could have an effect. Nutrition research is completely different from drug discovery because humans are already consuming different substances through diet as part of normal nutrition especially with a healthy lifestyle, rich in polyphenols. The ideal approach would be to take the opposite direction, from epidemiological studies to randomized controlled clinical trials, using standardized foods or supplements high in polyphenols or pure bioactive polyphenols, on well-defined cohorts and subsequently, if beneficial effects are highlighted, those components and their metabolites should be sought and the effects checked *in vitro*, at the molecular level, to validate the hypothesis of the mechanism of action. Nevertheless, multiple mechanisms of action are possible, and acting on many different targets even with lower affinity, may result in a combined effect, which could be sufficient to provide an overall CVD risk reduction.

Research should focus on assessing the polyphenol content of foods, in the form of databases that enable a more precise assessment of total polyphenol content and help practicians recommend practical changes in diet to improve CVD risk. Mobile applications could be developed to simplify the choices of those who want to increase their consumption of polyphenols. A series of studies with fruits that contain a high dose of polyphenols (blueberries, cherries) have made a big splash because they have shown that consuming an equivalent daily amount of 100 g reduces blood pressure. But how practical is it to use such means to control certain diseases? Unfortunately, doctors cannot prescribe blueberries, they can only recommend dietary changes. Also, what should we do with the patient's perception of the effectiveness of this intervention? Some patients accept a treatment that comes from a vial, in the form of a tablet, much more easily than a radical lifestyle change, hence the explosion of nutritional supplements on the market.

In the heyday of resveratrol, it was very fashionable to look for an active molecule responsible for all positive effects, "The Molecule", instead of doing intensive studies on the common grape pomace. Meanwhile, the study of the microbiota took a big leap and introduced new concepts and mechanisms of action which, along with the disappointing results of resveratrol, has led to a return to the study of grape products as a whole.

"An apple a day keeps the doctor away!" Popular wisdom anticipated the results of studies that have shown that in a fresh apple there are millions of bacteria that contribute to the diversity of our microbiota. The more diverse the microbiota, the lower the risk of diseases (allergies, obesity, depression, etc.). Filtered and pasteurized apple juice does not bring the same benefits; on the contrary, it has been associated with increased cardiovascular risk and the development of diabetes, through increased intake of fructose, as opposed to the consumption of whole fruit. Fermented foods, fresh fruit, and vegetables, therefore, bring more than just nutrients, vitamins, and minerals, and intensely processed foods lack these bacteria. The same can be extrapolated for grape and resveratrol: a whole complex of bioactive compounds offers a protective effect, not a dose of a pure substance, hygienically incapsulated.

A polyphenol-rich diet may have a pleiotropic effect on CVD risk factors thanks to the specific action of different polyphenol subclasses. In the case of grape pomace, we have the "proof of concept" and a least some of the mechanisms of action are known. We know that it is unlikely that we will find a bioactive molecule that will do it all and offer us all the benefits alone. Therefore, future studies should focus on a diet containing different classes of polyphenols rather than a specific food or phenolic compound.

Some questions still need answers:

- What is the minimum amount of polyphenols that bring benefits? Is there a linear relationship between polyphenol consumption and decreased cardiovascular risk? There is still inconclusive evidence on the effectiveness of polyphenols in the management of cardio-metabolic risk factors to recommend their use as supplements to reduce CVD and diabetes risk.
- Are we going back to testing grape pomace as such?
- Is grape pomace more economically and practically advantageous than other fruit or other more appetizing foods?
- Is the search for an anti-aging, CVD-protective, plant-originated "miracle pill" a futile endeavor?

## REFERENCES

Akbari, M., Tamtaji, O. R., Lankarani, et al. The effects of resveratrol on lipid profiles and liver enzymes in patients with metabolic syndrome and related disorders: A systematic review and meta-analysis of randomized controlled trials. *Lipids Health Dis.* 2020 Feb 17;19(1):25. doi: 10.1186/s12944-020-1198-x.

Álvarez, E., Rodiño-Janeiro, B. K., Jerez, M., Ucieda-Somoza, R., Núñez, M. J., González-Juanatey, J. R. Procyanidins from grape pomace are suitable inhibitors of human endothelial NADPH oxidase. *J Cell Biochem.* 2012 Apr; 113(4):1386-96. doi: 10.1002/jcb.24011.

Argani, H., Ghorbanihaghjo, A., Vatankhahan, H., Rashtchizadeh, N., Raeisi, S., Ilghami, H. The effect of red grape seed extract on serum paraoxonase activity in patients with mild to moderate hyperlipidemia. *Sao Paulo Med J.* 2016 May 13;134(3):234-9. doi: 10.1590/1516-3180.2015.01702312.

Arts, I. C., Hollman, P. C., Feskens, E. J., Bueno de Mesquita, H. B., Kromhout, D. Catechin intake might explain the inverse relation between tea consumption and ischemic heart disease: the Zutphen Elderly Study. *Am J Clin Nutr.* 2001 Aug;74(2):227-32.

Asbaghi, O., Nazarian, B., Reiner, Ž., Amirani, E., Kolahdooz, F., Chamani, M., & Asemi, Z. The effects of grape seed extract on glycemic control, serum lipoproteins, inflammation, and body weight: A systematic review and meta-analysis of randomized controlled trials. *Phytotherapy Research.* 2020, 34(2), 239–253. https://doi.org/10.1002/ptr.6518.

Biala, A., Tauriainen, E., Siltanen, A., Shi, J., Merasto, S., Louhelainen, M., Martonen, E., Finckenberg, P., Muller, D. N., Mervaala, E. Resveratrol induces mitochondrial biogenesis and ameliorates Ang II-induced cardiac remodeling in transgenic rats harboring human renin and angiotensinogen genes. *Blood Press.* 2010 Jun;19(3):196-205. doi: 10.3109/08037051.2010.481808.

Borghi, C., Tsioufis, K., Agabiti-Rosei, E., et al. Nutraceuticals and blood pressure control: a European Society of Hypertension position document. *J Hypertens.* 2020 May;38(5):799-812. doi: 10.1097/HJH.0000000000002353.

Cheng, C. K., Luo, J. Y., Lau, C. W., Chen, Z. Y., Tian, X. Y., & Huang, Y. (2020). Pharmacological basis and new insights of resveratrol action in the cardiovascular system. *British Journal of Pharmacology,* 177(6), 1258–1277. https://doi.org/10.1111/bph.14801.

di Castelnuovo, A., Rotondo, S., Iacoviello, L., Donati, M. B., & de Gaetano, G. (2002). Meta-analysis of wine and beer consumption in relation to vascular risk. *Circulation,* 105(24), 2836–2844. https://doi.org/10.1161/01.CIR.0000018653.19696.01.

Espín, J. C., González-Sarrías, A., Tomás-Barberán, F. A. The gut microbiota: A key factor in the therapeutic effects of (poly)phenols.

*Biochem Pharmacol.* 2017 Sep 1; 139:82-93. doi: 10.1016/j.bcp. 2017.04.033.

Feringa, H. H., Laskey, D. A., Dickson, J. E., Coleman, C. I. The effect of grape seed extract on cardiovascular risk markers: a meta-analysis of randomized controlled trials. *J Am Diet Assoc.* 2011 Aug;111(8):1173-81. doi: 10.1016/j.jada.2011.05.015.

Fogacci, F., Fogacci, S., Cicero, A. Resveratrol for High Blood Pressure: A Total Failure or the Need to Identify the Right Patient? *High Blood Press Cardiovasc Prev.* 2019 Oct;26(5):421-423. doi: 10.1007/s40292-019-00333-5.

Ghaedi, E., Moradi, S., Aslani, Z., Kord-Varkaneh, H., Miraghajani, M., & Mohammadi, H. (2019). Effects of grape products on blood lipids: A systematic review and dose-response meta-analysis of randomized controlled trials. *Food and Function,* 10(10), 6399–6416. https://doi.org/10.1039/c9fo01248f.

Gil-Sánchez, I., Ayuda-Durán, B., González-Manzano, S., et al. Chemical characterization and in vitro colonic fermentation of grape pomace extracts. *J Sci Food Agric.* 2017 Aug;97(10):3433-3444. doi: 10.1002/jsfa.8197.

Haghighatdoost, F., Gholami, A., & Hariri, M. (2020). Effect of grape polyphenols on selected inflammatory mediators: a systematic review and meta-analysis randomized clinical trials. *EXCLI Journal,* 19, 251–267. https://doi.org/10.17179/excli2020-1011.

Heidker, R. M., Caiozzi, G. C., & Ricketts, M.-L. (). Dietary procyanidins selectively modulate intestinal farnesoid X receptor-regulated gene expression to alter enterohepatic bile acid recirculation: elucidation of a novel mechanism to reduce triglyceridemia. *Molecular Nutrition & Food Research.* 2016, 60(4), 727–736. https://doi.org/10.1002/mnfr.201500795.

Hertog, M. G. L., Feskens, E. J. M., Kromhout, D., Hertog, M. G. L., Hollman, P. C. H., Hertog, M. G. L., & Katan, M. B. Dietary antioxidant flavonoids and risk of coronary heart disease: the Zutphen Elderly Study. *The Lancet.* 1993, 342(8878), 1007–1011. https://doi.org/10.1016/0140-6736(93)92876-U.

Hervert-Hernández, D., Pintado, C., Rotger, R., Goñi, I. Stimulatory role of grape pomace polyphenols on Lactobacillus acidophilus growth. *Int J Food Microbiol.* 2009 Nov 30;136(1):119-22. doi: 10.1016/j.ijfoodmicro.2009.09.016. Epub 2009 Sep 26.

http://retractionwatch.com/2012/01/11/uconn-resveratrol-researcher-dipak-das-fingered-in-sweeping-misconduct-case/

https://khn.org/news/a-fountain-of-youth-pill-sure-if-youre-a-mouse/

Iacopini, P., Baldi, M., Storchi, P., & Sebastiani, L. Catechin, epicatechin, quercetin, rutin and resveratrol in red grape: Content, in vitro antioxidant activity and interactions. *Journal of Food Composition and Analysis.* 2008, 21(8), 589–598. https://doi.org/10.1016/j.jfca.2008.03.011.

Koushki, M., Lakzaei, M., Khodabandehloo, H., Hosseini, H., Meshkani, R., & Panahi, G. Therapeutic effect of resveratrol supplementation on oxidative stress: A systematic review and meta-analysis of randomised controlled trials. *Postgraduate Medical Journal.* 2020, 96(1134), 197–205. https://doi.org/10.1136/postgradmedj-2019-136415.

Kruger, M. J., Davies N., Myburgh K. H., Lecour S. Proanthocyanidins, anthocyanins and cardiovascular diseases, *Food Research International*, 2014, 59, 41-52 https://doi.org/10.1016/j.foodres.2014.01.046.

Li, S. H., Zhao, P., Tian, H. B., Chen, L. H., & Cui, L. Q. Effect of grape polyphenols on blood pressure: A meta-analysis of randomized controlled trials. *PLoS ONE.* 2015, 10(9), e0137665. https://doi.org/10.1371/journal.pone.0137665.

Lupoli, R., Ciciola, P., Costabile, G., Giacco, R., di Minno, M. N. D., & Capaldo, B. Impact of Grape Products on Lipid Profile: A Meta-Analysis of Randomized Controlled Studies. *Journal of Clinical Medicine*. 2020, 9(2), 313. https://doi.org/10.3390/jcm9020313.

Manjeet, K. R., Ghosh, B. Quercetin inhibits LPS-induced nitric oxide and tumor necrosis factor-alpha production in murine macrophages. *Int J Immunopharmacol.* 1999 Jul;21(7):435-43.

Martinez-Micaelo, N., González-Abuín, N., Terra, X., Richart, C., Ardèvol, A., Pinent, M., & Blay, M. Omega-3 docosahexaenoic acid and procyanidins inhibit cyclo-oxygenase activity and attenuate NF-κB activation through a p105/p50 regulatory mechanism in macrophage inflammation. *Biochemical Journal.* 2012, 441(2), 653–663. https://doi.org/10.1042/BJ20110967.

Milder, I. E., Feskens, E. J., Arts I. C., Bueno-de-Mesquita H. B., Hollman P. C., Kromhout D. Intakes of 4 dietary lignans and cause-specific and all-cause mortality in the Zutphen Elderly Study. *Am J Clin Nutr.* 2006 Aug;84(2):400-5.

Mink, P. J., Scrafford, C. G., Barraj, L. M., Harnack, L., Hong, C. P., Nettleton, J. A., & Jacobs, D. R. Flavonoid intake and cardiovascular disease mortality: A prospective study in postmenopausal women. *American Journal of Clinical Nutrition.* 2007, 85(3), 895–909. https://doi.org/10.1093/ajcn/85.3.895.

Piepoli M. F., Hoes A. W., Agewall S., Albus C., Brotons C., Catapano A. L., Cooney M. T., Corrà U., Cosyns B., Deaton C., Graham I., Hall M. S., Hobbs F. D. R., Løchen M. L., Löllgen H., Marques-Vidal P., Perk J., Prescott E., Redon J., Richter D. J., Sattar N., Smulders Y., Tiberi M., van der Worp H. B., van Dis I., Verschuren W. M. M., Binno S; ESC Scientific Document Group. 2016 European Guidelines on cardiovascular disease prevention in clinical practice: The Sixth Joint Task Force of the European Society of Cardiology and Other Societies on Cardiovascular Disease Prevention in Clinical Practice (constituted by representatives of 10 societies and by invited experts) Developed with the special contribution of the European Association for Cardiovascular Prevention & Rehabilitation (EACPR). *Eur Heart J.* 2016 Aug 1;37(29): 2315-2381. doi: 10.1093/eurheartj/ehw106. Epub 2016 May.

Pimpão, R. C., Ventura, M. R., Ferreira, R. B., Williamson, G., & Santos, C. N. Phenolic sulfates as new and highly abundant metabolites in human plasma after ingestion of a mixed berry fruit purée. *British*

*Journal of Nutrition.* 2015, 113(3), 454–463. https://doi.org/10.1017/S0007114514003511.

Ravishankar, D., Albadawi, D. A. I., Chaggar, V. et al. Isorhapontigenin, a resveratrol analogue selectively inhibits ADP-stimulated platelet activation. *Eur J Pharmacol.* 2019 Nov 5;862:172627. doi: 10.1016/j.ejphar.2019.172627.

Rienks, J., Barbaresko, J., Nöthlings, U. Association of isoflavone biomarkers with risk of chronic disease and mortality: a systematic review and meta-analysis of observational studies. *Nutr Rev.* 2017 Aug 1;75(8):616-641. doi: 10.1093/nutrit/nux021.

Rotches-Ribalta, M., Andres-Lacueva, C., Estruch R, Escribano E, Urpi-Sarda M. Pharmacokinetics of resveratrol metabolic profile in healthy humans after moderate consumption of red wine and grape extract tablets. *Pharmacol Res.* 2012 Nov;66(5):375-82. doi: 10.1016/j.phrs.2012.08.001.

Sahebkar, A., Serban, C., Ursoniu, S., Wong, N. D., Muntner, P., Graham, I. M., … Banach, M Lack of efficacy of resveratrol on C-reactive protein and selected cardiovascular risk factors - Results from a systematic review and meta-analysis of randomized controlled trials. *International Journal of Cardiology.* 2015, 189(1), 47–55. https://doi.org/10.1016/j.ijcard.2015.04.008.

Semba, R. D., Ferrucci, L., Bartali, B. et al. Resveratrol levels and all-cause mortality in older community-dwelling adults. *JAMA Internal Medicine.* 2014, 174(7), 1077–1084. https://doi.org/10.1001/jamainternmed.2014.1582.

Sihag, S., Cresci, S., Li, A. Y., Sucharov, C. C., Lehman, J. J. PGC-1alpha and ERRalpha target gene downregulation is a signature of the failing human heart. *J Mol Cell Cardiol.* 2009 Feb;46(2):201-12. doi: 10.1016/j.yjmcc.2008.10.025.

Streppel, M. T., Ocké, M. C., Boshuizen, H. C., Kok, F. J., & Kromhout, D. Long-term wine consumption is related to cardiovascular mortality and life expectancy independently of moderate alcohol intake: The Zutphen Study. *Journal of Epidemiology and Community*

*Health.* 2009, 63(7), 534–540. https://doi.org/10.1136/jech.2008.082198.

Tabrizi, R., Tamtaji, O. R., Lankarani, K. B., et al. The effects of resveratrol supplementation on biomarkers of inflammation and oxidative stress among patients with metabolic syndrome and related disorders: A systematic review and meta-analysis of randomized controlled trials. *Food and Function* 2018, 9(12), 6116–6128. https://doi.org/10.1039/c8fo01259h.

Tang, Y.-L., & Chan, S.-W. (). A Review of the Pharmacological Effects of Piceatannol on Cardiovascular Diseases. *Phytotherapy Research.* 2014, 28(11), 1581–1588. https://doi.org/10.1002/ptr.5185.

Tebib, K., Besançon, P., Rouanet, J. M. Dietary grape seed tannins affect lipoproteins, lipoprotein lipases and tissue lipids in rats fed hypercholesterolemic diets. *J Nutr.* 1994 Dec;124(12):2451-7. DOI: 10.1093/jn/124.12.451.

World Health Organization. *Global status report on non-communicable diseases 2014* https://apps.who.int/iris/bitstream/handle/10665/148114/9789241564854_eng.pdf?sequence=1.

Xie, C., Kang, J., Chen, J. R., Nagarajan, S., Badger, T. M., & Wu, X. Phenolic acids are in vivo atheroprotective compounds appearing in the serum of rats after blueberry consumption. *Journal of Agricultural and Food Chemistry.* 2011, 59(18), 10381–10387. https://doi.org/10.1021/jf2025264.

Yilmazer-Musa, M., Griffith, A. M., Michels, A. J., Schneider, E., & Frei, B. Grape seed and tea extracts and catechin 3-gallates are potent inhibitors of α-amylase and α-glucosidase activity. *Journal of Agricultural and Food Chemistry.* 2012, 60(36), 8924–8929. https://doi.org/10.1021/jf301147n.

Yoo, M. Y., Oh, K. S., Lee, J. W., Seo, H. W., Yon, G. H., Kwon, D. Y., Kim, Y. S., Ryu, S. Y., Lee, B. H. Vasorelaxant effect of stilbenes from rhizome extract of rhubarb (Rheum undulatum) on the contractility of rat aorta. *Phytother Res.* 2007 Feb;21(2):186-9.

Zamora-Ros, R., Urpi-Sarda, M., Lamuela-Raventós, et al. High urinary levels of resveratrol metabolites are associated with a reduction in the prevalence of cardiovascular risk factors in high-risk patients. *Pharmacological Research.* 2012, 65(6), 615–620. https://doi.org/10.1016/j.phrs.2012.03.009.

Zhang, H., Liu, S., Li, L., Liu, S., Liu, S., Mi, J., Tian, G. The impact of grape seed extract treatment on blood pressure changes: A meta-analysis of 16 randomized controlled trials. *Medicine* (Baltimore). 2016 Aug;95(33):e4247. doi: 10.1097/MD.0000000000004247.

Zhu, X., Wu, C., Qiu, S., Yuan, X., Li L. Effects of resveratrol on glucose control and insulin sensitivity in subjects with type 2 diabetes: systematic review and meta-analysis. *Nutr Metab* (Lond). 2017 Sep 22;14:60. doi: 10.1186/s12986-017-0217-z.

In: Grape Pomace in Health …
Editor: Veronica Sanda Chedea
ISBN: 978-1-68507-409-8


*Chapter 7*

# GRAPE POMACE EFFECTS AND PREVENTION IN NON-ALCOHOLIC STEATOHEPATITIS

***George Saraci[1], Roxana Sechel[2], Lorena Ciumărnean[3], Antonia Eugenia Macarie[4], Sonia Irina Vlaicu[5], Mădălina Sava[6] and Ştefan Cristian Vesa[7,*]***

[1]"Iuliu Haţieganu" University of Medicine and Pharmacy, Cluj-Napoca, Romania

[2]Department of Pathology - Regional Institute of Gastroenterology and Hepatology, Cluj-Napoca, Romania

[3]Department of Internal Medicine, 4th Medical Clinic, "Iuliu Haţieganu," University of Medicine and Pharmacy, Cluj-Napoca, Romania

[4]Department of Geriatrics-Gerontology, "Iuliu Haţieganu," University of Medicine and Pharmacy, Cluj-Napoca, Romania

[5]Department of Internal Medicine, 1st Medical Clinic, "Iuliu Haţieganu" University of Medicine and Pharmacy, Cluj-Napoca, Romania

---

[*] Corresponding Author's E-mail: stefanvesa@gmail.com.

[6]Department of Dermatology, County Hospital, Oradea, Romania
[7]Department of Pharmacology, Toxicology and Clinical Pharmacology, "Iuliu Haţieganu" University of Medicine and Pharmacy

## ABSTRACT

Grape pomace (GP) has demonstrated its beneficial effects for the prevention and progress of NASH, from simple steatosis to steatohepatitis and even severe cirrhosis and its complications, as well as prevention in people with or without metabolic syndrome or associated disorders. GP contains high amounts of phenolic compounds that are a potential source of natural antioxidants with benefits in many diseases including atherosclerosis, cancer prevention and complementary treatment, oxidative stress, diabetes, degenerative, neurological, gastrointestinal, and metabolic disorders. The skin and the seeds are the main parts of the residue that make this product a unique formula. Fatty liver disease encompasses a wide spectrum of pathologies mainly characterized by fatty infiltration of liver cells in the absence of excessive alcohol intake or in the presence of moderate alcohol consumption. This spectrum includes simple fatty liver, fatty infiltration with elevated transaminase levels, fibrosis, and cirrhosis of the liver. It is assumed that most cases of liver cirrhosis of unknown origin are the direct consequence of NAFLD (Non-Alcoholic Fatty Liver Disease). There is a wide variety of drugs and supplements used in this condition. Among them, GP has occupied a unique place due to its beneficial effects on oxidative stress and lipid metabolic balance. The current chapter reviews the main challenges to obtain clinical and biochemical effects in Non-Alcoholic SteatoHepatitis (NASH) using GP products and presents the most recent advances regarding the effects of these kinds of products in hepatic steatosis. We also discuss potential toxicity and drug interactions, considering that NASH is often associated with other medical and metabolic disorders that require treatment with certain drugs.

**Keywords:** grape pomace, NASH, antioxidant effects, procyanidins, liver cirrhosis, polyphenols

# INTRODUCTION

Non-alcoholic fatty liver disease (NAFLD) is a very common condition characterized by increased triglycerides in the liver involving greater than 5% of the liver parenchyma. Its severe form, when inflammation and liver injury are present, is referred to as non-alcoholic steatohepatitis (NASH). From this point, the disease may evolve towards a normal status or inflammation, hepatocyte destruction, and regeneration lead to liver cirrhosis, a condition prone to the development of liver cancer and other life-threatening complications (ascites, esophageal varices, spontaneous bacterial peritonitis, hepatorenal and hepatopulmonary syndromes, portal encephalopathy, portal hypertension, and liver failure ao). In this material, the term NASH is used when referring to fat accumulation inside liver cells, with or without inflammation. Intervention is required especially when the condition evolves towards another stage (e.g., steatohepatitis) (Anstee 2019).

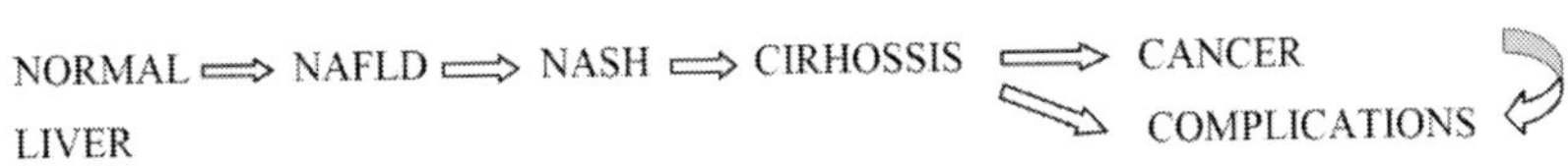


Figure 1. The spectrum of NAFLD (modified according to Anstee 2019).

Another distinguishing feature is the absence of excessive alcohol intake defined as less than 30 g per day for men and 20 g per day for women. Percentage of triglyceride charge of liver cells is also a subject of debate due to biopsy sampling bias and other sophisticated methods are not widely available (proton density fat fraction – more than 5% or proton magnetic resonance spectroscopy – more than 5.6%). Therefore, the main diagnostic approaches are represented by ultrasonography, elastography, or quantitative fat/water selective magnetic resonance (EASL 2016).

It is essential to make the difference between primary NASH (with or without obesity) and secondary NASH: drugs (methotrexate, amiodarone, nucleoside analogues, tamoxifen), Wilson disease, Hans Weber Christian disease, lipodystrophies, obesity, diabetes, dyslipidemia, celiac disease, parenteral nutrition, vinyl chloride, carbon tetrachloride, Kwashiorkor, sleep apnea ao (Adams 2010).

Metabolic syndrome (MS) is a collection of various elements strongly connected to insulin resistance and recent opinions consider that most cases of MS are also associated with primary NASH, while in the presence of NASH onc must search for MS in both obese and non-obese patients (Kaur 2019).

**Table 1. Definition of metabolic syndrome (modified according to Anguilar 2019)**

| Pathologic component | Discriminative value | |
|---|---|---|
| I - Hyperinsulinemia | Plasma insulin > 75% of normal population | |
| C - Hypercoagulation | Increased tendency to develop blood clots | |
| H – Arterial hypertension* | ≥ 130/85 mmHg, or medication for high blood pressure | |
| A - Atherosclerosis | Serum triglycerides* | > 150 mg/dl |
| | Serum HDL-Cholesterol* | < 40mg/dl men, <50 mg/dl women |
| D - Diabetes | Fasting glucose > 100 mg/dl or antidiabetic medication* | |
| O - Obesity | Waist circumference ≥ 94 cm men, ≥80 cm women* | |
| U - Hyperuricemia | Serum uric acid > 7.8 mg/dl men, > 6.8 mg/dl women | |

*Risk factors for the definition of MS – considering serum triglycerides and HDL Cholesterol a single item, with 3 risk factors out of 4 MS is considered diagnosed. Non-marked criteria are not included in nowadays definition but represent a certain association. In 1998, WHO introduced renal impairment as urine albumin > 20mcg/min or albumin/creatinine > 30 mg/g, while in 2003 AACE introduced risk factors for insulin resistance such as polycystic ovary syndrome, family history of diabetes, or sedentary lifestyle.

## NALD – Main Characteristics and Potential Evolution. Current Therapeutic Approaches

Diagnosis of the condition is usually provided by ultrasound examinations as an increase in hepatic echogenicity compared to similar echogenicity structures (e.g., kidney) (Table 2). Patients may accuse pain in the right upper quadrant of the abdomen or minimal fatigability, often without any symptoms. Laboratory tests show elevated liver enzymes (ASAT – aspartate aminotransferase and ALAT – alanine aminotransferase) usually related to the evolution of NASH. Moreover, the presence of elevated cholestatic enzyme levels (GGT – gamma-glutamyl transferase, AP – alkaline phosphatase, 5NT – 5 nucleotidase) may be observed. Other test results are usually normal. The gold standard for diagnosis has long been represented by liver biopsy showing lipid accumulation inside hepatocytes, pushing the nucleus aside, accompanied by portal inflammation and Mallory bodies (Romero Gomez 2020).

**Table 2. Ultrasonographic diagnosis and staging of NASH (modified after De Lucia Rolfe 2018)**

| Grade | Severity | Description |
|---|---|---|
| 1 (<33%) | mild | Increased echogenicity of liver parenchyma compared with kidney parenchyma |
| 2 (33-66%) | moderate | 1 + blurred appearance of portal vein branches inside liver parenchyma |
| 3 (>66%) | severe | 2 + posterior attenuation of the ultrasound beam with difficult visualization of the diaphragm |

Figure 2 shows lipid-loaded hepatocytes with the formation of micro and macrovesicles, inflammatory cells, predominantly lymphocytes, and rare neutrophils, arranged in groups around lipid vesicles forming lipogranulomas that mark the activity, intracytoplasmic bile pigment accumulation at 12 o'clock with regeneration aspects of adjacent hepatocytes - binuclear cells.

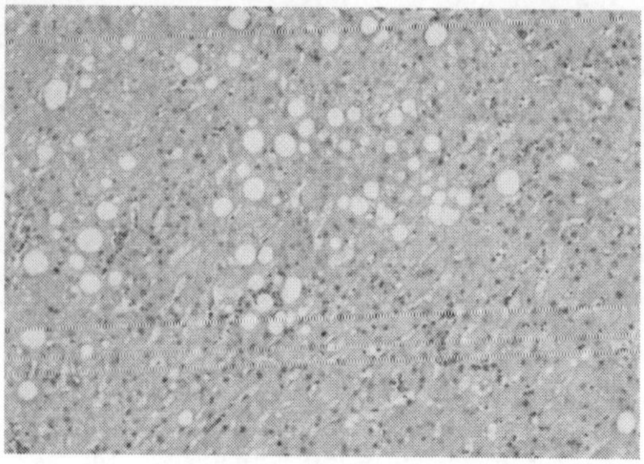

Figure 2. Liver biopsy H&E staining. 20x, NASH (Sechel collection).

In the current era of noninvasive approaches, there is a wide variety of tests and scores able to detect early stages of inflammation and fibrosis in the evolution of NASH. Some of them are evidence-based diagnostic and prognostic tests, while others are more difficult to assess and are only used for research purposes as they are not ready for routine use in clinical practice. These include NAFLD fibrosis score, Fibrotest, BAAT test, ELF and modified ELF score, Fibrometer, Fib 4, BARD and BARDI score, APRI score, BAAT score, PNFS score, Hepascore ao (Arulandan 2015). The first step in the assessment of NASH is the detection of steatosis while ruling out cirrhosis. The next step is the identification of inflammation and the possible presence of fibrosis in different stages. Therapy is recommended in every stage of the disease, but it is compulsory in the presence of inflammation and fibrosis (Sircana 2019). Among lifestyle changes and weight loss in obese individuals, drug therapies are the cornerstone of NASH regression, preventing its evolution towards cirrhosis. Several conventional and novel treatments proposed for NASH are further presented. Some are still experimental and need clinical validation in larger studies (Table 3).

In what concerns the current therapeutic strategies in NASH, despite the great number of potential drugs, clinical practice is focused on liver protectors, phospholipids, antioxidant supplements, and insulin sensitizers (Oseini 2017).

To understand new and potential therapies, one must have a little knowledge on the development of NASH, which is a very complex process encompassing liver changes together with metabolic, hormone, adipose, muscle, digestive, and microbiota functional alterations.

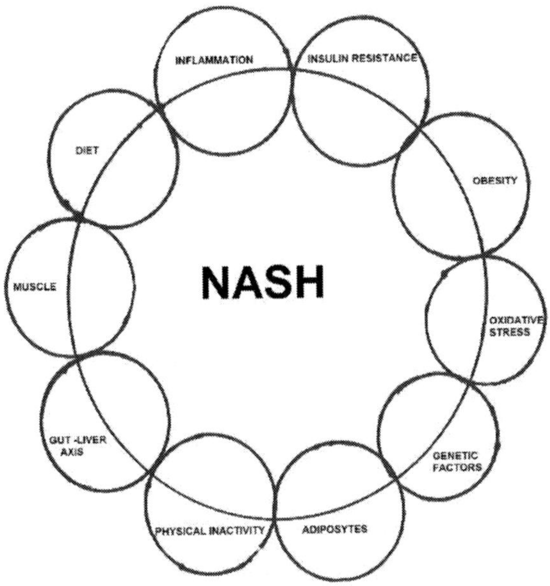


Figure 3. NASH spectrum (personal approach).

The main pathologic event is the increased amount of lipids inside liver cells (steatosis) triggered by various phenomena such as insulin resistance that stimulates gluconeogenesis and lipid synthesis or high fatty acids and carbohydrates intake. Insulin resistance may also elevate lipid levels in liver cells being accompanied by insulin resistance in adipocytes and muscle cells with subsequent release of fatty acids and reduced glucose uptake that will eventually provide the substrate for lipid synthesis in the liver (Maher 2016). Adipocytes die, adiponectin secretion is suppressed and as a result, lipid synthesis in the liver will not be correctly regulated and will also cause inflammation. High levels of TNF-α, IL6, IL1 will disrupt lipid metabolism in liver and adipose tissues and will convert simple steatosis into steatohepatitis.

**Table 3. Treatment for NASH (sources included in the first column). There are many studies for every potential drug and also for other unlisted drugs; the purpose of this synthesis was just to offer a perspective on the available therapies and not a systematic review on the subject**

| Author | Agent | Comments |
|---|---|---|
| Pan 2020 | SGLUT 2 | Lower levels of lipids in liver cells, decreased levels of inflammatory markers |
| Tahara 2020 | SGLUT 2 + Metformin | Murine model |
| Oliveira 2019 | N Acetylcysteine/ Ursodeoxycholic acid + Metformin | NAFLD activity score, ALT levels, histologic improvement |
| Banerjee 2019 | Sildenafil + Leucine + Metformin | Liver and adipose cell lines |
| Yang 2019 | Omega 3 fatty acids | Reduced inflammation in early stages but not advanced |
| Hegazy 2019 | Omega 6 fatty acids | Improved insulin sensitivity |
| Pan 2013 | Selenium | Decreased concentration with the progression of inflammation and fibrosis |
| Pham 2019 | NADH | Reduction of fibrosis progression rate |
| Xia 2016 | Myricetin | Regression of steatosis in a murine model |
| Hosseini 2020 | Resveratrol | Improved steatosis through changes in the Nrf2 pathway, reduced oxidative stress |
| Parafati 2018 | Polyphenols | Reduced inflammation, oxidative stress, lipid-lowering, insulin sensitizer, ao |
| Eslam 2019 | Obeticholic acid | Inflammation, balloon degeneration, fibrosis |
| Neokosmidis 2018 | Cenicriviroc | Inflammation, macrophage recruitment, fibrosis |
| Sahin 2020 | Silymarin | Reduced inflammation, protective effect |
| Alkhouri 2020 | Resmetirom | Improved lipid metabolism, less fat accumulation |

| Author | Agent | Comments |
|---|---|---|
| Iruarrizaga-Lejarreta 2017 | Arachidyl amido cholanoic acid | Less fat accumulation, increased glutathione levels |
| Choudhary 2019 | Saroglitazar | Histologic improvement, lipid metabolism |
| Van Meeteren 2020 | Elafibranor | NASH resolution, lipid changes, progression |

From this point, mitochondrial dysfunction increases oxidative stress and the amount of lipids and inflammation. Liver changes are also influenced by the dysfunction of intestinal cell junctions allowing antigens and bacteria to enter from the intestinal lumen and promote an imbalance of gut microbiota with depletion of short-chain fatty acids, diminished choline and bile acid pool together with toxin translocation and formation of endogenous alcohol (Petta 2016). These changes will worsen liver inflammation and stimulate stellate cells to produce collagen, opening the path towards fibrosis and cirrhosis. The entire process, including the progression of cirrhosis to hepatic carcinoma, is controlled by certain genes (PPARγ, PNPLA3, PLCG ao) (Liu 2020).

## Grape Pomace-Purifying Methods, Demonstrated Effects

GP is the moist-dry residue of *Vitis vinifera* and other related grape species obtained during the production of wine consisting of skin, seeds, and stems, demonstrating a wide range of beneficial effects in many disorders, in health promotion, prevention of various diseases, and antiaging properties. GP contains dietary fibers, carbohydrates, proteins, lipids, sodium, potassium, chlorine, calcium, phosphorus, magnesium, manganese, sulfur, copper, iron, selenium, cobalt, vitamin E, myristic, palmitic, stearic, palmitoleic, linoleic fatty acids, amino acids including arginine - the precursor of nitric oxide, polyphenols including flavonoids, anthocyanins, and the stilbene, resveratrol (Sousa 2014). The skin contains dietary fibers and phenolic compounds, while seeds contain unsaturated lipids, sterols, vitamins, and antioxidants. It is important to obtain a purified product to have a concentrated mass of compounds and to avoid virtual fungal and bacterial contamination, in this respect, the concentration of ochratoxin A and other biogenic amines are indicators of a purified product (Jiménez-Martínez 2018).

The presence of polyphenolic compounds provides GP with antioxidant, anti-inflammatory, anticancer, anti-aging, antimicrobial, insulinotropic, and anti-lipotropin properties, acting in various conditions. Some of them include oxidative stress, arterial hypertension, diabetes, metabolic syndrome, obesity, neoplasms, antiaging, antimicrobial, neurodegenerative conditions, macular disorders, chronic venous insufficiency, athletic performance, cognitive dysfunction, dyslipidemia, constipation, chronic fatigue syndrome, and hormonal dysfunction (Kalli 2018).

One of the major effects on atherosclerosis and metabolic disorders has recently been described and consists of the suppression of lecithin-like oxidized receptor 1 (LOX1) expressed by monocytes and endothelial cells, whose main actions are to transform macrophages into foam cells and continue the accumulation of lipids in the artery wall and to bind the oxidized LDL cholesterol. The extracellular domain of LOX1 suffers proteolytic cleavage resulting in the soluble form (SLOX) that can be quantified in serum levels to assess its vascular density and efficacy of various tested products or smoking cessation (Kattoor 2019).

## Grape Pomace – Action Mechanisms and Pharmacological Effects

GP has a great variety of beneficial effects in the treatment of NASH regardless of stage progression, from simple steatosis to steatohepatitis and even late stages of cirrhosis and its complications, as well as in prevention in people with or without metabolic syndrome or associated disorders. GP ameliorates all metabolic profiles including dyslipidemia, glucose tolerance, obesity, and modulates appetite (Van Hul 2018), predominantly through changes in the gut microbiota and by reducing inflammation (Anhê 2015). In cell culture experiments, which are predominant for these types of novel supplements, resveratrol reduces de novo synthesis of fatty acids, especially palmitic acids, and reduces the activity of acetyl-CoA carboxylase, so the incorporation of fatty acids into triglycerides was significantly diminished. This led to reduced accumulation of lipids in hepatocytes indicating that this approach may lead to the stabilization or regression of steatosis (Gnoni 2009). The same effects were obtained in animal models. In diet-induced obese mice, simple GP did not show expected results alone. Supplementation with an extract from *Schisandra chinensis* (omija fruit) was mandatory to obtain lower leptin, PAI 1, TNF α, IL6, IL1 serum levels. However, GP alone reduced the HDL cholesterol and the atherogenic index, while the GP plus omija group increased HDL cholesterol levels but reduced the atherogenic index. GP alone also decreased NF-κB activation in white adipose tissue (Cho 2013). Oxidative stress is an important step in the evolution of steatosis and steatohepatitis triggered by increased fatty acid levels in liver cells and induced beta-oxidation, mitochondrial dysfunction, and production of toxic lipids (Chen 2020). GP contains well-known and demonstrated substances that can act as antioxidants. GP supplements in pigs increased their antioxidant capacity assessed by serum glutathione levels, total antioxidant capacity, catalase activity, protein carbonyl activity, and thiobarbituric acid reactive substances. An interesting effect of growth inhibition of pathogenic bacteria by *Enterobacteriacae* family and *Campylobacter jejuni* was noticed, as well as an increased concentration of n-3 fatty acids and decreased n-6/n-3 fatty acids ratio (Kafantari 2018).

Macrophages are the core component in the process of tissue repair and also in the formation of the extracellular matrix including specific type 1 and 3 collagens involved in liver fibrogenesis and onset of cirrhosis. Activated macrophages may play an inflammatory role and stimulate fibrogenesis releasing MCP1, TNF α, IL6 chemokines, and other cytokines similarly as they promote the transformation into foam cell and continue the development and lesions in atherosclerotic plaque or they may switch the secretion to an anti-inflammatory pattern especially via IL 4 and other anti-inflammatory cytokines and prevent the mechanisms of inflammatory liver injury and fibrosis (Ginhoux 2014). Resveratrol from GP is believed to play a decisive role in reprogramming macrophages to switch from inflammatory to anti-inflammatory pattern increasing mRNA and IL10 secretion and thus inhibiting the onset of fibrosis in toxic-induced liver damage in animal models (Yu 2019).

Gastrointestinal peptides and neuropeptides are involved in metabolic processes like gluconeogenesis, fatty liver infiltration, or appetite regulation, with elevated levels in diabetes and metabolic syndrome, including GIP, CCK, YY peptide, GLP1, and nesfatin 1. The latter is secreted by various structures including the brain, liver, and gastrointestinal tract, and regulates food intake. Resveratrol and other compounds like GLP 1 receptor agonists, curcumin, ginsenoides, coffee, CCK receptor analogues have been proved to prevent the evolution of NASH towards cirrhosis and liver cancer in human subjects (Tarantino 2020). Resveratrol also inhibits the development of liver fibrosis by normalizing mitochondrial function assessed by mitochondrial membrane potential with flow cytometry analysis and expression of mitochondrial genome genes PGC-α and fibrosis-associated genes collagen I, collagen III, and α-SMA with western blot technique in murine models (Chen 2019). Stem therapy using autologous adipose-derived stem cells for diabetes and associated conditions like NASH is boosted by resveratrol by improving sirt 1 and survival signaling and oxidative damage in the diabetic liver (Chen 2020).

It is important to know resveratrol concentration in various GP products because the dose is highly essential for expected results and the prevention of unwanted effects. For instance, a three-month double-blind study compared lifestyle changes with 500 mg of resveratrol showing improved inflammatory status, steatosis, and ALAT levels in the resveratrol-treated group (Faghihzadeh 2015), while a study using 600 mg of resveratrol daily for 3 months versus placebo showed improved inflammatory status and ASAT and ALAT levels as well as insulin resistance through homeostasis model assessment as an index of insulin resistance (Chen 2015). On the other hand, an eight-week study on obese patients with 3000 mg of resveratrol daily increased ASAT and ALAT levels and did not significantly alter transcription of NQO1, PTP1B, IL6, or HO1 in peripheral blood mononuclear cells (Chachay 2014).

## PHARMACOKINETICS

The pharmacokinetic profile of grape pomace has not been intensively studied and there are definite deciphering mechanisms even though a few studies are showing individual variability. After administration of a certain dose in healthy volunteers, the main circulating metabolites were phenyl-gamma-valerolactones, hydroxybenzoic acids, simple phenols, hydroxyphenylpropionic acids, hydroxycinnamates, and catechin phase II conjugates (Castello 2018). To produce their effects, all the active compounds of GP must have an optimal bioavailability, which is dependent on metabolism and absorption in the gastrointestinal tract, as well as distribution in systemic circulation and cell environment and changes inside the cell (Chedea 2016). Last but not least, metabolism and changes in colon microbiota are also essential as this is the starting point for many of the beneficial effects in most conditions, especially in NASH (Kim 2015).

Resveratrol and other polyphenols from GP are absorbed in the small intestine through passive diffusion or facilitated by transmembrane transporters like integrins. To facilitate absorption, some investigators recommend mixing the product with alcohol to increase solubility at the cost of lowering its antiproliferative effect (Delmas 2000) or cyclodextrin or lipophilic molecules (Lopez, Nicolas 2006). After absorption, resveratrol is rapidly eliminated or metabolized so only a small amount circulates in free form or bound to albumin and other proteins and then transferred to cells with LDL-cholesterol or albumin receptors (Gambini

2015). To increase the bioavailability of polyphenols after oral intake, multiple types of delivery systems have been engineered: nanocrystals, liposomes, solid dispersion, micelles, nanoemulsions, and nanoparticles, each with advantages and disadvantages, rapid or sustained-release (Chimento 2019). After absorption in the small intestine, resveratrol is transferred to the liver via vena porta, and some is excreted in its native form into the bile, without any metabolism, reaching again the intestine from where, through the enterohepatic circuit, it returns to the liver circulating in the same manner as biliary acids. Here, it is metabolized and excreted at the vascular pole of hepatocytes into the systemic circulation, where it is bound to albumin and then transferred to LDL and albumin receptors of cells, while free forms attach to α-v-β3 integrin receptors. It enters the nucleus of the cell and modulates nuclear acids and protein synthesis (Delmas 2011). In the liver, resveratrol and other polyphenols are metabolized by adding glucuronide and sulphate groups resulting in products with lower biological activity: resveratrol-3-O-glucuronide, resveratrol-4-O-glucuronide, resveratrol-trisulphate, most of them trans isomers as cis-isomer is not a stable form (Zamora Ros 2006, Gambini 2015). Resveratrol and other polyphenols are mainly excreted in the urine, where 24-hour tests can indicate resveratrol concentrations, GP, or wine ingestion (Zamora-Ros 2016). An interesting study was performed aiming to investigate the pharmacokinetics, tissue distribution, and excretion in mice by measuring trans-resveratrol-3-O-glucuronide, trans-resveratrol-3-O-glucoside, and trans-resveratrol in plasma, tissue, bile, urine, and stools following intragastric administration of 75, 150, or 300 mg/kg of trans-resveratrol; resveratrol was rapidly absorbed and converted into metabolites mainly excreted in the urine, with the digestive tract showing the most extensive tissue distribution (Su 2019).

Altered pharmacokinetics and brain availability of catechin, epicatechin, quercetin, and resveratrol conjugated metabolites were demonstrated in diabetic rats after administration of GP assessed by plasma and brain concentrations (Chen 2017).

In healthy human volunteers, liquid chromatography coupled with electrospray ionization hybrid linear ion trap quadrupole-Orbitrap-mass spectrometry proved to be an efficient tool in characterizing absorption, metabolism, and excretion of polyphenols after oral administration of beverages enriched with GP (Sasot 2017).

After oral intake, GP has a very interesting modulatory action on gut microbiota to a healthier phenotype producing many of its effects by changes in microbiota without altering normal gut bacteria (Sánchez 2018). After chronic intake of GP, the concentration of acetic, propionic, and butyric acids was increased by up to 54% as an indicator of microbiota fermentative activity, together with increased ammonium concentrations as an indicator of the proteolytic activity of the microbiota. Bacteria groups like Lactobacillus and Bacteroides increased, while non-beneficial bacteria like Chlostydium decreased (Gil-Sánchez 2018).

## INDICATIONS

GP has many indications in various disorders and even in healthy individuals. In this section, we will only refer to the indications in NASH and other related liver diseases. In this case, the indications can be divided into 3 major categories: indications for the prevention of NASH, indications for the prevention of NASH evolution and complications, indication for complications, and other liver conditions that associate steatosis or resembling pathogenetic mechanisms.

Prevention of NASH (Perez-Ramirez 2020, Charytoniuk 2017):

- Healthy individuals
- Life extension
- Type 2 diabetes mellitus
- Impaired fasting glucose, impaired glucose resistance
- Metabolic syndrome
- Atherosclerosis and high cardiovascular risk profile
- Obesity

- High homocysteine levels

NASH (Cicero 2018, Martinez-Maqueda 2018):

- Reduce fatty liver infiltration
- Reduce progressive risk
- Reduce portal inflammation
- Protect from oxidative stress
- Restore mitochondrial function
- Reduce liver fibrosis
- Regression of fibrosis
- Protect from further lesions in cirrhosis
- Adjuvant in liver cancer
- Change in microbiota with the prevention of portal bacteremia
- Neurotransmission anomalies in portal encephalopathy
- Improve survival in liver cancer

Other liver conditions:

- Viral hepatitis; there are some controversies on this subject due to divergent opinions. For hepatitis C infection, most opinions are in favor of GP (Lee 2019), while for hepatitis B infections some authors found a beneficial effect (Deng 2017) and other studies suggest that resveratrol from GP could enhance HBV replication as the Sirt1-PGC-1α-PPARα pathway is an essential mechanism for the virus (Shi 2016).
- Alcoholic liver disease; GP has antioxidative, anti-inflammatory, iron chelation, pro-apoptosis, and/or antiproliferative effects (Tu 2019).
- Autoimmune hepatitis; GP has promising effects reducing infiltration of macrophages and T cells, enhancing the regenerative potential of hepatocytes by decreasing Ki67, PCNA, Cyclin D1, and Cdk2 expression (Huang 2017).

- Wilson's disease; normalization of serum copper and zinc levels (Majewski 2020).
- Hemochromatosis; decreasing liver and heart injuries by reversing the acetylation of Forkhead fox-O-1 (FoxO1) transcription factor (Das 2016).
- Alpha 1-antitrypsin deficiency and Tyrosinemia; GP can reduce inflammation and could be a potential adjuvant (Nishiumi 2012), but so far there has been no study for GP or its components in these conditions (https://www.ncbi.nlm.nih.gov/pubmed/April 2020).
- Hepatocellular carcinoma; through its components, GP acts on both preventing the evolution of cirrhosis following NASH and viral injuries (Rawat 2018). Resveratrol also has many antitumoral actions: changes of cyclins and cyclin-dependent kinases with inhibition of G0/G1 cell cycle phase, induces apoptosis by activating p53, TNF-α, and mitochondrial pathways (Ko 2017).
- Primary sclerosing cholangitis, biliary cholangitis, obstructive jaundice, cystic fibrosis, and other cholestatic disorders; GP regulates farnesoid X receptor pathway involved in the enterohepatic circulation of bile acids (Ding 2018).
- Biliary lithiasis; resveratrol proved to relax gallbladder muscle and alleviate biliary colic associated with nitric oxide, ATP-sensitive potassium channel, and large-conductance calcium-activated potassium channel pathways (Tsai 2017).

## Adverse Reactions and Toxicity

Most GP products and derivatives show no side effects and would not be an issue in healthy individuals, but in people with certain conditions, under medication, or prone to diseases, this aspect should be taken into account. As producers do not alert consumers about potential adverse reactions of GP and there are not many studies concerning this matter, it would be advisable to refer to this section as precautions rather than toxicity and adverse reactions (Timmers 2011). On the other hand, the vast majority of studies does not focus on adverse reactions and insist on product advantages. For example, a study assessing the cosmetic benefits of GP performed on healthy volunteers aged 35-65, evaluated serum and skin antioxidant capacity in Carratelli units along with skin moisture, elasticity and surface, and the intensity of age spots. Effects were spectacular 60 days after administration, but the study did not collect data regarding side effects nor did it use a QoL questionnaire to detect virtual changes (Buonocore 2012).

A study performed on nonhuman pregnant primates demonstrated the benefits of resveratrol for the mother, placenta, and fetus through increased uterine blood flow, improved glucose tolerance, placental inflammation, and liver steatosis. However, the fetal pancreatic mass was enlarged by 42%, with a 12-fold increase in proliferation by Ki67 immunohistochemistry. Therefore, the authors strongly discouraged resveratrol use during pregnancy (Roberts 2014). On embryos and larvae of zebrafish (*Danio rerio*), the toxic effect of resveratrol was dependent on concentration, with LC50 (96h) of 75.3 mg/l in fish embryo toxicity test and LC50 (168h) of 51.4 mg/l in the short-term chronic ecotoxicity test along with a plethora of multiorgan malformations (Cavalcante 2017).

A study on VAF rats aiming to detect the side effects of resveratrol in 50-3000 mg/kg doses indicated no toxicity up to 1500 mg/kg. Subjects with higher doses presented: sudden death, severe weight loss, increased serum alanine aminotransferase, alkaline phosphatase, and bilirubin with no histological changes in the liver, low albumin, and hemoglobin with decreased albumin/globulin ratio and elevated BUN and creatinine levels. Kidney lesions were predominant: glomerular necrosis, papillary necrosis, tubule dilatation, ulceration of pelvic epithelium, pelvic inflammation, papillary fibrosis, hyperplasia of the pelvic epithelium, diffuse epithelial hyperplasia of the urinary bladder, changes that were considered to be the cause of death (Crowell 2004).

Toxicity and adverse reactions are dose-dependent and there is a difference in establishing the dose and tissue concentration between animal and human studies, as well as between in vivo and in vitro studies (Zupancic 2015). At high tissue concentration, especially o-quinone metabolites, may enhance tissue inflammation and oxidative stress, act as cytotoxic agents, induce cell death by changes in mitochondrial redox potential, damage endothelial cell and increase cardiovascular mortality, induce DNA breaks and disrupt DNA synthesis and repair, induce cell necrosis in tissues without harmful effects at the low dose, similarly to how it destroys malignant cells when used in optimal concentrations (Shaito 2020).

In inflammation and oxidative stress, including NASH and other similar conditions, resveratrol shows a biphasic response: at lower and medium doses it has antioxidant and protective effects, while at high doses it has pro-oxidative, inflammatory, and cytotoxic effects (Shaito 2020). In human subjects, resveratrol is well tolerated at doses up to 1g per day (normal dose up to 500 mg/day). Doses greater than 1 g/day may induce nephrotoxicity and gastrointestinal toxicity: nausea, abdominal pain, diarrhea, flatulence, but this is not an important issue as GP mostly contains 100-350 mg of resveratrol (Poulsen 2013, la Porte 2010, actafarma.com).

The most controversial aspects of the adverse reactions are not necessarily related to dose toxicity, but the interaction with the endocrine system, especially sex hormones. These have a major influence on hormone-dependent cancers like breast and prostate cancers, liver cancers with estrogen receptors, and liver cirrhosis with altered estrogen metabolism (Simons 2014). Resveratrol can block androgen and estrogen receptors modulating various gene expressions and pathways involved in cancer like p38 MACK/CK2, p53 NFIY, ERα promoter, MCF 7, CYP17A1, P13K, ERK 1, IGF 1, inducing tumor regression and growth (De Amicis 2019). However, resveratrol and other compounds from GP can act both as agonists and antagonists on estrogen receptors, so caution should be taken in people at risk for the development of hormone-dependent cancers or in men with low testosterone / high estrogen levels or patients with liver cirrhosis or liver impairment and doses must be kept low (Gehm 1997, Hendler 2008). Ultimately, contamination with ochratoxin and bacterial metabolites may cause gastrointestinal and allergic symptoms (Gil-Serna 2018).

## Drug Interactions

The issue of drug interactions in what concerns GP compounds, especially resveratrol, is another dose-related problem as doses less than 1g/day may not have a significant impact and doses higher than 1 g/day are demonstrated to inhibit cytochrome P450 isoenzyme CYP3A4, CYP2C9, and CYP2D6 and activate CYP1A2 (Detampe 2012). Substrates like alprazolam, amlodipine, atorvastatin, cyclosporin, diazepam, estradiol, simvastatin, verapamil are metabolized by CYP3A4 so resveratrol might increase serum concentrations of these drugs. The same effect was noticed for CYP2D6 isoenzyme metabolized substances: amitriptyline, carvedilol, codeine, donepezil, haloperidol, metoprolol, paroxetine, risperidone, tramadol (Lynch 2007). The CYP1A2 isoenzyme is responsible for metabolizing caffeine, clozapine, theophylline, flutamide, mexiletine, mirtazapine, olanzapine, rasagiline, triamterene, and zolmitriptan, so in this case, the administration of GP could determine a more rapid metabolism and a higher dose (Faber 2005). A real problem in today's medicine is the inhibition of CYP2C9, involved in the metabolism of warfarin, effects observed in doses of 1 g/day that could lead to hemorrhagic complications (Rao 2019).

Statins, the most commonly prescribed drugs for cholesterol-related disorders and NASH, have a stronger effect when administered with resveratrol in terms of both cholesterol-lowering and anti-proliferative actions. Induction of Trx-1 induces the expression of HO-1 with angiogenic and cardio-protective roles (Penumathsa 2007). In what concerns the new cholesterol-lowering PPCSK 9 we found no data in the literature about possible interactions.

Regarding the interaction with the renin-angiotensin-aldosterone system, it has been demonstrated that resveratrol suppressed the expression of ACE, angiotensin 1, and AT1R while stimulating the expression of ACE 2, angiotensin 1-7, and AT2R, but these effects were mostly studied on animal models in deciphering the mechanism of aging (Jang 2018). In human endothelial cells, GP compounds reduced ACE activity, but the study showed no effect for resveratrol, and the effect was validated by flavonoids in a dose-dependent manner (Persson 2013).

Silymarin, generally prescribed for hepatoprotection in NASH, does not seem to interact with GP, but have synergic actions that may allow dose reduction: antioxidant, anti-inflammatory, mitochondria optimizer, partial activator of estrogen receptors, reduction of TNFα, IL 6, IL 1, and antifibrotic action (Cicero 2018).

The interaction of GP with PPAR γ like fibrates and thiazolidinediones is also favorable in NASH as both drug categories validate their action at the mitochondrial level, polyphenols, and PPAR γ by inhibiting reactive oxygen species and pro-inflammatory cytokines, while the latter also enhances NO production (Morel 2014).

GP does not affect GLUT 2 in the intestine and kidney, so there is no possibility to interact with SGLUT 2 (dapagliflozin empagliflozin, canagliflozin, ertugliflozin), but may synergically reduce GLUT 2 in the liver, increasing liver glycogen and SIRT 1 (Yonamine 2016).

Both resveratrol and metformin aim to reduce insulin resistance and it has been demonstrated that when administered together they had a better effect on insulin resistance and subsequently in NASH than when administered alone (Frendo-Cumbo 2016).

Resveratrol acts together with 5FU in CD 133 positive colorectal cancer, as resveratrol added to culture cell lines treated with 5FU showed a dramatic apoptosis rate and the mechanism seems to be the modulation of BAX tumor suppression gene (Huang 2019).

Resveratrol can influence the TGF-β/Smad signaling pathway for tamoxifen in breast cancer, thus resensitizing these cells to tamoxifen (Shi 2013).

Nitrates are widely prescribed in cardiovascular disease and portal hypertension and tolerance to these substances may be an issue. Resveratrol proved to restore tolerance to nitrates in an isolated internal mammary artery model in vitro through the inhibition of NAD(P)-derived superoxide production in the endothelium (Coskun 2006).

Resveratrol combined with omega 3 fatty acids has synergistic effects on inflammation and lipid metabolism reducing PGE2, IL6, IL 8, omega 3 fatty acids acting predominantly on chronic inflammation, while resveratrol is capable of reducing inflammation from early stages so this combination might be a promising approach in NASH (Kakoti 2015).

The combination of resveratrol with vitamin D modulates estrogen receptor signaling mechanisms and inhibits ovarian cancer cell proliferation acting together on many pathways, the most important being the up-regulation of the powerful p21 suppressor gene resulting in the G0/G1 cell cycle phase arrest (Uberti 2017).

GP may interact with various drugs, foods, or supplements in the intestine, and its antioxidant properties could enhance gut microbiota modulation for several probiotics, an effect that is also of great interest in NASH (Dos Santos 2017).

## Future Perspectives and Studies

Most animal and human studies on this matter compared the effect of GP on diet-induced NASH or in NASH that had already been confirmed. It would be interesting to find out if GP can prevent NASH and not only to improve the confirmed disease or to prevent the progression to fibrosis, cirrhosis, and cancer.

The majority of the studies are performed on animal models or cell lines and these studies must be validated in humans. From the studies involving human subjects, there are a lot of GP compounds, but they mostly focus on resveratrol, which is an essential compound with many effects. It would be interesting to assess the effects of GP as a whole, keeping in mind that it contains other substances besides resveratrol, with effects that are not assessed in those studies. As previously shown, many studies were performed with GP as a meal supplement in animals used for human consumption, with a lot of positive metabolic changes in terms of animal health, milk, and meat quality, which is a great achievement for producers and consumers. Still, there is a need for further studies to determine whether these effects are reproducible in human subjects and what are the long term effects on the consumer. Many double-blind studies might be pictured, for example, one group receiving evidence-based medical treatment and another GP alone, but these kinds of studies are not possible due to ethical implications. If we just compare groups with conventional treatment to groups with additional GP, we could reach certain conclusions, but we will still not be able to determine their separate effects on biological and histological changes and so we can only recommend GP as a supplement and not as medicine with specific indications. Another aspect would be the various production and purifying methods for obtaining GP. As we do not have a standard product and every production company has its own recipe and dosing, we cannot compare studies with GP as they might use a different product. This issue could be solved if every producer registers their product and present the exact dose and composition.

## CONCLUSION

NASH is a complex condition with a wide spectrum of clinical and pathological manifestations from simple liver fatty infiltration to portal inflammation, degeneration of liver cells, and fibrosis. It has been demonstrated that it is associated with other metabolic disorders, especially metabolic syndrome and cardiovascular diseases. It might progress toward liver cirrhosis, with the entire series of complications and hepatocellular carcinoma. It is apparently a benign condition with little or no clinical manifestation at the beginning, but its evolution brings about severe conditions with limited therapeutic resources and high medical and social costs, and human sufferings. Many therapeutic approaches have been tested, some with clear and consistent results, others with questionable benefits or anecdotal evidence. GP, a semisolid residue obtained during the process of winemaking, seems to have many properties able to lower lipid deposits in liver cells, decrease inflammation and impede portal collagen synthesis with subsequent fibrosis and cirrhosis. It also has effects on confirmed cirrhosis and even on hepatocellular carcinoma. It also showed notable effects in metabolic syndrome and other disorders related to NASH. Unfortunately, there are not many studies on humans for this product, which is mainly used as a supplement, usually in healthy individuals or to treat and prevent other conditions or in anti-aging therapies. Many of its beneficial actions have been undoubtedly demonstrated in animal models or experiments using cell cultures or in vivo/in vitro microbiology studies. Many of its effects are linked to changes in gut microbiota. Like any other therapy, it also has several adverse reactions and drug interactions, but much less than conventional medicines.

In conclusion, GP is a solid approach to NASH and its related conditions, but further studies are mandatory to prove its properties from an evidence-based medicine perspective.

## REFERENCES

Adams LA, Feldstein AE. Nonalcoholic steatohepatitis: risk factors and diagnosis. *Expert Review of Gastroenterology & Hepatology* 2010, 4(5), 623–635 https://doi.org/10.1586/egh.10.56.

Aguilar-Salinas CA, Viveros-Ruiz T. Recent advances in managing/understanding the metabolic syndrome. F1000Res 2019;8:F1000 *Faculty Rev*-370. 3. doi:10.12688/f1000research.17122.1.

Alkhouri, N. (2020). Thyromimetics as emerging therapeutic agents for nonalcoholic steatohepatitis: rationale for the development of resmetirom (MGL-3196). *Expert Opinion on Investigational Drugs,* 29(2), 99–101. https://doi.org/10.1080/13543784.2020.1708899.

Anhê FF, Roy D, Pilon G, Dudonné S, Matamoros S, Varin TV, Garofalo C, Moine Q, Desjardins Y, Levy E, Marette A. A polyphenol-rich cranberry extract protects from diet-induced obesity, insulin resistance, and intestinal inflammation in association with increased Akkermansia spp. population in the gut microbiota of mice. *Gut* 2015, 64:872–883. doi:10.1136/gutjnl-2014-307142.

Anstee QM, Reeves HL, Kotsiliti E, Govaere O, & Heikenwalder M. From NASH to HCC: current concepts and future challenges. *Nature Reviews Gastroenterology & Hepatology* 2019, 16(7), 411–428. https://doi.org/10.1038/s41575-019-0145-7.

Arulanandan A, Loomba R. Non-invasive Testing for NASH and NASH with Advanced Fibrosis: Are We There Yet? *Curr Hepatol Rep.* 2015; 14(2):109–118. doi:10.1007/s11901-015-0263-9.

Banerjee J, Bruckbauer A, Thorpe T, Zemel MB. Biphasic Effect of Sildenafil on Energy Sensing is Mediated by Phosphodiesterases 2 and 3 in Adipocytes and Hepatocytes. *Int. J. Mol. Sci.* 2019, 20, 2992.

Buonocore D, Lazzeretti A, Tocabens P, et al. Resveratrol-procyanidin blend: nutraceutical and antiaging efficacy evaluated in a placebo controlled, double-blind study. *Clin Cosmet Investig Dermatol* 2012; 5:159–165. doi:10.2147/CCID.S36102.

Castello F, Costabile G, Bresciani L, et al. Bioavailability and pharmacokinetic profile of grape pomace phenolic compounds in humans. *Arch Biochem Biophys* 2018; 646:1–9. doi:10.1016/j.abb.2018.03.021.

Cavalcante AK, Lopes-Ferreira M, Rogero S, Rogero JR. Evaluation of resveratrol toxicity in the embryolarval stage of Danio rerio fish. *Ecotoxicology and Environmental Contamination* 2017, 12:133–139. https://doi.org/10.5132/eec.2017.01.15.

Chachay VS, Macdonald GA, Martin JH, Whitehead JP, O'Moore-Sullivan TM, Lee P, Franklin M, Klein K, Taylor PJ, Ferguson M, Coombes JS, Thomas GP, Cowin GJ, Kirkpatrick CMJ, Prins JB, Hickman IJ. Resveratrol does not benefit patients with nonalcoholic fatty liver disease. Clinical Gastroenterology and Hepatology : *The*

*Official Clinical Practice Journal of the American Gastroenterological Association* 2014, 12(12):2092–2096. https://doi.org/10.1016/j.cgh.2014.02.024.

Charytoniuk T, Drygalski K, Konstantynowicz-Nowicka K, Berk K, Chabowski A. Alternative treatment methods attenuate the development of NAFLD: A review of resveratrol molecular mechanisms and clinical trials. *Nutrition* (Burbank, Los Angeles County, Calif.) 2017, 34:08–117. https://doi.org/10.1016/j.nut.2016.09.001.

Chedea, V; Pop, R. Procyanidins-Bioavailability and Metabolization; in *Procyanidins: Characterisation, Antioxidant Properties and Health Benefits*, Chedea V.S. Ed. Nova Science Pub Inc, New York USA, 2016; pp. 91–128.

Chen S, Zhao X, Ran L, Wan J, Wang X, Qin Y, Shu F, Gao Y, Yuan L, Zhang Q, Mi M. Resveratrol improves insulin resistance, glucose and lipid metabolism in patients with non-alcoholic fatty liver disease: a randomized controlled trial. Digestive and Liver Disease : *Official Journal of the Italian Society of Gastroenterology and the Italian Association for the Study of the Liver* 2015, 47(3):226–232. https://doi.org/10.1016/j.dld.2014.11.015.

Chen TT, Peng, S, Wang Y, Hu Y, Shen Y, Xu Y, Yin J, Liu C, Cao J. Improvement of Mitochondrial Activity and Fibrosis by Resveratrol Treatment in Mice with *Schistosoma japonicum* Infection. *Biomolecules* 2019, 9(11). https://doi.org/10.3390/biom9110658.

Chen TY, Ferruzzi MG, Wu QL, et al. Influence of diabetes on plasma pharmacokinetics and brain bioavailability of grape polyphenols and their phase II metabolites in the Zucker diabetic fatty rat. *Mol Nutr Food Res* 2017; 61(10):10.1002/mnfr.201700111. doi:10.1002/mnfr.201700111.

Chen, TS, Lai CH, Shen CY, Pai PY, Chen, RJ, PadmaViswanadha V, Yang CK, Chen MC, Lin YM, Huang CY. Orally administered resveratrol enhances the therapeutic effect of autologous transplanted adipose-derived stem cells on rats with diabetic hepatopathy. *Biotechnic & Histochemistry: Official Publication of the Biological*

*Stain Commission* 2020, 95(1):37–45. https://doi.org/10.1080/10520295.2019.1631481.

Chen, Z, Tian R, She Z, Cai J, Li H. Role of oxidative stress in the pathogenesis of nonalcoholic fatty liver disease. *Free Radical Biology & Medicine* 2020, 152:116–141. https://doi.org/10.1016/j.freeradbiomed.2020.02.025.

Chimento A, De Amicis F, Sirianni R, et al. Progress to Improve Oral Bioavailability and Beneficial Effects of Resveratrol. *Int J Mol Sci* 2019; 20(6):1381. doi:10.3390/ijms20061381.

Cho SJ, Jung UJ, Park HJ, Kim HJ, Park YB, Kim SR, Choi MS. Combined Ethanol Extract of Grape Pomace and Omija Fruit Ameliorates Adipogenesis, Hepatic Steatosis, and Inflammation in Diet-Induced Obese Mice. *Evidence-Based Complementary and Alternative Medicine* 2013, 212139. https://doi.org/10.1155/2013/212139.

Choudhary NS, Kumar N, Duseja A. Peroxisome Proliferator-Activated Receptors and Their Agonists in Nonalcoholic Fatty Liver Disease. *J Clin Exp Hepatol.* 2019 Nov-Dec;9(6):731-739. doi: 10.1016/j.jceh.2019.06.004.

Cicero AFG, Colletti A, Bellentani S. Nutraceutical Approach to Non-Alcoholic Fatty Liver Disease (NAFLD): The Available Clinical Evidence. *Nutrients* 2018, 10(9). https://doi.org/10.3390/nu10091153.

Coskun B, Soylemez S, Parlar A, Tulga U, Fehmi K, Akar F. Effect of Resveratrol on Nitrate Tolerance in Isolated Human Internal Mammary Artery, *Journal of Cardiovascular Pharmacology* 2006, 47(3):437-445.

Crowell JA, Korytko PJ, Morrissey RL, Booth TD, Levine BS. Resveratrol-associated renal toxicity. *Toxicol Sci* 2004; 82(2):614–619. doi:10.1093/toxsci/kfh263.

Das SK, DesAulniers J, Dyck JRB, Kassiri Z, Oudit GY (2016). Resveratrol mediates therapeutic hepatic effects in acquired and genetic murine models of iron-overload. *Liver International: Official*

*Journal of the International Association for the Study of the Liver* 2016, 36(2), 246–257. https://doi.org/10.1111/liv.12893.

De Amicis F, Chimento A, Montalto FI, Casaburi I, Sirianni R, Pezzi V. Steroid Receptor Signallings as Targets for Resveratrol Actions in Breast and Prostate Cancer. *Int J Mol Sci.* 2019; 20(5):1087. Published 2019 Mar 3. doi:10.3390/ijms20051087.

De Lucia Rolfe E, Brage S, Sleigh A, et al. Validity of ultrasonography to assess hepatic steatosis compared to magnetic resonance spectroscopy as a criterion method in older adults. *PLoS One* 2018; 13(11):e0207923. doi:10.1371/journal.pone.0207923.

Delmas D et al. 2000. Inhibitory effect of resveratrol on the proliferation of human and rat hepatic derived cell lines. *Oncol. Rep* 2000. 7: 847–852.

Delmas D, Aires V, Limagne E, et al. Transport, stability, and biological activity of resveratrol. *Ann N Y Acad Sci* 2011; 1215:48–59. doi:10.1111/j.1749-6632.2010.05871.x.

Deng JJ, Kong KE, Gao WW, et al. Interplay between SIRT1 and hepatitis B virus X protein in the activation of viral transcription. *Biochim Biophys Acta Gene Regul Mech* 2017; 1860(4):491–501. doi:10.1016/j.bbagrm.2017.02.007.

Detampel P, Beck M, Krähenbühl S, Huwyler J. Drug interaction potential of resveratrol. *Drug Metab Rev* 2012; 44(3):253–265. doi:10.3109/03602532.2012.700715.

Ding, L, Zhang B, Li J, Yang L, Wang Z. Beneficial effect of resveratrol on αnaphthyl isothiocyanate induced cholestasis via regulation of the FXR pathway. *Molecular Medicine Reports* 2018; 17.1: 1863-1872.

Dos Santos KM, de Oliveira IC, Lopes MA, Cruz AP, Buriti FC, Cabral LM. Addition of grape pomace extract to probiotic fermented goat milk: the effect on phenolic content, probiotic viability and sensory acceptability. *J Sci Food Agric* 2017;97(4):1108–1115. doi:10.1002/jsfa.7836.

EASL–EASD–EASO Clinical Practice Guidelines for the management of non-alcoholic fatty liver disease. *Journal of Hepatology* 2016, 64(6): 1388 – 1402.

Eslam M, Alvani R, Shiha G. Obeticholic acid: towards first approval for NASH. *Lancet.* 2019 Dec 14;394(10215):2131-2133. doi: 10.1016/S0140-6736(19)32963-0.

Faber MS, Jetter A, Fuhr U. Assessment of CYP1A2 activity in clinical practice: why, how, and when? *Basic Clin Pharmacol Toxicol* 2005; 97:125-134.

Faghihzadeh F, Adibi P, Hekmatdoost A. The effects of resveratrol supplementation on cardiovascular risk factors in patients with non-alcoholic fatty liver disease: A randomised, double-blind, placebo-controlled study. *Br. J. Nutr* 2015; 114:796–803. doi: 10.1017/S0007 11451500243.

Frendo-Cumbo S, MacPherson RE, Wright DC. Beneficial effects of combined resveratrol and metformin therapy in treating diet-induced insulin resistance. *Physiol Rep.* 2016; 4(15):e12877. doi:10.14814/ phy2.12877.

Gambini J, Inglés M, Olaso G, et al. Properties of Resveratrol: In Vitro and In Vivo Studies about Metabolism, Bioavailability, and Biological Effects in Animal Models and Humans. *Oxid Med Cell Longev.* 2015; 2015:837042. doi:10.1155/2015/837042.

Gehm BD, McAndrews JM, Chien PY, Jameson JL. Resveratrol, a polyphenolic compound found in grapes and wine, is an agonist for the estrogen receptor. *Proc Natl Acad Sci U S A* 1997; 94(25):14138–14143. doi:10.1073/pnas.94.25.14138.

Gil-Sánchez I, Cueva C, Sanz-Buenhombre M, Guadarrama A, Moreno-Arribas MV, Bartolomé B. Dynamic gastrointestinal digestion of grape pomace extracts: Bioaccessible phenolic metabolites and impact on human gut microbiota. *Journal of Food Composition and Analysis* 2018, 68:41–52. https://doi.org/https://doi.org/10. 1016/j.jfca.2017.05.005.

Gil-Serna J, Vázquez C, González-Jaén M, Patino B. Wine Contamination with Ochratoxins: A Review. *Beverages* 2020, 4, 6. https://doi.org/10.3390/beverages4010006.

Ginhoux F, Jung S. Monocytes and macrophages: developmental pathways and tissue homeostasis *Nat. Rev. Immunol* 2014, 14 (6):392-404.

Gnoni GV, Paglialonga G. Resveratrol inhibits fatty acid and triacylglycerol synthesis in rat hepatocytes. *European Journal of Clinical Investigation* 2009, 39(3):211–218. https://doi.org/10.1111/j.1365-2362.2008.02077.x.

Hegazy M, Elsayed NM, Ali HM, Hassan HG, Rashed L. Diabetes Mellitus, Nonalcoholic Fatty Liver Disease, and Conjugated Linoleic Acid (Omega 6): What Is the Link? *Journal of Diabetes Research*, 2019, 5267025. https://doi.org/10.1155/2019/5267025.

Hendler SS, Rorvik DR, eds, eds. *PDR for Nutritional Supplements*. 2nd edition ed: Thomson Reuters; 2008.

Hosseini H, Teimouri M, Shabani M, Koushki M, Babaei Khorzoughi R, Namvarjah F, Izadi P, Meshkani R. Resveratrol alleviates non-alcoholic fatty liver disease through epigenetic modification of the Nrf2 signaling pathway. *Int J Biochem Cell Biol.* 2020 Feb;119:105667. doi: 10.1016/j.biocel.2019.105667. Epub 2019 Dec 12.

Huang L, Zhang S, Zhou J & Li X. Effect of resveratrol on drug resistance in colon cancer chemotherapy. *RSC Adv* 2019, 9(5), 2572–2580. https://doi.org/10.1039/C8RA08364A.

Huang TH, Chen CC, Liu HM, Lee TY, Shieh SH. Resveratrol Pretreatment Attenuates Concanavalin A-induced Hepatitis through Reverse of Aberration in the Immune Response and Regenerative Capacity in Aged Mice. *Scientific Reports* 2017, 7(1):2705. https://doi.org/10.1038/s41598-017-02881-z.

Iruarrizaga-Lejarreta M, Varela-Rey M, Fernández-Ramos D, et al. Role of Aramchol in steatohepatitis and fibrosis in mice. *Hepatol Commun.* 2017;1(9):911–927. doi:10.1002/hep4.1107.

Jang IA, Kim EN, Lim JH, et al. Effects of Resveratrol on the Renin-Angiotensin System in the Aging Kidney. *Nutrients.* 2018; 10(11):1741. Published 2018 Nov 12. doi:10.3390/nu10111741.

Jiménez-Martínez MD, Gil-Muñoz R, Gómez-Plaza E, Bautista-Ortín AB. Performance of purified grape pomace as a fining agent to reduce the levels of some contaminants from wine. *Food Additives & Contaminants: Part A* 2018, 35(6):1061–1070. https://doi.org/10.1080/19440049.2018.1459050.

Kafantaris I, Stagos D, Kotsampasi B, Hatzis A, Kypriotakis A, Gerasopoulos K, Makri S, Goutzourelas N, Mitsagga, C, Giavasis I, Petrotos K, Kokkas S, Goulas P, Christodoulou V, Kouretas D. Grape pomace improves performance, antioxidant status, fecal microbiota and meat quality of piglets. Animal : *An International Journal of Animal Bioscience* 2018, 12(2):246–255. https://doi.org/10.1017/S1751731117001604.

Kakoti BB, Hernandez-Ontiveros DG, Kataki MS, Shah K, Pathak Y, Panguluri SK. Resveratrol and Omega-3 Fatty Acid: Its Implications in Cardiovascular Diseases. *Front Cardiovasc Med.* 2015; 2:38. Published 2015 Dec 11. doi:10.3389/fcvm.2015.00038.

Kalli E, Lappa I, Bouchagier P, Tarantilis PA, Skotti E. (2018). Novel application and industrial exploitation of winery by-products. *Bioresources and Bioprocessing* 2018, 5(1):46. https://doi.org/10.1186/s40643-018-0232-6.

Kattoor AJ, Goel A, Mehta JL. LOX-1: Regulation, Signaling and Its Role in Atherosclerosis. *Antioxidants (Basel).* 2019; 8(7):218. doi:10.3390/antiox8070218.

Kaur JA. Comprehensive review on metabolic syndrome *Cardiol Res Pract* 2014;2014:943162. doi:10.1155/2014/943162.

Kim H, Kim DH, Seo KH, et al. Modulation of the intestinal microbiota is associated with lower plasma cholesterol and weight gain in hamsters fed chardonnay grape seed flour. *J Agric Food Chem.* 2015; 63(5):1460–1467. doi:10.1021/jf5026373.

Ko JH, Sethi G, Um JY, et al. The Role of Resveratrol in Cancer Therapy. *Int J Mol Sci* 2017; 18(12):2589. Published 2017 Dec 1. doi:10.3390/ijms18122589.

la Porte C, Voduc N, Zhang G, et al. Steady-State pharmacokinetics and tolerability of trans-resveratrol 2000 mg twice daily with food, quercetin and alcohol (ethanol) in healthy human subjects. *Clin Pharmacokinet* 2010; 49(7):449–454. doi:10.2165/11531820-000000000-00000.

Lee S, Mailar K, Kim MI, et al. Plant-Derived Purification, Chemical Synthesis, and In Vitro/In Vivo Evaluation of a Resveratrol Dimer, Viniferin, as an HCV Replication Inhibitor. *Viruses* 2019; 11(10):890. Published 2019 Sep 23. doi:10.3390/v11100890.

Liu J, Lin B, Chen Z, et al. Identification of key pathways and genes in nonalcoholic fatty liver disease using bioinformatics analysis. *Arch Med Sci*. 2020; 16(2):374–385. Published 2020 Mar 2. doi:10.5114/aoms.2020.93343.

Lopez-Nicolas JM et al. Determination of stoichiometric coefficients and apparent formation constants for beta-cyclodextrin complexes of trans-resveratrol using reversed-phase liquid chromatography. *J. Chromatogr A* 2006, 1135: 158–165.

Lynch T, Price A. The effect of cytochrome P450 metabolism on drug response, interactions, and adverse effects. *Am Fam Physician* 2007; 76(3):391–396.

Maher JJ. Pathogenesis of NAFLD and NASH. In: Chalasani N., Szabo G. (eds) *Alcoholic and Non-Alcoholic Fatty Liver Disease*. Springer, Cham, 2016.

Majewski M, Ognik K, Thoene M, Rawicka A, Juskiewicz, J. Resveratrol modulates the blood plasma levels of Cu and Zn, the antioxidant status and the vascular response of thoracic arteries in copper deficient Wistar rats. *Toxicology and Applied Pharmacology* 2020, 390:114877. https://doi.org/10.1016/j.taap.2020.114877.

Martinez-Maqueda D, Zapatera B, Gallego-Narbon A, Vaquero MP, Saura-Calixto F, Perez-Jimenez J. A 6-week supplementation with grape pomace to subjects at cardiometabolic risk ameliorates insulin sensitivity, without affecting other metabolic syndrome markers. *Food & Function* 2018, 9(11):6010–6019. https://doi.org/10.1039/c8fo01323c.

Morel J, Singer M. Statins, fibrates, thiazolidinediones and resveratrol as adjunctive therapies in sepsis: could mitochondria be a common target? *Intensive Care Med Exp*. 2014;2(1):9. doi:10.1186/2197-425X-2-9.

Neokosmidis G, Tziomalos K. Role of cenicriviroc in the management of nonalcoholic fatty liver disease. *World J Gastroenterol* 2018; 24(48): 5415-5417.

Nishiumi S, Mukai R, Ichiyanagi T, Ashida H. Suppression of lipopolysaccharide and galactosamine-induced hepatic inflammation by red grape pomace. *Journal of Agricultural and Food Chemistry* 2012, 60(36), 9315–9320. https://doi.org/10.1021/jf302298n.

Oseini AM, Sanyal AJ. Therapies in non-alcoholic steatohepatitis (NASH). *Liver Int*. 2017; 37 Suppl 1(Suppl 1):97–103. doi:10.1111/liv.13302.

Pan D, Huang H. Hair Selenium Levels in Hepatic Steatosis Patients. Biological Trace Element Research 2013, 152(3), 305–309. https://doi.org/10.1007/s12011-013-9624-9.

Pan, CS, Stanley TL. Effect of Weight Loss Medications on Hepatic Steatosis and Steatohepatitis: A Systematic Review. *In Frontiers in Endocrinology* 2020 Vol. 11, p. 70). https://www.frontiersin.org/article/10.3389/fendo.2020.00070.

Parafati M, Lascala A, La Russa D, Mignogna C, Trimboli F, Morittu VM, Riillo C, Macirella R, Mollace V, Brunelli E, Janda, E. Bergamot Polyphenols Boost Therapeutic Effects of the Diet on Non-Alcoholic Steatohepatitis (NASH) Induced by "Junk Food": Evidence for Anti-Inflammatory Activity. *Nutrients* 2018, 10, 1604.

Penumathsa SV, Thirunavukkarasu M, Koneru S, et al. Statin and resveratrol in combination induces cardioprotection against myocardial infarction in hypercholesterolemic rats. *J Mol Cell Cardiol*. 2007; 42(3):508–516. doi:10.1016/j.yjmcc.2006.10.018.

Perez-Ramirez IF, de Diego EH, Riomoros-Arranz M, Reynoso-Camacho R, Saura-Calixto F, Perez-Jimenez J. Effects of acute intake of grape/pomegranate pomace dietary supplement on glucose metabolism and oxidative stress in adults with abdominal obesity. *International Journal of Food Sciences and Nutrition* 2020, 71(1):94–105. https://doi.org/10.1080/09637486.2019.1607831.

Persson I. Red wine, white wine, rosé wine, and grape juice inhibit angiotensin-converting enzyme in human endothelial cells. *Int J Nutr Pharmacol Neurol Dis* 2013; 3:17-23.

Petta S, Gastaldelli A, Rebelos E, Bugianesi E, Messa P, Miele L, Svegliati-Baroni G, Valenti L, Bonino F. Pathophysiology of Non Alcoholic Fatty Liver Disease. *Int. J. Mol. Sci*. 2016, 17, 2082.

Pham TX, Bae M, Kim MB, Lee Y, Hu S, Kang H, Park YK, Lee JY. Nicotinamide riboside, an NAD+ precursor, attenuates the development of liver fibrosis in a diet-induced mouse model of liver fibrosis. *Biochim Biophys Acta Mol Basis Dis.* 2019 Sep 1;1865(9):2451-2463. doi: 10.1016/j.bbadis.2019.06.009. Epub 2019 Jun 11.

Poulsen MM, Vestergaard PF, Clasen BF, et al. High-dose resveratrol supplementation in obese men: an investigator-initiated, randomized, placebo-controlled clinical trial of substrate metabolism, insulin sensitivity, and body composition. *Diabetes* 2013; 62(4):1186–1195. doi:10.2337/db12-0975.

Rao M. Pharmacogenomics in Palliative Medicine. *Indian J Palliat Care* 2019;25(2):169–171. doi:10.4103/IJPC.IJPC_46_19.

Rawat D, Shrivastava S, Naik RA, Chhonker SK, Mehrotra A, Koiri RK. An Overview of Natural Plant Products in the Treatment of Hepatocellular Carcinoma. *Anticancer Agents Med Chem* 2018; 18(13):1838–1859. doi:10.2174/1871520618666180604085612.

Roberts VH, Pound LD, Thorn SR, et al. Beneficial and cautionary outcomes of resveratrol supplementation in pregnant nonhuman primates. *FASEB J* 2014; 28(6):2466–2477. doi:10.1096/fj.13-245472.

Romero-Gomez M. *NAFLD and NASH Biomarkers in Detection, Diagnosis, and Monitoring.* Springer Switzerland 2020.

Sahin E, Bagci R, Bektur Aykanat NE, Kacar S, Sahinturk V. Silymarin attenuated nonalcoholic fatty liver disease through the regulation of endoplasmic reticulum stress proteins GRP78 and XBP-1 in mice. *J Food Biochem.* 2020 Mar 18:e13194. doi: 10.1111/jfbc.13194.

Sánchez I, Esteban-Fernández A, Llano D, Sanz-Buenhombre M, Guadarrana, A, Salazar N, Gueimonde M, Reyes-Gaviláne C, Gómez L, Bermejo M, Bartolomé B, Moreno-Arribas MV. Supplementation with grape pomace in healthy women: Changes in biochemical parameters, gut microbiota and related metabolic biomarkers. *Journal of Functional Foods* 2018, 45:34–46. https://doi.org/10.1016/j.jff.2018.03.031.

Sasot G, Martínez-Huélamo M, Vallverdú-Queralt A, Mercader-Martí M, Estruch R, Lamuela-Raventós RM. Identification of phenolic metabolites in human urine after the intake of a functional food made from grape extract by a high resolution LTQ-Orbitrap-MS approach. *Food Res Int.* 2017; 100(Pt 3):435–444. doi:10.1016/j.foodres.2017.01.020.

Shaito A, Posadino AM, Younes N, et al. Potential Adverse Effects of Resveratrol: A Literature Review. *Int J Mol Sci* 2020; 21(6):2084. Published 2020 Mar 18. doi:10.3390/ijms21062084.

Shi XP, Miao S, Wu Y, et al. Resveratrol sensitizes tamoxifen in antiestrogen-resistant breast cancer cells with epithelial-mesenchymal transition features. *Int J Mol Sci.* 2013;14(8):15655–15668. Published 2013 Jul 26. doi:10.3390/ijms140815655.

Shi Y, Li Y, Huang C, et al. Resveratrol enhances HBV replication through activating Sirt1-PGC-1α-PPARα pathway. *Sci Rep* 2016; 6:24744. Published 2016 Apr 21. doi:10.1038/srep24744.

Simons SS Jr, Edwards DP, Kumar R. Minireview: dynamic structures of nuclear hormone receptors: new promises and challenges. *Mol Endocrinol* 2014; 28(2):173–182. doi:10.1210/me.2013-1334.

Sircana A, Paschetta E, Saba F, Molinaro F, Musso G. Recent Insight into the Role of Fibrosis in Nonalcoholic Steatohepatitis-Related Hepatocellular Carcinoma. *Int J Mol Sci.* 2019; 20(7):1745. Published 2019 Apr 9. doi:10.3390/ijms20071745.

Sousa EC, Uchoa-Thomaz AMA, Carioca JOB, Morais SM de, Lima A de, Martins CG, Alexandrino CD, Ferreira PAT, Rodrigues ALM, Rodrigues SP, Silva J do N, Rodrigues L. Chemical composition and bioactive compounds of grape pomace (*Vitis vinifera* L.), Benitaka variety, grown in the semiarid region of Northeast Brazil. *Food Science and Technology* 2014, 34:135–142. http://www.scielo.br/scielo.php?script=sci_arttext&pid=S0101-20612014000100020&nrm=iso.

Su M, Dong C, Wan J, Zhou M. Pharmacokinetics, tissue distribution and excretion study of trans-resveratrol-3-O-glucoside and its two metabolites in rats. *Phytomedicine* 2019; 58:152882. doi:10.1016/j.phymed.2019.152882.

Tahara A, Takasu T. Therapeutic Effects of SGLT2 Inhibitor Ipragliflozin and Metformin on NASH in Type 2 Diabetic Mice. *Endocrine Research* 2020, 0(0):1–15. https://doi.org/10.1080/07435800.2020.1713802.

Tarantino G, & Balsano C. Gastrointestinal peptides and nonalcoholic fatty liver disease. Current Opinion in Endocrinology, *Diabetes, and Obesity* 2020, 27(1):11–15. https://doi.org/10.1097/MED.0000000000000514.

Timmers S, Konings E, Bilet L, et al. Calorie Restriction-like Effects of 30 Days of Resveratrol Supplementation on Energy Metabolism and Metabolic Profile in Obese Humans. *Cell Metabolism* 2011; 14: 612-622.

Tsai CC. Lee MC, Tey SL, Liu CW, Huang SC (2017). Mechanism of resveratrol-induced relaxation in the human gallbladder. *BMC Complementary and Alternative Medicine* 2017, 17(1), 254. https://doi.org/10.1186/s12906-017-1752-x.

Tu Y, Zhu S, Wang J, Burstein E, Jia D. Natural compounds in the chemoprevention of alcoholic liver disease. *Phytotherapy Research* 2019: PTR, 33(9), 2192–2212. https://doi.org/10.1002/ptr.6410.

Uberti F, Morsanuto, V, Aprile S et al. Biological effects of combined resveratrol and vitamin D3 on ovarian tissue. *J Ovarian Res* 2017, 10, 61. https://doi.org/10.1186/s13048-017-0357-9.

Van Hul M, Geurts L, Plovier H, Druart C, Everard A, Stahlman M, Rhimi M, Chira K, Teissedre PL, Delzenne NM, Maguin E, Guilbot A, Brochot A, Gerard P, Backhed F, Cani PD. Reduced obesity, diabetes, and steatosis upon cinnamon and grape pomace are associated with changes in gut microbiota and markers of gut barrier. *American Journal of Physiology. Endocrinology and Metabolism* 2018, 314(4), E334–E352. https://doi.org/10.1152/ajpendo.00107.2017.

Westerouen Van Meeteren MJ, Drenth JPH, Tjwa ETTL. Elafibranor: a potential drug for the treatment of nonalcoholic steatohepatitis (NASH). *Expert Opinion on Investigational Drugs* 2020, 29(2), 117–123. https://doi.org/10.1080/13543784.2020.1668375.

Xia SF, Le GW, Wang P, QiuYY, Jiang YY, Tang X. Regressive Effect of Myricetin on Hepatic Steatosis in Mice Fed a High-Fat Diet. *Nutrients* 2016, 8, 799.

Yang J, Fernández-Galilea M, Martínez-Fernández L, González-Muniesa P, Pérez-Chávez A, Martínez JA, Moreno-Aliaga MJ Oxidative Stress and Non-Alcoholic Fatty Liver Disease: Effects of Omega-3 Fatty Acid Supplementation. *Nutrients* 2019, 11, 872.

Yonamine CY, Pinheiro-Machado E, Michalani ML, et al. Resveratrol improves glycemic control in insulin-treated diabetic rats: participation of the hepatic territory. *Nutr Metab* (Lond). 2016; 13:44. Published 2016 Jun 29. doi:10.1186/s12986-016-0103-0.

Yu B, Qin SY, Hu BL, Qin QY, Jiang HX, Luo W. Resveratrol improves CCL4-induced liver fibrosis in mouse by upregulating endogenous IL-10 to reprogramme macrophages phenotype from M(LPS) to M(IL-4). *Biomedicine & Pharmacotherapy = Biomedecine & Pharmacotherapie* 2019, 117, 109110. https://doi.org/10.1016/j.biopha.2019.109110.

Zamora-Ros R, Rothwell JA, Achaintre D, et al. Evaluation of urinary resveratrol as a biomarker of dietary resveratrol intake in the European Prospective Investigation into Cancer and Nutrition (EPIC) study. *Br J Nutr.* 2017; 117(11):1596–1602. doi:10.1017/S0007114517001465.

Zamora-Ros R, Urpí-Sardà M, Lamuela-Raventós RM, Estruch R, Vázquez-Agell M, Serrano-Martínez M, Jaeger W, Andres-Lacueva C. Diagnostic performance of urinary resveratrol metabolites as a biomarker of moderate wine consumption. *Clin Chem* 2006;52 (7):1373-80.

Zupancic S, Lavric Z, Kristl J. Stability and solubility of trans-resveratrol are strongly influenced by pH and temperature. *Eur. J. Pharm. Biopharm* 2015, 93, 196–204.

In: Grape Pomace in Health …
Editor: Veronica Sanda Chedea
ISBN: 978-1-68507-409-8


*Chapter 8*

# PHYTOCHEMICALS FROM GRAPE POMACE: BIOLOGICAL EFFECT AND POTENTIAL APPLICATION IN CANCER

***Oana Zanoaga[1], Cornelia Braicu[1,*], Ancuţa Jurj[1], Lajos Raduly[1], Laura Pop[1], Andreea Nutu[1] and Ioana Berindan-Neagoe[1]***

[1]Research Center for Functional Genomics,
Biomedicine and Translational Medicine,
"Iuliu Hațieganu" University of Medicine and Pharmacy,
Cluj-Napoca, Cluj, Romania

## ABSTRACT

Grape pomace is a cheap and rich source of phenolic compounds with potentially beneficial effects on human health due to their antioxidant, antimicrobial, antiviral, anti-inflammatory, and anticancer properties.

* Corresponding Author's E-mail: braicucornelia@yahoo.com.

The possible use of grape pomacc as a chemopreventive and chemotherapeutic agent has considerable potential and could be of great interest in the cancer research field. In this manuscript, we summarize the existing knowledge on the anticancer activity of grape pomace.

**Keywords**: grape pomace, grape extract, phytochemicals, cancer

## INTRODUCTION

According to The World Health Organization, cancer is the second leading cause of death worldwide, being responsible for an estimated 9.6 million deaths in 2018. Moreover, due to the occurrence of side effects of conventional therapies, the development of effective and safe alternative therapies became more and more necessary.

In recent years, the residue obtained from the processing of different fruits such as grape, apple, and orange peels, rich in bioactive phytochemicals was proposed as a source to be exploited for the development of novel nutraceuticals. It has been demonstrated that mild-to-moderate amounts of red wine can produce a high beneficial effect (Lippi et al., 2010). Grape pomace is a by-product obtained during wine production consisting of skins, seeds, and stems that have a high content of phytochemical compounds, such as phenolic acids, flavonoids, and anthocyanins (Guaita and Bosso 2019, Brezoiu et al., 2019, Peixoto et al., 2018, Xia et al., 2010).

In this chapter, we summarized recent advancements in the research of grape pomace (GP- the residual of grapes after winemaking) with application in cancer therapy, with a focus on the most relevant findings on cell culture and animal-based studies.

## BIOACTIVE PHYTOCHEMICALS - CLASSIFICATION, THE MAIN SOURCES AND IMPLICATION IN CANCER

Phytochemicals are natural biologically active agents, that proved to have protective effects on human health (Braicu et al., 2017). These beneficial effects occur mainly due to their capacity to balance antioxidants and free radicals. In the last decade there has been a significant increase of interest in the role of natural phytochemicals on human health (Yu and Ahmedna 2013). Epidemiological evidence demonstrates clearly that a diet rich in phytochemicals is related to important beneficial effects, with impact on cardiovascular disease, neurodegenerative disease, or cancer (Cojocneanu Petric et al., 2015).

The French paradox is a phenomenon that refers to the decrease in the rate of cardiovascular mortality in France compared to the United States, despite high consumption of dietary cholesterol and saturated fat (Lippi et al., 2010). In this regard, many studies that were performed to identify the nutritional/epidemiologic support between this association were based on red wine cardioprotective activity by mediating anti-platelet activity. The benefits of red wine are based on thrombus formation *in vivo* (Galinski, Zwicker, and Kennedy 2016), collagen inhibition, as well as epinephrine- or ADP-stimulated platelet aggregation (Polagruto et al., 2007). Red wine components, such as resveratrol and flavonoids, were found to decrease oxidative stress, to increase the levels of high-density lipoprotein cholesterol, and thereby, the cholesterol efflux in blood vessels. Due to those beneficial effects, red wine may be considered a nonpharmacological alternative to prevent the development and progression of cardiovascular disease. Moreover, specific cellular signaling mechanisms, biochemical changes at cellular and plasma levels, and interactions between genomic components are involved (Lippi et al., 2010).

**Table 1. Main phytochemical classes, biological source, and their biological role**

| Phytochemical classes | Phytochemical subclasses | Compounds (Examples) | Source | Therapeutic effects | References |
|---|---|---|---|---|---|
| Phenolics | Phenolic acids | Hydroxy-benzoic acids (gallic, vanillic, syringic and protocatechuic), hydroxyl-cinnamic acids (p-cumaric, caffeic, ferulic and synaptic) | Cereals, legumes, oilseeds, fruits, vegetables, beverages herbs, and grape pomace | Antioxidant, antimicrobial, antiviral, anti-inflammatory, anti-diabetes | (Li et al., 2009, Kumar and Goel 2019, Yu and Ahmedna 2013, Gerardi et al., 2020) |
| | Stilbene | Resveratrol, Pterostilbene | Berries, peanuts, grapes, and grape pomace | Antioxidant, anti-inflammatory, anti-tumoral-induced cell death by apoptosis and autophagy | (Sirerol et al., 2016, Yu and Ahmedna 2013, Gerardi et al., 2020) |
| | Coumarins | Brodifacoum, Bromadiolone, Difenacoum, Auraptene, Ensaculin, Phenprocoumon | Tonka bean, vanilla grass, sweet woodruff, sweet grass, cinnamon, strawberries, black currants, apricots, and cherries | Antimicrobial, antiviral, anti inflammatory, antidiabetes, antioxidant | (Poumale et al., 2013, Pinto and Silva 2017, Venkata Sairam et al., 2016) |
| | Tannins | Gallotannins, Ellagitannins, Proanthocyanidins | Tea, coffee, pomegranates, persimmons, most berries, chocolate grapes, and grape pomace | Antioxidant, antimicrobial, anti tumoral, cardio-protective | (Smeriglio et al., 2017, Yu and Ahmedna 2013, Gerardi et al., 2020) |
| | Lignans | Honokiol | Berries, fruits, vegetables, and whole grains | Antioxidant, antimicrobial, induced apoptosis, and autophagy | (Lin et al., 2016) |

| Phytochemical classes | Phytochemical subclasses | | Compounds (Examples) | Source | Therapeutic effects | References |
|---|---|---|---|---|---|---|
| | Flavonoids | Flavones | Diosmetin, Luteolin, Apigenin | Green tea, parsley, chamomile, rooibos tea | Anti-inflammatory, anti-oxidant, antiviral, induced apoptosis, inhibited angiogenesis | (Ren et al., 2003, Panche, Diwan, and Chandra 2016) |
| | | Flavonols | Myricetin, Kaempferol, Quercetin, Galangin, Fisetin | Apples, onions, leek | Induced apoptosis, enhanced chemosensitivity, anti-oxidant activity, antiproliferative and proapoptotic effects | (Younas et al., 2018, Ren et al., 2003, Panche, Diwan, and Chandra 2016) |
| | | Flavanones | Naringenin, Hesperitin, Eriodictyol, Silibinin | Yerba santa, lemon juice, orange juice | The chemoprotective effect, cytotoxic and pro-apoptotic activities, suppressive effects on new tumors | (Panche, Diwan, and Chandra 2016) |
| | | Flavanols | Epicatechin, Catechin, Epigallocatechi, Epigallocatechin Gallate | Green tea, pears, apples, cocoa, grapes, and grape pomace | Inhibition of EMT, antioxidant effect, inhibition of proliferation and tumorigenesis, pro-apoptotic | (Younas et al., 2018, Yu and Ahmedna 2013, Gerardi et al., 2020) |
| | | Isoflavones | Glycitein, Genistein, Daidzein | Soy products | Modulation of NK cell activity, cells apoptosis, cell cycle arrest | (Younas et al., 2018, Ren et al., 2003, Panche, Diwan, and Chandra 2016) |
| | | Anthocyanidins | Peonidin, Petunidin, Pelargonidin, Malvidin, Delphinidin, | Blackberries, blueberries, grapes, and grape pomace | Anti-inflammatory, pro-apoptotic antiproliferative effect | (Younas et al., 2018, Yu and Ahmedna 2013, Gerardi et al., 2020) |

## Table 1. (Continued)

| Phytochemical classes | Phytochemical subclasses | Compounds (Examples) | Source | Therapeutic effects | References |
|---|---|---|---|---|---|
| Alkaloids | Vinorelbine, Vincristine, Vindesine, Camptothecin, Vinblastin, Berberine, Sanguinarine, Evodiamine, Piperine, Matrine And Tetrandrine, Nitidine chloride, Khasuanine A, Bisleuconothine A, Subtidine, Fascaplysin, Piperlongumine | | Madagascar periwinkle plants | Antiproliferation, drug resistance, and antimetastasis effects | (Lu et al., 2012, Moudi et al., 2013) |
| | | | Plants (Solanaceae, and Fumariaceae), bacteria, fungus, and insects | Anti-oxidant, anti-fungal, anti-inflammatory, and analgesic functions | (Zhai et al., 2016) |
| Terpenes | Carotenoids (Crocetin, Lutein, Lycopene, β-carotene) | | Carrot, sweet potatoes, saffron, spinach, tomato, wetter melon, grapes | Inhibition of proliferation and metastasis, cell cycle arrest | (Gonzalez-Vallinas et al., 2013) |
| | Non-catotenoids (Anethole, Bisacurone, Carnosol, Ginsenoside, Limonene, Lupeol, Ursolic acid) | | Tumeric, ginseng, citrus fruits, mango, rosemary, basil | Antioxidant, anti-inflammatory, pro-apoptotic, DNA damage repair | (Gonzalez-Vallinas et al., 2013) |
| Organosulfur compounds | Indoles, Isothiocyanates, Allylic sulfur compounds | | Brussels sprouts, broccoli, mustard, papaya, garlic, and Allium species | Antioxidant, anti-inflammatory, antitumoral | (Petropoulos, Di Gioia, and Ntatsi 2017, Putnik et al., 2019) |

The Asian paradox refers to the decreased rates of heart disease and cancer among Asian people despite high rates of cigarette smoking. Some studies revealed that the consumption of 1.2 L of green tea provides an increase in levels of polyphenols and other antioxidants (Sumpio et al., 2006). These components play an important role and have the capability to improve cardiovascular health, such as improving cholesterol levels, as well as blood platelets coagulation prevention. Green tea prevents the oxidation of low-density lipoprotein (LDL cholesterol) by reducing the buildup of plaque in arteries. Moreover, low-density cholesterol can be reduced using green tea enriched in theaflavin extract with other dietary approaches (Nugala et al., 2012). More studies were performed in this area to investigate the effects of phytochemicals in the oncology domain. In their study, Kinure et al., observed that 1-theanine, an amino acid found in green tea, might cause anti-stress effects through the inhibition of cortical neuron excitation (Kimura et al., 2007). Also, the presence of antioxidants in green tea may prevent, but also reduce the severity of rheumatoid arthritis (Kim et al., 2008).

Phytochemicals have pleiotropic effects in the cell, interfering with multiple signaling pathways with minimal toxic side-effects, thus disturbing many aspects of cellular fate through multiple mechanisms, such as impairing proliferation, dedifferentiation invasion, migration, angiogenesis, and metastasis (Surh 2003, Cojocneanu Petric et al., 2015, Bishayee and Sethi 2016). However, the most important activities of natural compounds are related to their modulation of cell apoptosis and autophagy (Budisan et al., 2017, Moosavi et al., 2018). Apoptosis and autophagy are two important natural barriers that restrict malignant cells from surviving and disseminating, as an effect of phytochemicals exposure (Braicu et al., 2017, Budisan et al., 2017).

Phytochemicals have the potential to affect cancer cells preferentially, and understanding these mechanisms is necessary for the development of efficient anticancer drugs. At the molecular level, natural phytochemicals proved to have the capacity to interfere with key oncogenic mechanisms due to their antioxidant and anti-inflammatory features and to their capacity of mimicking the chemical structure and activity of the natural hormones (Cojocneanu Petric et al., 2015). These natural bioactive agent compounds can target coding and non-coding genes with an impact on physiological and pathological processes (Budisan et al., 2017). Table 1 summarizes the main phytochemical classes, their biological source, and their biological role.

## Phytochemicals Target Cancer Hallmarks

Phytochemicals, by targeting specific cell signaling pathways, have the potential to affect cancer cells preferentially. Among the signaling pathways targeted by phytochemical compounds, the most illustrative are represented by the mitogen-activated protein kinase (MAPK) pathways, the oncogenic protein kinase B (AKT) pathway, and proteins associated with the cell cycle progression (Lee, Bode, and Dong 2011). MEK1 was proven to be an important target for MAPK signaling disruption and a key component of oncogenic RAS signaling (Lee, Bode, and Dong 2011). RAS stimulation promoted the activation of inflammation-related proteins such as p38, ERKs, and JUN N-terminal kinase (JNKs), resulting in the generation of downstream signaling effectors. Activation of PI3K and AKT due to activation of RAS, SRC, and FYN is correlated with the translocation of p27 from the nucleus to the cytosol, and with protein degradation. P27 is a cell cycle inhibitor involved in the development of CDK-cyclin complexes to induce cell cycle progression (Lee, Bode, and Dong 2011).

## Biological Effects of Grape Pomace

### Antioxidant Activity

Agro-industrial residues could be a completely safe alternative source of natural antioxidants (González-Centeno et al., 2013). In this regard, *in vitro*, and *in vivo* studies found that a daily diet rich in red wine grape pomace (RWGP) has beneficial effects on antioxidant and metabolic activity (Rodriguez Lanzi et al., 2016, Urquiaga et al., 2015, Hernández-Salinas et al., 2015, Veskoukis et al., 2012). A comparative study between the phenolic composition and antioxidant properties of grape pomace byproducts and those of their corresponding stems, revealed that stems have a higher phenolic and tannins amount and a powerful antioxidant activity (González-Centeno et al., 2013). Polyphenol-rich grape pomace extract has higher antioxidant and chemopreventive properties due to removal of DPPH• and ABTS•+ radicals and inhibition of DNA damage induced by peroxyl and hydroxyl radicals (Veskoukis et al., 2012).

## Anti-Inflammatory Activity

Nowadays, the anti-inflammatory activity of the grape pomace extracts was observed to be enhanced by an increase in the phenolic content (Bucić-Kojić et al., 2020). Expression of inflammatory molecules such as TNF-α and IL-1 β decreased in microglia cells as a result of grape pomace treatment and in response to lipopolysaccharide (LPS) (Tu et al., 2018). Also, high levels of TNF-α have been identified in patients with coronary atherosclerosis (Bertrand and Tardif 2017, Klinghammer et al., 2013). The systemic inflammatory status can be modulated by RWGP supplementation that can reduce TNF-α circulating levels related to the anti-inflammatory properties of polyphenols and anthocyanins from RWGP composition (Rivera et al., 2019). Grape seed polyphenols exhibited a significant anti-inflammatory activity through the decrease of NF-kB transactivation and JNK/ERK activation in macrophages (Sakurai et al., 2010). Treatment with Aglianico grape pomace extracts had produced anti-inflammatory activity in an *in vivo* rheumatoid arthritis model, while also being correlated with a reduction in serum levels of IL-17, IL-1b, and IL-17–triggering cytokines (Parisi et al., 2020).

## Antimicrobial Activity

Throughout the years, there has been increased interest in the investigation of grape pomace's inhibitory activity on multiple pathogenic microorganisms. Thus, the combination of certain components from grape pomace extracts such as luteolin, gallic acid, and quercetin with different classes of antibiotics, such as tetracycline, βlactam, amphenicol quinolone, and fluoroquinolone, inhibited the growth of *S. aureus* and *E. coli* (Sanhueza et al., 2017). The grape-stem extracts have proven to be efficient against Gram-positive (*L. monocytogenes, S. aureus, and Enterococcus faecalis*) and Gram-negative (*Pseudomonas aeruginosa*) bacteria due to their high content of phenols and flavonoids (Leal et al., 2020). The seeds from red grape pomace (Peixoto et al., 2018) as well as those from white grape pomace (Olejar et al., 2019) presented the highest antibacterial activities against Gram-positive bacteria compared to the Gram-negative ones.

Grape pomace extracts from a mixture of Chilean grape varieties (Cabernet Sauvignon, Carmènere, and Syrah) had an inhibitory effect against the phytopathogenic fungus *Botrytis cinerea* (Mendoza et al., 2013). Natural extracts obtained from grape pomace (GPE) and grape seeds (GSE) can provide fungicidal and fungistatic protection against *Rhizopus microsporus*, *Fusarium graminearum*, *Alternaria infectoria,* and *Cladosporium herbarum* (Alexa, Poiana, and Sumalan 2012).

Grape seed extract inhibited hepatitis C virus replication and virus-induced inflammation by decreasing cellular COX-2 expression through the inactivation of NF-κB and ERK/JNK MAPK signaling pathways (Sullivan-Nelson, Kuller, and Zacur 1989).

## Anticancer Activity

Cell death is a fundamental cellular response that has a crucial role in a variety of biological processes, controlling the development, the multicellular organisms' immune response and the tissue homeostasis by eliminating unwanted cells. According to the literature, most studies have focused on three major types of cell death: apoptosis (type I), cell death associated with autophagy (type II), and necrosis (type III). In mammalian cells, the apoptotic response was observed to be mediated by either an intrinsic or an extrinsic pathway, depending on the origin of the death stimuli, and was almost caspase-dependent. Although necrosis has been considered for a long time to be an accidental and uncontrolled form of cell death, scientific evidence supports the claim that necrotic cell death in some cases can be as well controlled and programmed as caspase-dependent apoptosis (Yuan, Najafov, and Py 2016). Autophagy is foremost a survival mechanism that is activated in cells subjected to nutrient or growth factor deprivation.

These unique molecules are often considered a valuable support as models for the development of more efficacious analogs and prodrugs.

The beneficial effect of the natural phytochemicals in reducing the risk of chronic disease, including cancer, was demonstrated in several epidemiological studies.

Grape's pomace anticancer effect has been studied using different techniques. Thus, the most commonly used test was the MTT assay that measures cytotoxicity or cytostatic activity of potential medicinal agents. Nuclear magnetic resonance (NMR) allows the simultaneous identification and absolute quantification of different compounds (Hong et al., 2011), being often used for metabolic profiling of vine extracts and vinified products.

There is growing evidence pointing that grape pomace, due to its composition, has anti-cancer activity. Thus, an important number of investigations recommend consumption of grape components, epidemiological studies demonstrating the correlation with a decreased risk of certain cancers as can be seen in Table 2. The bioactive agents from grape pomace were found to prevent carcinogenesis and cancer progression. The antitumoral effects of grape pomace components were identified in both *in vitro* and *in vivo* models (Table 2). Grape pomace phytochemicals reduce cell proliferation, specifically activation of apoptosis by targeting key oncogenes, and also promote cell cycle arrest on cell culture and rodent models.

Muscadine grapes treatment in prostate cancer cell lines induced a reduction in Akt activity through a reduction in Akt transcription. Furthermore, the extract was observed to increase proteosome degradation of Akt and to alter the levels of DJ-1, the regulator of PTEN (Hudson et al., 2007). Ethanol extracts of the ground and freeze-dried pomace were found to inhibit HeLa and mouse mammary 4T1 cells, for both in culture and transplanted tumors in mice (Morré and Morré 2006). Also, this study demonstrated the use of the tNOX protein as a potential flavonoid target in cancer and evaluated the anti-cancer activity of grapes and grape extracts.

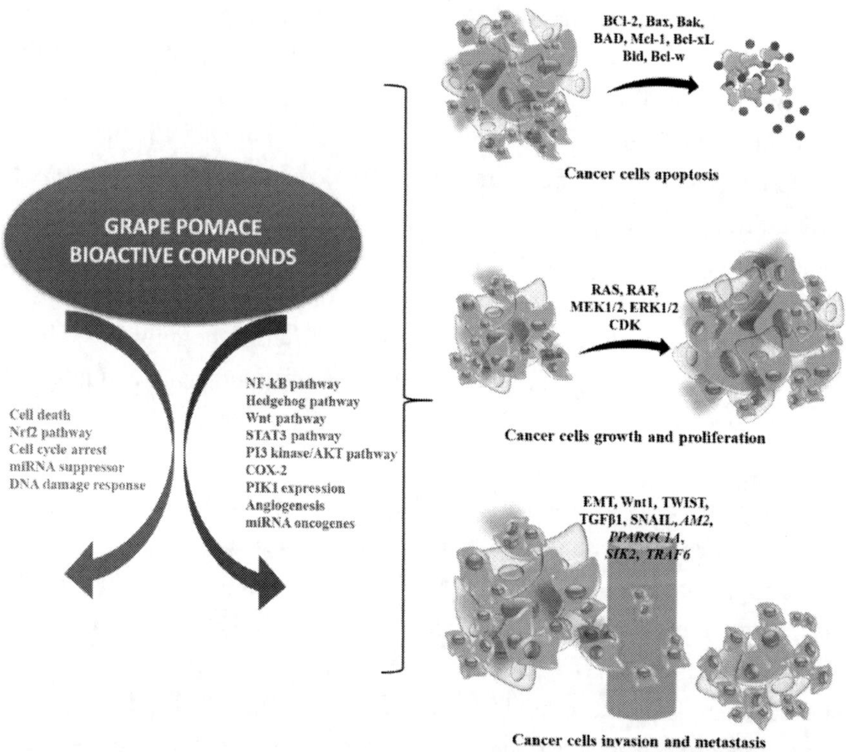


Figure 1. The main biological effect and the target genes of grape pomace.

A purified white grape pomace extract (100 μg/ml) inhibited colon adenocarcinoma cell growth (Jara-Palacios et al., 2015) in colon cancer cells Caco-2. The inhibition process was observed to be due to a combination of antiproliferative activity and via a direct initiation of cell death. Furthermore, in colorectal cancer HT-29 cells, red wine pomace seasonings extracts were found to have dose-dependent anti-proliferative effects that can help to attenuate cancer progression and also anti-genotoxic effects, preventing mutagenesis and blocking tumor initiation and progression (Del Pino-García et al., 2017). Furthermore, the seasoning derived from seedless wine pomace was observed to have the strongest effect before digestion, while the seasonings containing wine pomace seeds increased their chemopreventive ability during digestion.

The purified white grape pomace extract (PWGPE) has induced apoptosis in acute lymphoblastic leukemia Jurkat (León-González et al., 2017), the apoptosis process being correlated with mitochondrial depolarization and caspase-3 cleavage. Therefore, the generation of $H_2O_2$ was identified as a key event in the cytotoxic process of PWGPE, depending on ROS production and regulation of epigenetic gene silencing.

NMR techniques and DNA microarray on blood samples from female C57BL/6J mice demonstrated that a diet rich in lyophilized red grape pomace may help reduce the risk of colon cancer due to the presence of alterations in the tumor suppressor genes and proto-oncogenes expression. Also, the genes modulation was found from different pathways, including apoptosis, lipid biosynthesis, cell cycle, and energy metabolism (Lizarraga et al., 2011). Tinta Cao and Chardonnay grape pomace extracts inhibited the proliferation of Caco-2 and HT-29 cancer cells by triggering apoptosis.

An increase of caspase-3 expression and in DNA fragmentation was also observed after the pomace treatment. The Caco-2 and HT-29 cells treatment with a crude and a purified extract obtained from white and red pomace and grape seeds, reduced cell viability and proliferation, specifically in the case of Caco-2 (Pérez-Ortiz et al., 2019).

**Table 2. The main biological effects of the grape pomace in *in vitro/in vivo* studies**

| Cancer type | Study type | Extraction method | Biological effect | References |
|---|---|---|---|---|
| Human cervical cancer | *in vitro* | Ethanol | Inhibition of Hela cells proliferation | (Morré and Morré 2006) |
| | *in vitro* | Ethanol | Induction of apoptosis and inhibition of cell growth | (Morré and Morré 2006) |
| Mammary carcinoma | *in vivo* | Ethanol | Growth inhibition of 4T1 mammary tumors *in situ* in mice. | (Morré and Morré 2006) |
| Colon cancer | *in vitro* | Methanol | Inhibition of Caco-2 cells growth | (Jara-Palacios et al., 2015) |
| | *in vitro* | Methanol | Antiproliferative activities and attenuation of oxidative DNA damage | (Del Pino-García et al., 2017) |
| | *in vivo* | lyophilization | Expression of tumor suppressor genes and proto-oncogenes alterations in female C57BL/6J mice | (Lizarraga et al., 2011) |
| | *in vitro* | Acetone | Inhibition of Caco-2 and HT-29 human colon cancer cell proliferation through the induction of apoptosis | |
| | *in vitro* | ethanol/water solution (50:50 v/v) | Inhibition of cell proliferation and decrease of Myc expression in Caco-2. | (Pérez-Ortiz et al., 2019) |
| Leukemia | *in vitro* | Methanol | Increase of apoptosis and decrease of pro-survival factors (Bcl-2) in Jurkat leukemia cells | (León-González et al., 2017) |
| Breast cancer | *in vitro* | acetone/methanol/water/formic acid (40:40:20:0.1, v/v/v/v) | Induction of apoptosis and S-phase arrest in MDA-MB-231 cells | (Luo, Wei, et al., 2017) |
| | *in vitro* | Methanol | Apoptosis activation via caspases and cell cycle arrest | (Luo, Song, et al., 2017) |
| Human hepatocarcinoma | *in vitro* | ethanol | Decrease of HepG2 cell proliferation and viability | (de Sales et al., 2018) |

A downregulation of Myc gene expression in HT-29 cells and upregulation of Ptg2 in Caco-2 cells were identified. The phenolic fractions from the muscadine grape "Noble" pomace have the potential to be used as an antitumoral agent in breast cancer (Luo, Wei, et al., 2017), these fraction having superior antitumoral activity than the fraction obtained from "Cabernet Sauvignon" (Luo, Wei, et al., 2017). This effect can be explained by the different phytochemical's composition and concentration, having different biological active properties. Thereby, in MDA-MB-231 cells, the extracts from grape pomace have induced inhibition of cell proliferation correlated with the induction of S-phase arrest and apoptosis. Bcl-2 expression was significantly downregulated while Bax expression was upregulated in the treatment groups compared with the control group (Luo, Wei, et al., 2017).

In human hepatocarcinoma cells, Pinot noir grape pomace extract has induced early metabolic changes targeted to mitochondria (de Sales et al., 2018). After long-term incubation of hepatocarcinoma cells with grape pomace extract, significant cytotoxic effects and cell death mainly by necrosis were observed. Furthermore, in the same study, grape pomace was found to be non-toxic on human fibroblasts cells.

A fraction from muscadine grape 'Noble' pomace extracts containing a mixture of anthocyanidins and ellagic acids was identified to have the strongest anti-oxidative activity and the most powerful capacity to induce apoptosis via caspase activation and cell cycle arrest by downregulation of cyclin A and upregulation of p21 (Luo, Song, et al., 2017).

## Clinical Trials on Grape Extract Phytochemicals in Cancer

In the last decades, many studies started to focus on the investigation of natural compounds ability to counteract many biological processes, especially the development of cancer. The phytochemicals derived from diet are considered important, as they can be attractive alternatives for cancer chemoprevention. In this regard, phytochemicals such as resveratrol, genistein, folate, and curcumin have undergone extensive mechanistic and preclinical efficacy investigation. Generally, new anticancer drugs are designed to act on specific targets, meanwhile, phytochemicals exert a plethora of actions without having a specific target (Scott et al., 2009).

The literature search on various databases found a reduced number of clinical trials assessing the effects of grape products. A clinical trial (www.ClinicalTrials.gov Identifier: NCT02760160) reveals promising results by using the oral grape powder to prevent non-melanoma skin cancers (NMSCs) and sun damage.

Another clinical trial (www.ClinicalTrials.gov Identifier: NCT00566553) using Grape Seed Extract in postmenopausal women did not act as an estrogen mimetic (Wahner-Roedler et al., 2014), despite the encouraging preclinical data (Eng et al., 2003). The clinical study NCT03087903 failed to show the efficacy of orally-administered IH636-grape seed pro-anthocyanidin extract in patients with breast induration following radiotherapy for breast cancer (Brooker et al., 2006).

On prostate cancer, there is a clinical trial (www.ClinicalTrials.gov Identifier: NCT03087903) focused on studying the grape seed extract effect in asymptomatic non-metastatic prostate cancer patients with rising PSA-, and that trial is expected to have encouraging data. Another clinical trial (www.ClinicalTrials.gov Identifier: NCT00578396) aims to determine the minimum quantity of resveratrol-rich fresh red grapes required to display signs of prevention, this study being on recruiting phase.

More promising results in a clinical trial (NCT00256334) were revealed in the case of resveratrol and grape seed powder, these agents exhibiting colon cancer prevention activity, by targeting Wnt signaling in colonic mucosa and colon cancer (Nguyen et al., 2009). Unfortunately, there is no clinical trial available able to demonstrate the beneficial effect of grape pomace.

## Conclusion

In summary, concerning cancer prevention and treatment, grape components, including grape pomace have acquired attention, and most investigations in preclinical studies demonstrated their potential application as an anticancer or adjuvant system. Even though some studies showed the very promising potential of grape pomace extracts as an anticancer agent, they are not sustained by clinical trials, and also there is a high degree of inconsistency within the studies related to the health outcomes.

Yet, many papers were focused on their *in vitro* activities and mechanisms. Since the absorption of these phenolic compounds can be inadequate, the studies to determine the dose responses of the extracts and their components are required to be performed in animals and humans, in order to demonstrate the *in vivo* mechanisms of action. The possible use of grape pomace in cancer prevention or therapy has considerable potential, and additional studies into this challenging domain are warranted.

## References

Alexa, E., M. A. Poiana, and R. M. Sumalan. 2012. "Mycoflora and ochratoxin a control in wheat grain using natural extracts obtained from wine industry by-products." *Int J Mol Sci* 13 (4):4949-67. doi: https://10.3390/ijms13044949.

Bertrand, M. J., and J. C. Tardif. 2017. "Inflammation and beyond: new directions and emerging drugs for treating atherosclerosis." *Expert Opin Emerg Drugs* 22 (1):1-26. doi: https://10.1080/14728214.2017.1269743.

Bishayee, A., and G. Sethi. 2016. "Bioactive natural products in cancer prevention and therapy: Progress and promise." *Semin Cancer Biol* 40-41:1-3. doi: https://10.1016/j.semcancer.2016.08.006.

Braicu, C., N. Mehterov, B. Vladimirov, V. Sarafian, S. M. Nabavi, A. G. Atanasov, and I. Berindan-Neagoe. 2017. "Nutrigenomics in cancer: Revisiting the effects of natural compounds." *Semin Cancer Biol* 46:84-106. doi: https://10.1016/j.semcancer.2017.06.011.

Brezoiu, A. M., C. Matei, M. Deaconu, A. M. Stanciuc, A. Trifan, A. Gaspar-Pintiliescu, and D. Berger. 2019. "Polyphenols extract from grape pomace. Characterization and valorisation through encapsulation into mesoporous silica-type matrices." *Food Chem Toxicol* 133:110787. doi: https://10.1016/j.fct.2019.110787.

Brooker, S., S. Martin, A. Pearson, D. Bagchi, J. Earl, L. Gothard, E. Hall, L. Porter, and J. Yarnold. 2006. "Double-blind, placebo-controlled, randomised phase II trial of IH636 grape seed proanthocyanidin extract (GSPE) in patients with radiation-induced breast induration." *Radiother Oncol* 79 (1):45-51. doi: https://10.1016/j.radonc.2006.02.008.

Bucić-Kojić, A., F. Fernandes, T. Silva, M. Planinić, M. Tišma, G. Šelo, D. Šibalić, D. M. Pereira, and P. B. Andrade. 2020. "Enhancement of the anti-inflammatory properties of grape pomace treated by Trametes versicolor." *Food Funct* 11 (1):680-688. doi: https://10.1039/c9fo02296a.

Budisan, L., D. Gulei, O. M. Zanoaga, A. I. Irimie, C. Sergiu, C. Braicu, C. D. Gherman, and I. Berindan-Neagoe. 2017. "Dietary Intervention by Phytochemicals and Their Role in Modulating Coding and Non-Coding Genes in Cancer." *Int J Mol Sci* 18 (6). doi: https://10.3390/ijms18061178.

Cojocneanu, P., R., C. Braicu, L. Raduly, O. Zanoaga, N. Dragos, P. Monroig, D. Dumitrascu, and I. Berindan-Neagoe. 2015. "Phytochemicals modulate carcinogenic signaling pathways in breast and hormone-related cancers." *Onco Targets Ther* 8:2053-66. doi: https://10.2147/OTT.S83597.

de Sales, N. F. F., L. Silva da Costa, T. I. A. Carneiro, D. A. Minuzzo, F. L. Oliveira, L. M. C. Cabral, A. G. Torres, and T. El-Bacha. 2018. "Anthocyanin-Rich Grape Pomace Extract (*Vitis vinifera* L.) from Wine Industry Affects Mitochondrial Bioenergetics and Glucose

Metabolism in Human Hepatocarcinoma HepG2 Cells." *Molecules* 23 (3). doi: https://10.3390/molecules23030611.

Del Pino-García, R., M. D. Rivero-Pérez, M. L. González-SanJosé, M. Ortega-Heras, J. García Lomillo, and P. Muñiz. 2017. "Chemopreventive Potential of Powdered Red Wine Pomace Seasonings against Colorectal Cancer in HT-29 Cells." *J Agric Food Chem* 65 (1):66-73. doi: https://10.1021/acs.jafc.6b04561.

Eng, E. T., J. Ye, D. Williams, S. Phung, R. E. Moore, M. K. Young, U. Gruntmanis, G. Braunstein, and S. Chen. 2003. "Suppression of estrogen biosynthesis by procyanidin dimers in red wine and grape seeds." *Cancer Res* 63 (23):8516-22.

Galinski, C. N., J. I. Zwicker, and D. R. Kennedy. 2016. "Revisiting the mechanistic basis of the French Paradox: Red wine inhibits the activity of protein disulfide isomerase *in vitro*." *Thromb Res* 137:169-173. doi: https://10.1016/j.thromres.2015.11.003.

Gerardi, G., M. Cavia-Saiz, M. D. Rivero-Pérez, M. L. González-SanJosé, and P. Muñiz. 2020. "The dose-response effect on polyphenol bioavailability after intake of white and red wine pomace products by Wistar rats." *Food Funct* 11 (2):1661-1671. doi: https://10.1039/c9fo01743g.

González-Centeno, M. R., M. Jourdes, A. Femenia, S. Simal, C. Rosselló, and P. L. Teissedre. 2013. "Characterization of polyphenols and antioxidant potential of white grape pomace byproducts (*Vitis vinifera* L.)." *J Agric Food Chem* 61 (47):11579-87. doi: https://10.1021/jf403168k.

Gonzalez-Vallinas, M., M. Gonzalez-Castejon, A. Rodriguez-Casado, and A. Ramirez de Molina. 2013. "Dietary phytochemicals in cancer prevention and therapy: a complementary approach with promising perspectives." *Nutr Rev* 71 (9):585-99. doi: https://10.1111/nure.12051.

Guaita, M., and A. Bosso. 2019. "Polyphenolic Characterization of Grape Skins and Seeds of Four Italian Red Cultivars at Harvest and after Fermentative Maceration." *Foods* 8 (9). doi: https://10.3390/foods8090395.

Hernández-Salinas, R., V. Decap, A. Leguina, P. Cáceres, D. Perez, I. Urquiaga, R. Iturriaga, and V. Velarde. 2015. "Antioxidant and anti hyperglycemic role of wine grape powder in rats fed with a high fructose diet." *Biol Res* 48:53. doi: https://10.1186/s40659-015-0045-4.

Hong, Y. S., C. Cilindre, G. Liger-Belair, P. Jeandet, N. Hertkorn, and P. Schmitt-Kopplin. 2011. "Metabolic influence of Botrytis cinerea infection in champagne base wine." *J Agric Food Chem* 59 (13):7237-45. doi: https://10.1021/jf200664t.

http://agris.fao.org/agris-search/search.do?recordID=DJ2012073192.

http://www.uaiasi.ro/revagrois/PDF/2012-1/paper/2012-55(1)-5-en.pdf.

Hudson, T. S., D. K. Hartle, S. D. Hursting, N. P. Nunez, T. T. Wang, H. A. Young, P. Arany, and J. E. Green. 2007. "Inhibition of prostate cancer growth by muscadine grape skin extract and resveratrol through distinct mechanisms." *Cancer Res* 67 (17):8396-405. doi: https://10.1158/0008-5472.Can-06-4069.

Jara-Palacios, M. J., D. Hernanz, T. Cifuentes-Gomez, M. L. Escudero-Gilete, F. J. Heredia, and J. P. Spencer. 2015. "Assessment of white grape pomace from winemaking as source of bioactive compounds, and its antiproliferative activity." *Food Chem* 183:78-82. doi: https://10.1016/j.foodchem.2015.03.022.

Kim, H. R., R. Rajaiah, Q. L. Wu, S. R. Satpute, M. T. Tan, J. E. Simon, B. M. Berman, and K. D. Moudgil. 2008. "Green tea protects rats against autoimmune arthritis by modulating disease-related immune events." *J Nutr* 138 (11):2111-6. doi: https://10.3945/jn.108.089912.

Kimura, K., M. Ozeki, L. R. Juneja, and H. Ohira. 2007. "L-Theanine reduces psychological and physiological stress responses." *Biol Psychol* 74 (1):39-45. doi: https://10.1016/j.biopsycho.2006.06.006.

Klinghammer, L., K. Urschel, I. Cicha, P. Lewczuk, D. Raaz-Schrauder, S. Achenbach, and C. D. Garlichs. 2013. "Impact of telmisartan on the inflammatory state in patients with coronary atherosclerosis-influence on IP-10, TNF-α and MCP-1." *Cytokine* 62 (2):290-6. doi: https://10.1016/j.cyto.2013.02.001.

Kumar, N., and Nidhi Goel. 2019. "Phenolic acids: Natural versatile molecules with promising therapeutic applications." *Biotechnology Reports* 24:e00370. doi: https://doi.org/10.1016/j.btre.2019.e00370.

Leal, C., R. A. Santos, R. Pinto, M. Queiroz, M. Rodrigues, M. José Saavedra, A. Barros, and I. Gouvinhas. 2020. "Recovery of bioactive compounds from white grape (*Vitis vinifera* L.) stems as potential antimicrobial agents for human health." *Saudi J Biol Sci* 27 (4):1009-1015. doi: https://10.1016/j.sjbs.2020.02.013.

Lee, K. W., A. M. Bode, and Z. Dong. 2011. "Molecular targets of phytochemicals for cancer prevention." *Nat Rev Cancer* 11 (3):211-8. doi: https://10.1038/nrc3017.

León-González, A. J., M. J. Jara-Palacios, M. Abbas, F. J. Heredia, and V. B. Schini-Kerth. 2017. "Role of epigenetic regulation on the induction of apoptosis in Jurkat leukemia cells by white grape pomace rich in phenolic compounds." *Food Funct* 8 (11):4062-4069. doi: https://10.1039/c7fo00263g.

Li, L., Claudia Harflett, Michael H. Beale, and Jane L. Ward. 2009. "Chapter 5 - Phenolic Acids." In *Healthgrain Methods*, edited by Peter R. Shewry and Jane L. Ward, 41-52. AACC International Press.

Lin, C. J., T. L. Chen, Y. Y. Tseng, G. J. Wu, M. H. Hsieh, Y. W. Lin, and R. M. Chen. 2016. "Honokiol induces autophagic cell death in malignant glioma through reactive oxygen species-mediated regulation of the p53/PI3K/Akt/mTOR signaling pathway." *Toxicol Appl Pharmacol* 304:59-69. doi: https://10.1016/j.taap.2016.05.018.

Lippi, G., M. Franchini, E. J. Favaloro, and G. Targher. 2010. "Moderate red wine consumption and cardiovascular disease risk: beyond the "French paradox." *Semin Thromb Hemost* 36 (1):59-70. doi: https://10.1055/s-0030-1248725.

Lizarraga, D., M. P. Vinardell, V. Noé, J. H. van Delft, G. Alcarraz-Vizán, S. G. van Breda, Y. Staal, U. L. Günther, J. B. Carrigan, M. A. Reed, C. J. Ciudad, J. L. Torres, and M. Cascante. 2011. "A lyophilized red grape pomace containing proanthocyanidin-rich dietary fiber induces genetic and metabolic alterations in colon mucosa of female C57BL/6J mice." *J Nutr* 141 (9):1597-604. doi: https://10.3945/jn.110.133199.

Lu, J. J., J. L. Bao, X. P. Chen, M. Huang, and Y. T. Wang. 2012. "Alkaloids isolated from natural herbs as the anticancer agents." *Evid Based Complement Alternat Med* 2012:485042. doi: https://10.1155/2012/485042.

Luo, J., S. Song, Z. Wei, Y. Huang, Y. Zhang, and J. Lu. 2017. "The comparative study among different fractions of muscadine grape 'Noble' pomace extracts regarding anti-oxidative activities, cell cycle arrest and apoptosis in breast cancer." *Food Nutr Res* 61 (1):1412795. doi: https://10.1080/16546628.2017.1412795.

Luo, J., Z. Wei, S. Zhang, X. Peng, Y. Huang, Y. Zhang, and J. Lu. 2017. "Phenolic Fractions from Muscadine Grape "Noble" Pomace can Inhibit Breast Cancer Cell MDA-MB-231 Better than those from European Grape "Cabernet Sauvignon" and Induce S-Phase Arrest and Apoptosis." *J Food Sci* 82 (5):1254-1263. doi: https://10.1111/1750-3841.13670.

Mendoza, L., Karen Yañez, Marcela Vivanco, Ricardo Melo, and Milena Cotoras. 2013. "Characterization of extracts from winery by-products with antifungal activity against *Botrytis cinerea*." *Industrial Crops and Products* 43:360-364. doi: https://doi.org/10.1016/j.indcrop.2012.07.048.

Moosavi, M. A., A. Haghi, M. Rahmati, H. Taniguchi, A. Mocan, J. Echeverria, V. K. Gupta, N. T. Tzvetkov, and A. G. Atanasov. 2018. "Phytochemicals as potent modulators of autophagy for cancer therapy." *Cancer Lett* 424:46-69. doi: https://10.1016/j.canlet.2018.02.030.

Morré, D. M., and D. J. Morré. 2006. "Anticancer activity of grape and grape skin extracts alone and combined with green tea infusions." *Cancer Lett* 238 (2):202-9. doi: https://10.1016/j.canlet.2005.07.011.

Moudi, M., R. Go, C. Y. Yien, and M. Nazre. 2013. "Vinca alkaloids." *Int J Prev Med* 4 (11):1231-5.

Nguyen, A. V., M. Martinez, M. J. Stamos, M. P. Moyer, K. Planutis, C. Hope, and R. F. Holcombe. 2009. "Results of a phase I pilot clinical trial examining the effect of plant-derived resveratrol and grape powder on Wnt pathway target gene expression in colonic mucosa and colon cancer." *Cancer Manag Res* 1:25-37.

Nugala, B., A. Namasi, P. Emmadi, and P. M. Krishna. 2012. "Role of green tea as an antioxidant in periodontal disease: The Asian paradox." *J Indian Soc Periodontol* 16 (3):313-6. doi: https://10.4103/0972-124x.100902.

Olejar, K. J., A. Ricci, S. Swift, Z. Zujovic, K. C. Gordon, B. Fedrizzi, A. Versari, and P. A. Kilmartin. 2019. "Characterization of an Antioxidant and Antimicrobial Extract from Cool Climate, White Grape Marc." *Antioxidants (Basel)* 8 (7). doi: https://10.3390/antiox 8070232.

Panche, A. N., A. D. Diwan, and S. R. Chandra. 2016. "Flavonoids: an overview." *J Nutr Sci* 5:e47. doi: https://10.1017/jns.2016.41.

Parisi, V., A. Vassallo, C. Pisano, G. Signorino, F. Cardile, M. Sorrentino, F. Colelli, A. Fucci, E. L. D'Andrea, N. De Tommasi, A. Braca, and M. De Leo. 2020. "A Herbal Mixture from Propolis, Pomegranate, and Grape Pomace Endowed with Anti-Inflammatory Activity in an *In Vivo* Rheumatoid Arthritis Model." *Molecules* 25 (9). doi: https://10.3390/molecules25092255.

Peixoto, C. M., M. I. Dias, M. J. Alves, R. C. Calhelha, L. Barros, S. P. Pinho, and Icfr Ferreira. 2018. "Grape pomace as a source of phenolic compounds and diverse bioactive properties." *Food Chem* 253:132-138. doi: https://10.1016/j.foodchem.2018.01.163.

Pérez-Ortiz, J. M., L. F. Alguacil, E. Salas, I. Hermosín-Gutiérrez, S. Gómez-Alonso, and C. González-Martín. 2019. "Antiproliferative and cytotoxic effects of grape pomace and grape seed extracts on colorectal cancer cell lines." *Food Sci Nutr* 7 (9):2948-2957. doi: https://10.1002/fsn3.1150.

Petropoulos, S., F. Di Gioia, and G. Ntatsi. 2017. "Vegetable Organosulfur Compounds and their Health Promoting Effects." *Curr Pharm Des* 23 (19):2850-2875. doi: https://10.2174/138161 2823666170111100531.

Pinto, D., and A. M. S. Silva. 2017. "Anticancer Natural Coumarins as Lead Compounds for the Discovery of New Drugs." *Curr Top Med Chem* 17 (29):3190-3198. doi: https://10.2174/156802661866171215095750.

Polagruto, J. A., H. B. Gross, F. Kamangar, K. Kosuna, B. Sun, H. Fujii, C. L. Keen, and R. M. Hackman. 2007. "Platelet reactivity in male smokers following the acute consumption of a flavanol-rich grapesced extract." *J Med Food* 10 (4):725-30. doi: https://10.1089/jmf.2007.402.

Poumale, H., Martial Poumale, Rebecca Hamm, Yanqing Zang, Yoshihito Shiono, and Victor Kuete. 2013. "8 - Coumarins and Related Compounds from the Medicinal Plants of Africa." In *Medicinal Plant Research in Africa*, edited by Victor Kuete, 261-300. Oxford: Elsevier.

Putnik, P., D. Gabric, S. Roohinejad, F. J. Barba, D. Granato, K. Mallikarjunan, J. M. Lorenzo, and D. Bursac Kovacevic. 2019. "An overview of organosulfur compounds from Allium spp.: From processing and preservation to evaluation of their bioavailability, antimicrobial, and anti-inflammatory properties." *Food Chem* 276:680-691. doi: https://10.1016/j.foodchem.2018.10.068.

Ren, W., Z. Qiao, H. Wang, L. Zhu, and L. Zhang. 2003. "Flavonoids: promising anticancer agents." *Med Res Rev* 23 (4):519-34. doi: https://10.1002/med.10033.

Rivera, K., F. Salas-Pérez, G. Echeverría, I. Urquiaga, S. Dicenta, D. Pérez, P. de la Cerda, L. González, M. E. Andia, S. Uribe, C. Tejos, G. Martínez, D. Busso, P. Irarrázaval, and A. Rigotti. 2019. "Red Wine Grape Pomace Attenuates Atherosclerosis and Myocardial Damage and Increases Survival in Association with Improved Plasma Antioxidant Activity in a Murine Model of Lethal Ischemic Heart Disease." *Nutrients* 11 (9). doi: https://10.3390/nu11092135.

Rodriguez Lanzi, C., D. J. Perdicaro, A. Antoniolli, A. R. Fontana, R. M. Miatello, R. Bottini, and M. A. Vazquez Prieto. 2016. "Grape pomace and grape pomace extract improve insulin signaling in high-fat-fructose fed rat-induced metabolic syndrome." *Food Funct* 7 (3):1544-53. doi: https://10.1039/c5fo01065a.

Sakurai, T., K. Kitadate, H. Nishioka, H. Fujii, T. Kizaki, Y. Kondoh, T. Izawa, H. Ishida, Z. Radák, and H. Ohno. 2010. "Oligomerized grape seed polyphenols attenuate inflammatory changes due to antioxidative properties in coculture of adipocytes and macrophages." *J Nutr Biochem* 21 (1):47-54. doi: https://10.1016/j.jnutbio.2008.10.003.

Sanhueza, L., R. Melo, R. Montero, K. Maisey, L. Mendoza, and M. Wilkens. 2017. "Synergistic interactions between phenolic compounds identified in grape pomace extract with antibiotics of different classes against *Staphylococcus aureus* and *Escherichia coli*." *PLoS One* 12 (2):e0172273. doi: https://10.1371/journal.pone.0172273.

Scott, E. N., A. J. Gescher, W. P. Steward, and K. Brown. 2009. "Development of dietary phytochemical chemopreventive agents: biomarkers and choice of dose for early clinical trials." *Cancer Prev Res (Phila)* 2 (6):525-30. doi: https://10.1158/1940-6207.Capr-08-0223.

Sirerol, J. A., M. L. Rodriguez, S. Mena, M. A. Asensi, J. M. Estrela, and A. L. Ortega. 2016. "Role of Natural Stilbenes in the Prevention of Cancer." *Oxid Med Cell Longev* 2016:3128951. doi: https://10.1155/2016/3128951.

Smeriglio, A., Davide Barreca, Ersilia Bellocco, and Domenico Trombetta. 2017. "Proanthocyanidins and hydrolysable tannins: occurrence, dietary intake and pharmacological effects." *British journal of pharmacology* 174 (11):1244-1262. doi: https://10.1111/bph.13630.

Sullivan-Nelson, M., J. A. Kuller, and H. A. Zacur. 1989. "Clinical use of oral contraceptives administered vaginally: a case report." *Fertil Steril* 52 (5):864-6.

Sumpio, B. E., A. C. Cordova, D. W. Berke-Schlessel, F. Qin, and Q. H. Chen. 2006. "Green tea, the "Asian paradox," and cardiovascular disease." *J Am Coll Surg* 202 (5):813-25. doi: https://10.1016/j.jamcollsurg.2006.01.018.

Surh, Y. J. 2003. "Cancer chemoprevention with dietary phytochemicals." *Nat Rev Cancer* 3 (10):768-80. doi: https://10.1038/nrc1189.

Tu, S., F. Xiao, X. Min, H. Chen, X. Fan, and K. Cao. 2018. "Catechin Attenuates Coronary Heart Disease in a Rat Model by Inhibiting Inflammation." *Cardiovasc Toxicol* 18 (5):393-399. doi: https://10.1007/s12012-018-9449-z.

Urquiaga, I., S. D'Acuña, D. Pérez, S. Dicenta, G. Echeverría, A. Rigotti, and F. Leighton. 2015. "Wine grape pomace flour improves blood pressure, fasting glucose and protein damage in humans: a randomized controlled trial." *Biol Res* 48 (1):49. doi: https://10.1186/s40659-015-0040-9.

Venkata Sairam, K., B. M. Gurupadayya, R. S. Chandan, D. K. Nagesha, and B. Vishwanathan. 2016. "A Review on Chemical Profile of Coumarins and their Therapeutic Role in the Treatment of Cancer." *Curr Drug Deliv* 13 (2):186-201. doi: https://10.2174/1567201812666150702102800.

Veskoukis, A. S., A. Kyparos, M. G. Nikolaidis, D. Stagos, N. Aligiannis, M. Halabalaki, K. Chronis, N. Goutzourelas, L. Skaltsounis, and D. Kouretas. 2012. "The antioxidant effects of a polyphenol-rich grape pomace extract *in vitro* do not correspond *in vivo* using exercise as an oxidant stimulus." *Oxid Med Cell Longev* 2012:185867. doi: https://10.1155/2012/185867.

Wahner-Roedler, D. L., Brent A. Bauer, Laura L. Loehrer, Stephen S. Cha, Tanya L. Hoskin, and Janet E. Olson. 2014. "The effect of grape seed extract on estrogen levels of postmenopausal women: a pilot study." *Journal of dietary supplements* 11 (2):184-197. doi: https://10.3109/19390211.2013.859220.

Xia, E. Q., G. F. Deng, Y. J. Guo, and H. B. Li. 2010. "Biological activities of polyphenols from grapes." *Int J Mol Sci* 11 (2):622-46. doi: https://10.3390/ijms11020622.

Younas, M., Christophe Hano, Nathalie Giglioli-Guivarc'h, and Bilal Haider Abbasi. 2018. "Mechanistic evaluation of phytochemicals in breast cancer remedy: current understanding and future perspectives." *RSC Advances* 8 (52):29714-29744. doi: https://10.1039/C8RA04879G.

Yu, J., and Mohamed Ahmedna. 2013. "Functional components of grape pomace: their composition, biological properties and potential applications." *International Journal of Food Science & Technology* 48 (2):221-237. doi: https://10.1111/j.1365-2621.2012.03197.x.

Yuan, J., A. Najafov, and B. F. Py. 2016. "Roles of Caspases in Necrotic Cell Death." *Cell* 167 (7):1693-1704. doi: https://10.1016/j.cell.2016.11.047.

Zhai, H., S. Hu, T. Liu, F. Wang, X. Wang, G. Wu, Y. Zhang, M. Sui, H. Liu, and L. Jiang. 2016. "Nitidine chloride inhibits proliferation and induces apoptosis in colorectal cancer cells by suppressing the ERK signaling pathway." *Mol Med Rep* 13 (3):2536-42. doi: https://10.3892/mmr.2016.4827.

# EDITOR'S CONTACT INFORMATION

***Veronica Sanda Chedea***
Senior Scientist,
Research Station for Viticulture and Enology,
Blaj, (SCDVV Blaj), Romania
chedeaveronica@yahoo.com

# INDEX

## B



## C

## F



## G



## H

## M



## N

## O



## P



## Q



## R

## U



## V



## W